in print 59—

30⁰⁰

Handbook of Functional Neuroimaging of Cognition

Handbook of Functional Neuroimaging of Cognition

edited by Roberto Cabeza and Alan Kingstone

A Bradford Book
The MIT Press
Cambridge, Massachusetts
London, England

This book was set in Times New Roman in QuarkXPress by Asco Typesetters, Hong Kong, and was printed and bound in the United States of America.

Library of Congress Cataloging-in-Publication Data
Handbook of functional neuroimaging of cognition / edited by Roberto Cabeza and Alan Kingstone.
    p.   cm.
"A Bradford book."
   Includes bibliographical references and index.
   ISBN 0-262-03280-5
   1. Cognitive neuroscience—Handbooks, manuals, etc. 2. Brain—Tomography—Handbooks, manuals, etc. 3. Brain—Magnetic resonance imaging—Handbooks, manuals, etc.
I. Cabeza, Roberto. II. Kingstone, Alan.
QP360.5 .H36   2000
612.8′2′028—dc21   00-022253

Contents

Preface   vii

I   HISTORY AND METHODS   1

1   **Functional Neuroimaging: A Historical and Physiological Perspective**   3
Marcus E. Raichle

2   **Functional Neuroimaging Methods: PET and fMRI**   27
Randy L. Buckner and Jessica M. Logan

3   **Functional Neuroimaging: Network Analyses**   49
L. Nyberg and A. R. McIntosh

II   COGNITIVE DOMAINS   73

4   **Functional Neuroimaging of Attention**   75
Todd C. Handy, Joseph B. Hopfinger, and George R. Mangun

5   **Functional Neuroimaging of Visual Recognition**   109
Nancy Kanwisher, Paul Downing, Russell Epstein, and Zoe Kourtzi

6   **Functional Neuroimaging of Semantic Memory**   153
Alex Martin

7   **Functional Neuroimaging of Language**   187
Jeffrey Binder and Cathy J. Price

8   **Functional Neuroimaging of Episodic Memory**   253
John D. E. Gabrieli

9   **Functional Neuroimaging of Working Memory**   293
Mark D'Esposito

III   SPECIAL POPULATIONS   329

10   **Functional Neuroimaging of Cognitive Aging**   331
Roberto Cabeza

11   **Functional Neuroimaging of Neuropsychologically Impaired Patients**   379
Cathy J. Price and Karl J. Friston

Contributors   401
Index   403

Preface

In the late spring of 1998, a conference was held in the wonderful and rustic town of Banff, Alberta, situated deep in the heartland of the Canadian Rockies. There, over the course of three days and two nights, cognitive neuroscientists gathered to discuss and argue about issues that concerned the functional neuroimaging of cognitive processes. A great deal of data was presented, and a plethora of views were advanced. At times, people were convinced by the data and interpretations being put forward, but just as often, people were skeptical. So, the discussions and arguments would begin again. All in all, it was tremendous fun, and a very stimulating weekend!

Now, typically that would be the end of the story. Usually, when a intense meeting comes to a close, the participants brush themselves off, pick up their things, and head off for home; more tired than when they first arrived, and, hopefully, a little wiser as well. But this conference would prove to be very different. The discussions and arguments had highlighted to all that there was a very real need to put together a book on the functional neuroimaging of cognition. This book would have to do at least two things. It would have to provide a historical perspective on the issues and imaging results in a number of different cognitive domains. And for each domain, it would have to articulate where things stood currently, and where they might be heading. That is the goal of the present handbook.

The handbook was written with two types of readers in mind: those who are relatively new to functional neuroimaging and/or cognitive neuroscience, and those who are seeking to expand their understanding of cognitive and brain systems. It is our hope, and intention, that this unique combination of depth and breadth will render the book suitable for both the student and the established scientist alike. With a balanced blend of theoretical and empirical material, the handbook should serve as an essential resource on the functional neuroimaging of cognitive processes, and on the latest discoveries obtained through positron emission tomography (PET) and functional magnetic resonance imaging (fMRI). Indeed, in recent years the field of functional neuroimaging of cognition has literally exploded. From less than a dozen papers in 1994, the number of publications in this area increased to about 70 in 1995, and to more than 300 in 1999 (Cabeza & Nyberg, 2000, *Journal of Cognitive Neuroscience*, 12, 1–47). This handbook provides the reader with a comprehensive but concise account of this rapidly growing literature.

During its rapid development, functional neuroimaging has transformed itself several times, in terms of methods, topics of research, and subject populations. The handbook reviews and evaluates the progress of functional neuroimaging research along these three dimensions. The first part covers the history and methods of PET and fMRI, including physiological mechanisms (chapter 1), event-related paradigms (chapter 2), and network analysis techniques (chapter 3). The second part covers PET and fMRI findings in specific cognitive domains: attention (chapter 4), visual recognition (chapter 5), semantic memory (chapter 6), language (chapter 7), episodic memory (chapter 8), and working memory (chapter 9). The third and final part addresses the effects of aging on brain activity during cognitive performance (chapter 10) and research with neuropsychologically impaired patients (chapter 11).

We are grateful to a great number of individuals who had a part in making this handbook a reality. Michael Gazzaniga supported our idea for this book and brought it to the attention of Michael Rutter at The MIT Press. Michael Rutter and Katherine Almeida have been instrumental in all phases of development of this project from its initiation to the production of the volume. And, of course, the authors needed to carry the project forth. In editing this handbook, we had substantial help from several anonymous reviewers, and generous support from the Alberta Heritage Foundation for Medical Research. Last but not least, we are thankful to our wives for their love, patience, and support.

I HISTORY AND METHODS

1 Functional Neuroimaging: A Historical and Physiological Perspective

Marcus E. Raichle

INTRODUCTION

Since 1990 cognitive neuroscience has emerged as a very important growth area in neuroscience. Cognitive neuroscience combines the experimental strategies of cognitive psychology with various techniques to examine how brain function supports mental activities. Leading this research in normal humans are the new techniques of functional brain imaging: positron emission tomography (PET) and magnetic resonance imaging (MRI), along with event-related potentials (ERPs) obtained from electroencephalography (EEG) or magnetoencephalography (MEG).

The signal used by PET is based on the fact that changes in the cellular activity of the brain of normal, awake humans and unanesthetized laboratory animals are invariably accompanied by changes in local blood flow (for a review see Raichle, 1987). This robust, empirical relationship has fascinated scientists for well over a century, but its cellular basis remains largely unexplained despite considerable research.

More recently it has been appreciated that these changes in blood flow are accompanied by much smaller changes in oxygen consumption (Fox & Raichle, 1986; Fox et al., 1988). This leads to changes in the actual amount of oxygen remaining in blood vessels at the site of brain activation (i.e., the supply of oxygen is not matched precisely with the demand). Because MRI signal intensity is sensitive to the amount of oxygen carried by hemoglobin (Ogawa et al., 1990), this change in blood oxygen content at the site of brain activation can be detected with MRI (Ogawa et al., 1992; Kwong et al., 1992; Bandettini et al., 1992; Frahm et al., 1992).

Studies with PET and MRI and magnetic resonance spectroscopy (MRS) have brought to light the fact that metabolic changes accompanying brain activation do not appear to follow exactly the time-honored notion of a close coupling between blood flow and the oxidative metabolism of glucose (Roy & Sherrington, 1890; Siesjo, 1978). Changes in blood flow appear to be accompanied by changes in glucose utilization that exceed the increase in oxygen consumption (Fox et al., 1988; Blomqvist et al., 1994), suggesting that the oxidative metabolism of glucose may not supply all of the energy demands encountered transiently during brain activation. Rather, glycolysis alone may provide the energy needed for the transient changes in brain activity associated with cognition and emotion.

Because of the prominent role of PET and MRI in the study of human brain function in health and disease, it is important to understand what we currently know about the biological basis of the signals they monitor. Individuals using these tools or considering the results of studies employing them should have a working knowledge of their biological basis. This chapter reviews that information, which is, at times, conflicting and incomplete.

While it is easy to conclude that much of this work transpired since 1990 or so because of its recent prominence in the neuroscience literature, in truth work on these relationships and the tools to exploit them has been developing for more than a century. In order to place present work in its proper perspective, a brief historical review of work on the relationships between brain function, blood flow, and metabolism is included.

Before beginning, it is useful to consider the intended goal of functional localization with brain imaging. This may seem self-evident to most. Nevertheless, interpretations frequently stated or implied about functional imaging data suggest that, if one is not careful, functional brain imaging could be viewed as no more than a modern version of phrenology.

It is Korbinian Brodmann (Brodmann, 1909) whose perspective I find appealing. He wrote: "Indeed, recently theories have abounded which, like phrenology, attempt to localize complex mental activity such as memory, will, fantasy, intelligence or spatial qualities such as appreciation of shape and position to circumscribed cortical zones." He went on to say, "These mental faculties are notions used to designate extraordinarily involved complexes of mental functions. One cannot think of their taking place in any other way than through an infinitely complex and involved interaction and cooperation of numerous elementary activities. In each particular case [these] supposed elementary functional loci are active in differing numbers, in differing degrees and in differing combinations. Such activities are always the result of the function of a large number of suborgans distributed more or less widely over the cortical surface" (for these English translations see Garey, 1994: 254–255).

With this prescient admonition in mind, the task of functional brain imaging becomes clear: identify regions and their temporal relationships associated with the performance of a well-designed task. The brain instantiation of the task will emerge from an understanding of the elementary operations performed within such a network. The great strength of functional brain imaging is that it is *uniquely* equipped to undertake such a task and can do so in the brain of most interest to us, the human brain.

FUNCTIONAL NEUROIMAGING: A HISTORICAL AND PHYSIOLOGICAL PERSPECTIVE

Historical Background

The quest for an understanding of the functional organization of the normal human brain, using techniques to assess changes in brain circulation, has occupied mankind for more than a century. One has only to consult William James's monumental two-volume text, *Principles of Psychology* (1890: I, 97), to find reference to changes in brain blood flow during mental activities. He references primarily the work of the Italian physiologist Angelo Mosso (1881), who recorded the pulsation of the human cortex in patients with skull defects following neurosurgical procedures. Mosso showed that these pulsations increased regionally during mental activity and concluded—correctly, we now know—that brain circulation changes selectively with neuronal activity.

No less a figure than Paul Broca was interested in the circulatory changes associated with mental activities as manifested by changes in brain temperature (Broca, 1879). Though best known for his seminal observations on the effect of lesions of the left frontal operculum on language function (Broca, 1861), Broca also studied the effects of various mental activities, especially language, on the localized temperature of the scalp of medical students (Broca, 1879). While such measurements might seem unlikely to yield any useful information, the reported observations, unbiased by preconceived notions of the functional anatomy of the cortex, were remarkably perceptive. Also active in the study of brain temperature and brain function in normal humans were Mosso (1894) and Hans Berger (1901). Berger later abandoned his efforts in this area in favor of the development of the electroencephalogram.

Despite a promising beginning, including the seminal animal experimental observations of Roy and Sherrington (1890), which suggested a link between brain circulation and metabolism, interest in this research virtually ceased during the first quarter of the twentieth century. Undoubtedly, this was due in part to a lack of tools sophisticated enough to pursue this line of research. In addition, the work of Leonard Hill, Hunterian Professor of the Royal College of Surgeons in England, was very influential (Hill, 1896). His eminence as a physiologist overshadowed the inadequacy of his own experiments that led him to conclude that no relationship existed between brain function and brain circulation.

There was no serious challenge to Hill's views until a remarkable clinical study was reported by John Fulton in the journal *Brain* (Fulton, 1928). At the time of the report Fulton was a neurosurgery resident under Harvey Cushing at the Peter Bent Brigham Hospital in Boston. A patient presented to Cushing's service with gradually decreasing vision due to an arteriovenous malformation of the occipital cortex. Surgical removal of the malformation was attempted but unsuccessful, leaving the patient with a bony defect over primary visual cortex. Fulton elicited a history of a cranial bruit audible to the patient whenever he engaged in a visual task. Based on this history, Fulton pursued a detailed investigation of the behavior of the bruit, which he could auscultate and record over occipital cortex. Remarkably consistent changes in the character of the bruit could be appreciated, depending upon the visual activities of the patient. Opening the eyes produced only modest increases in the intensity of the bruit, whereas reading produced striking increases. The changes in cortical blood flow related to the complexity of the visual task and the attention of the subject to that task anticipated findings and concepts that have only recently been addressed with modern functional imaging techniques (Shulman, Corbetta, et al., 1997).

At the end of World War II, Seymour Kety and his colleagues opened the next chapter in studies of brain circulation and metabolism. Working with Lou Sokoloff and others, Kety developed the first quantitative methods for measuring *whole* brain blood flow and metabolism in humans. The introduction of an in vivo tissue auto-radiographic measurement of regional blood flow in laboratory animals by Kety's group (Landau et al., 1955; Kety, 1960) provided the first glimpse of quantitative changes in blood flow in the brain related directly to brain function. Given the later importance of derivatives of this technique to functional brain imaging with both PET and fMRI it is interesting to note the (dis)regard the developers had for this technique as a means of assessing brain functional organization. Quoting from the comments of William Landau to the members of the American Neurological Association meeting in Atlantic City (Landau et al., 1955): "Of course we recognize that this is a very secondhand way of determining physiological activity; it is rather like trying to measure what a factory does by measuring the intake of water and the output of sewage. This is only a problem of plumbing and only secondary inferences can be made about function. We would not suggest that this is a substitute for electrical recording in terms of easy evaluation of what is going on." With the introduction of the deoxyglucose technique for the regional measurement of glucose metabolism in laboratory animals (Sokoloff et al., 1977) and its later adaptation for PET (Reivich et al., 1979), enthusiasm was much greater for the potential of such measurements to enhance our knowledge of brain function (Raichle, 1987).

Soon after Kety and his colleagues introduced their quantitative methods for measuring whole brain blood flow and metabolism in humans, David Ingvar, Neils Lassen, and their colleagues introduced methods applicable to man that permitted regional blood flow measurements to be made by using scintillation detectors arrayed like a helmet over the head (Lassen et al., 1963). They demonstrated directly in normal human subjects that blood flow changes regionally during changes in brain functional activity. The first study of functionally induced regional changes in blood flow using these techniques in normal humans, reported by Ingvar and Risberg at an early meeting on brain blood and metabolism (Ingvar & Risberg, 1965), was greeted with cautious enthusiasm and a clear sense of its potential importance for studies of human brain function by Seymour Kety (1965). However, despite many studies of functionally induced changes in regional cerebral blood that followed (Raichle, 1987; Lassen et al., 1978), this approach was not embraced by most neuroscientists or cognitive scientists. It is interesting to note that this indifference disappeared almost completely in the 1980s, a subject to which we will return shortly.

Godfrey Hounsfield (1973) introduced X-ray computed tomography (CT), a technique based upon principles presented by Alan Cormack (1963; see also Cormack, 1973). Overnight the way in which we look at the human brain changed. Immediately, researchers envisioned another type of tomography, positron emission tomography (PET), which created in vivo autoradioagrams of brain function (Ter-Pogossian et al., 1975; Hoffman et al., 1976). A new era of functional brain mapping began. The autoradiographic techniques for the measurement of blood flow (Landau et al., 1955, Kety, 1960) and glucose metabolism (Sokoloff et al., 1977) in laboratory animals could now be used safely on humans (Reivich et al., 1979; Raichle et al., 1983). Additionally, quantitative techniques were developed (Frackowiak et al., 1980; Mintun et al., 1984) and, importantly, validated (Mintun et al., 1984; Altman et al., 1991) for the measurement of oxygen consumption.

Soon it was realized that highly accurate measurements of brain function in humans could be performed with PET (Posner & Raichle, 1994). Though this could be accomplished with measurements of either blood flow or metabolism (Raichle, 1987), blood flow became the favored technique because it could be measured quickly (<1 min) using an easily produced radiopharmaceutical ($H_2^{15}O$) with a short half-life (123 sec), which allowed many repeat measurements in the same subject.

The study of human cognition with PET was greatly aided in the 1980s by the involvement of cognitive psychologists, whose experimental designs for dissecting human behaviors using information-processing theory fit extremely well with the emerging functional brain imaging strategies (Posner & Raichle, 1994). It may well have been the combination of cognitive science and systems neuroscience with brain imaging that lifted this work from a state of indifference and obscurity in the neuroscience community in the 1970s to its current place of prominence in cognitive neuroscience.

As a result of collaboration among neuroscientists, imaging scientists, and cognitive psychologists, a distinct behavioral strategy for the functional mapping of neuronal activity emerged. This strategy was based on a concept introduced by the Dutch physiologist Franciscus C. Donders in 1868 (reprinted in Donders, 1969). Donders proposed a general method to measure thought processes based on a simple logic. He subtracted the time needed to respond to a light (say, by pressing a key) from the time needed to respond to a particular color of light. He found that discriminating color required about 50 msec. In this way, Donders isolated and measured a mental process

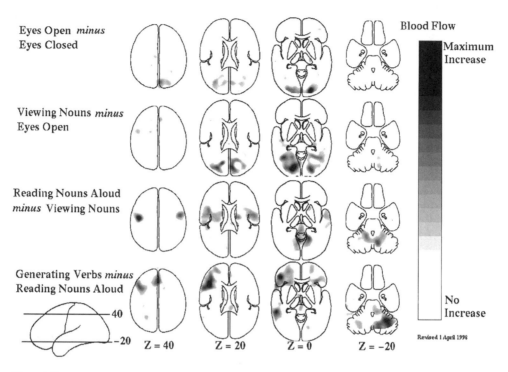

Figure 1.1
Four different hierarchically organized conditions are represented in these mean blood flow difference images obtained with PET. All of the changes shown in these images represent *increases* over the control state for each task. A group of normal subjects performed these tasks, involving common English nouns (Raichle et al., 1994; Petersen et al., 1988, Petersen et al., 1989), to demonstrate the spatially distributed nature of the processing by task elements going on in the normal human brain during a simple language task. Task complexity was increased from simply opening the eyes (row 1) through passive viewing of nouns on a television monitor (row 2); reading aloud the nouns as they appear on the screen (row 3); and saying aloud an appropriate verb for each noun as it appeared on the screen (row 4). These horizontal images are oriented with the front of the brain on top and the left side to the reader's left. Z=40, Z=20, and Z=−20 indicate millimeters above and below a horizontal plane through the brain (Z=0).

for the first time by subtracting a *control state* (responding to a light) from a *task state* (discriminating the color of the light). An example of the manner in which this strategy has been adopted for functional imaging is illustrated in figure 1.1.

One criticism of this approach has been that the time necessary to press a key after a decision to do so has been made is affected by the nature of the decision process itself. By implication, the nature of the processes underlying key press, in this example, may have been altered. Although this issue (known in cognitive science jargon as the *assumption of pure insertion*) has been the subject of continuing discussion in cognitive psychology, it finds its resolution in functional brain imaging, where changes in any process are directly signaled by changes in observable brain states. Events occur-

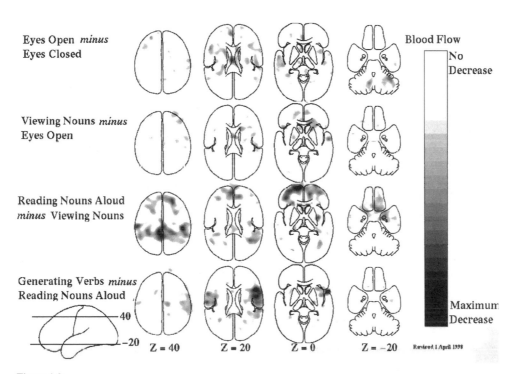

Eyes Open *minus* Eyes Closed

Viewing Nouns *minus* Eyes Open

Reading Nouns Aloud *minus* Viewing Nouns

Generating Verbs *minus* Reading Nouns Aloud

Blood Flow
No Decrease

Maximum Decrease

Z = 40   Z = 20   Z = 0   Z = -20   Revised 1 April 1998

Figure 1.2
Hierarchically organized subtractions involving the same task conditions as shown in figure 1.1, the difference being that these images represent areas of *decreased* activity in the task condition as compared to the control condition. Note that the major decreases occurred when subjects read the visually presented nouns aloud as compared to viewing them passively as they appeared on the television monitor (row 3), and when they said aloud an appropriate verb for each noun as it appeared on the television monitor as compared to reading the noun aloud (row 4). Combining the information available in figures 1.1 and 1.2 provides a fairly complete picture of the interactions between tasks and brain systems in hierarchically organized cognitive tasks studied with functional brain imaging. (From Raichle et al., 1994.)

ring in the brain are not hidden from the investigator, as they are in the purely cognitive experiments. Careful analysis of the changes in the functional images reveals whether processes (e.g., specific cognitive decisions) can be added or removed without affecting ongoing processes (e.g., motor processes). Processing areas of the brain that become inactive during the course of a particular cognitive paradigm are illustrated in figure 1.2. Examining the images in figures 1.1 and 1.2 together yields a more complete picture of the changes taking place in the cognitive paradigm illustrated in these two figures. Clearly, some areas of the brain active at one stage in a hierarchically designed paradigm can become inactive as task complexity is increased. Changes of this sort are hidden from the view of the cognitive scientist, but they become obvious when brain imaging is employed.

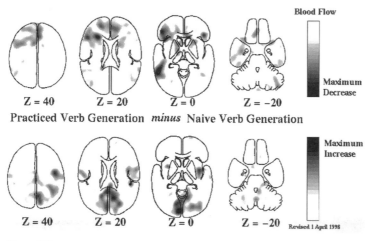

Figure 1.3
Practice-induced changes in brain systems involve both the disappearance of activity in systems initially supporting task performance (row 1) and the appearance of activity in other systems concerned with practiced performance (row 2). In this example, generating verbs aloud for visually presented nouns (see also row 4 of figures 1.1 and 1.2 for changes during the naive performance of the task), subjects acquired proficiency on the task after 10 min of practice. This improved performance was associated with a disappearance of activity in areas of frontal and temporal cortex and the right cerebellum (row 1) and the appearance of activity in sylvian-insular and occipital cortex (row 2). These images were created by subtracting the naive performance of verb generation from the practiced performance of the task. More details on these changes can be obtained from Raichle et al. (1994).

A final caveat with regard to certain cognitive paradigms is that the brain systems involved do not necessarily remain constant through many repetitions of the task. Though simple habituation might be suspected when a task is tedious, this is not the issue referred to here. Rather, when a task is *novel* and, more important, conflicts with a more habitual response to the presented stimulus, major changes can occur in the systems allocated to the task. A good example relates to the task shown in figures 1.1 and 1.2 (row 4), where subjects are asked to generate an appropriate verb for visually presented nouns rather than simply to read the noun aloud, as they had been doing (Raichle et al., 1994). In this task, regions uniquely active when the task is first performed (figure 1.1, row 4, and figure 1.3, row 1) are *replaced* by regions active when the task has become well practiced (figure 1.3, row 2). Such changes have both practical and theoretical implications when it comes to the design and interpretation of cognitive activation experiments. Functional brain imaging obviously provides a unique perspective that is unavailable in the purely cognitive experiment.

Finally, another technology emerged contemporaneously with PET and CT. This was magnetic resonance imaging (MRI). MRI is based upon yet another set of physical principles that have to do with the behavior of hydrogen atoms or protons in a magnetic field. These principles were discovered independently by Felix Block (1946) and Edward Purcell and his colleagues in 1946 (Purcell et al., 1946), and expanded to imaging by Paul Lauterbur (1973). Initially MRI provided superb anatomical information, and inherent in the data was important metabolic and physiological information. An opening for MRI in the area of functional brain imaging emerged when it was discovered that during changes in neuronal activity there are local changes in the amount of oxygen in the tissue (Fox & Raichle, 1986; Fox et al., 1988). By combining this observation with a much earlier observation by Pauling and Coryell (1936) that changing the amount of oxygen carried by hemoglobin changes the degree to which hemoglobin disturbs a magnetic field, Ogawa et al. (1990) were able to demonstrate that in vivo changes in blood oxygenation could be detected with MRI. The MRI signal (technically known as T2* or "tee-two-star") arising from this unique combination of brain physiology (Fox & Raichle, 1986) and nuclear magnetic resonance physics (Pauling & Coryell, 1936; Thulborn et al., 1982) became known as the blood oxygen level dependent (BOLD) signal (Ogawa et al., 1990). There quickly followed several demonstrations of BOLD signal changes in normal humans during functional brain activation (Ogawa et al., 1992; Kwong et al., 1992; Bandettini et al., 1992; Frahm et al., 1992), which gave birth to the rapidly developing field of functional MRI (fMRI).

In the discussion that follows, it is important to keep in mind that when a BOLD signal is detected, blood flow to a region of brain has changed out of proportion to the change in oxygen consumption (Kim & Ugurbil, 1997). When blood flow changes more than oxygen consumption, in either direction, there is a reciprocal change in the amount of deoxyhemoglobin present locally in the tissue, thus changing the local magnetic field properties. As you will see, both increases and decreases in the BOLD signal occur in the normal human brain.

Metabolic Requirements of Cognition

While many had assumed that behaviorally induced *increases* in local blood flow would be reflected in local increases in the *oxidative* metabolism of glucose (Siesjo, 1978), evidence from brain imaging studies with PET (Fox & Raichle, 1986; Fox et al., 1988) and fMRI (Kim & Ugurbil, 1997) have indicated otherwise. Fox and his colleagues (Fox & Raichle, 1986; Fox et al., 1988) demonstrated that in normal, awake adult humans, stimulation of the visual or somatosensory cortex results in dramatic increases in blood flow but minimal increases in *oxygen consumption*. Increases in *glucose utilization* occur in parallel with blood flow (Blomqvist et al., 1994; Fox et al., 1988), an observation fully anticipated by the work of others (Sokoloff et al.,

1977; Yarowsky et al., 1983). However, changes in blood flow and glucose utilization were much in excess of the changes in oxygen consumption, an observation contrary to most popularly held notions of brain energy metabolism (Siesjo, 1978). These results suggested that the additional metabolic requirements associated with increased neuronal activity might be supplied largely through glycolysis alone.

Another element of the relationship between brain circulation and brain function which was not appreciated prior to the advent of functional brain imaging is that regional blood flow and the fMRI BOLD signal not only increase in some areas of the brain appropriate to task performance but also decrease from a resting baseline in other areas (Shulman et al., 1997b), as shown in figure 1.2. An appreciation of how these decreases arise in the context of an imaging experiment is diagrammatically represented in figure 1.4. The possible physiological implications of these changes are discussed below.

Physiologists have long recognized that individual neurons in the cerebral cortex can either increase or decrease their activities from a resting, baseline firing pattern, depending upon task conditions. Examples abound in the neurophysiological literature (Georgopoulos et al., 1982). A parsimonious view of these decreases in neuronal activity is that they reflect the activity of inhibitory interneurons acting within local neuronal circuits of the cerebral cortex. Because inhibition is energy requiring (Ackerman et al., 1984), it is impossible to distinguish inhibitory from excitatory cellular activity on the basis of changes in either blood flow or metabolism. Thus, on this view a local increase in *inhibitory activity* would be as likely to increase blood flow and the fMRI BOLD signal as would a local increase in *excitatory activity*. How, then, might decreases in blood flow or the fMRI BOLD signal arise?

To understand the possible significance of the decreases in blood flow in functional imaging studies, it is important to distinguish *two separate conditions* in which they might arise.[1] The less interesting and more usually referred to circumstance arises when two images are compared: one contains a regional increase in blood flow due to some type of task activity (e.g., hand movement that produces increases in contralateral motor cortex blood flow) and a control image that does not (in this example, no hand movement). In our example, subtracting the image associated with no hand movement from the image associated with hand movement reveals the expected increase in blood flow in motor cortex. Simply reversing the subtraction produces an image with a decrease in the same area. While this example may seem trivial and obvious, such subtraction reversals are often presented in the analysis of very complex tasks and in such a manner as to be quite confusing even to those working in the field. A diagrammatic representation of how this occurs is presented in figure 1.4.

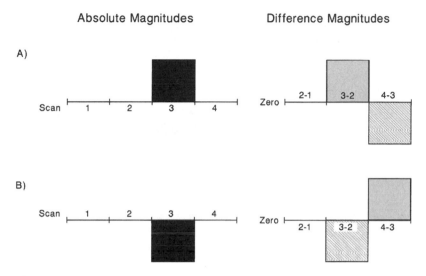

Figure 1.4
Functional images obtained with positron emission tomography (PET) and functional magnetic resonance imaging (fMRI) represent comparisons between two conditions usually referred to as a *control state* and a *task state*. The *task state* is designed to contain specific mental operations of interest. Because the *task state* invariably contains additional mental operations not of interest, a *control state* is selected which contains those operations to be ignored yet does not contain the operations of interest in the task state. Depending on the actual changes in brain activity in each state and the comparison made between states, the resulting changes depicted in the functional image will have either a positive (figure 1.1) or negative (figure 1.2) sign. This figure is designed to illustrate how the sign (i.e., positive or negative change) arises from the primary image data. Absolute changes (Absolute Magnitudes) are represented on the left for a hypothetical area in the brain as monitored by either PET or fMRI. The horizontal axis on the left represents 4 states studied in the course of a hypothetical imaging experiment. An Absolute Magnitude above the horizontal axis (*A*) represents an increase over the other states studied while an Absolute Magnitude below this axis (*B*) represents a decrease. The comparisons (i.e., 2.1, 3.2, and 4.3) leading to the functional images themselves are shown on the right (Difference Magnitudes). It should be appreciated from this figure that the sign of the change in the functional image is dependent on both the change in activity within an area during a particular task (Absolute Magnitudes) and the particular comparison subsequently made between states (Difference Magnitudes). These general principles should be kept in mind when evaluating data of the type shown in figures 1.1 to 1.3.

The second circumstance (figure 1.4) in which decreases in blood flow and the fMRI BOLD signal appear is not due to the above type of data manipulation (i.e., an *active* task image subtracted from a passive state image). Rather, blood flow and the fMRI BOLD signal actually decrease from the passive baseline state (i.e., the activity in a region of brain has not been first elevated by a task). The usual baseline conditions from which this occurs consist of lying quietly but fully awake in an MRI or PET scanner with eyes closed or passively viewing a television monitor and its image, be it a fixation point or a more complex stimulus (figure 1.2, row 3). In the examples discussed by Shulman and colleagues (1997b) areas of the medial orbital frontal cortex, the posterior cingulate cortex, and precuneus consistently showed decreased blood flow when subjects actively processed a wide variety of visual stimuli as compared to a passive baseline condition (compare with the example shown in figure 1.2).

The hypothesis one is led to consider, regarding these rather large area reductions in blood flow, is that a large number of neurons reduce their activity together (for one of the few neurophysiological references to such a phenomenon see, Creutzfeldt et al., 1989). Such group reductions could not be mediated by a local increase in the activity of inhibitory interneurons, since this would be seen as an increase in activity by PET and fMRI. Rather, such reductions are likely mediated through the action of diffuse projecting systems like dopamine, norepinephrine, and serotonin, or through a reduction in thalamic inputs to the cortex. The recognition of such changes probably represents an important contribution of functional brain imaging to our understanding of cortical function, and should stimulate increased interest in the manner in which brain resources are allocated on a large systems level during task performance.

The metabolic accompaniments of these functionally induced decreases in blood flow from a passive baseline condition were not initially explored, and it was tacitly assumed that such reductions would probably be accompanied by coupled reductions in oxygen consumption. Therefore, it came as a surprise that the fMRI BOLD signal, based on tissue oxygen availability, detected both increases and decreases during functional activation (figure 1.5). Decreases in the BOLD signal during a task state as compared to a passive, resting state have been widely appreciated by investigators using fMRI although, surprisingly, formal publications on the subject have yet to appear.

Complementing these observations from functional brain imaging on the relationship between oxygen consumption and blood flow during decreases are earlier quantitative metabolic studies of a phenomenon known as cerebellar diaschisis (Martin & Raichle, 1983; Yamauchi et al., 1992). In this condition, there is a reduction in blood flow and metabolism in the hemisphere of the cerebellum contralateral to an injury to the cerebral cortex, usually a stroke. Of particular interest is the fact that blood flow

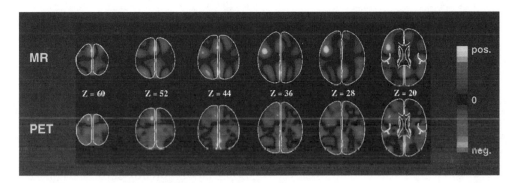

Figure 1.5
Functional magnetic resonance images (fMRI; top row) of the BOLD signal (Ogawa et al., 1990) and positron emission tomography (PET; bottom row) images of blood flow change. These images were obtained during the performance of a task in which subjects viewed three-letter word stems and were asked to speak aloud (PET) or think silently (fMRI) the first word to come to mind whose first three letters corresponded to the stems (e.g., see *cou*, say or think *couple*; Buckner et al., 1995). The color scale employed in these images shows activity increases in reds and yellows and activity decreases in greens and blues. Note that both PET and fMRI show similar increases as well as decreases. The fMRI images were blurred to the resolution of the PET images (18-mm FWHM) to facilitate comparison. (See color plate 1.)

is reduced significantly more than oxygen consumption (Martin & Raichle, 1983; Yamauchi et al., 1992). The changes in the cerebellum are thought to reflect a reduction in neuronal activity within the cerebellum due to reduced input from the cerebral cortex. One can reasonably hypothesize that similar, large-scale reductions in systems-level activity are occurring during the course of normal functional brain activity (Shulman, Fiez, et al., 1997).

Taken together, the data we have at hand suggest that blood flow changes more than oxygen consumption in the face of increases as well as decreases in local neuronal activity (figure 1.6). Glucose utilization also changes more than oxygen consumption during increases in brain activity (at present we have no data on decreases in glucose utilization) and may equal the changes in blood flow in both magnitude and spatial extent (Blomqvist et al., 1994; Fox et al., 1988). Though surprising to many, these results were not entirely unanticipated.

Experimental studies of epilepsy in *well-oxygenated, passively ventilated* experimental animals[2] (Plum et al., 1968) had indicated that blood flow increased in excess of the oxygen requirements of the tissue. During the increased neuronal activity of a seizure discharge increase in the brain venous oxygen content was routinely observed (Plum et al., 1968). Because of the increase in blood pressure associated with the seizure discharge, the fact that blood flow exceeded the oxygen requirements of the tissue was attributed to a loss of cerebral autoregulation (Plum et al., 1968). A similar con-

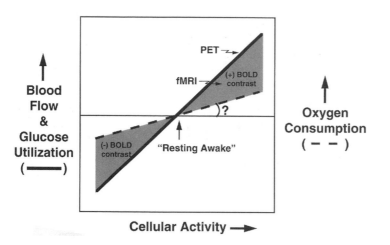

Figure 1.6
A summary of currently available data on the relationship of blood flow, glucose utilization and oxygen consumption to the cellular activity of the brain during changes in functional activity is shown in this figure. The changes occurring in blood flow and glucose utilization exceed changes in oxygen consumption. The degree to which oxygen consumption actually changes, if at all, remains to be determined. Positron emission tomography (PET) measures the changes in blood flow. Functional magnetic resonance imaging (fMRI) measures a blood oxygen level dependent (BOLD; Ogawa et al. 1990) signal or contrast that arises when changes in blood flow exceed changes in tissue oxygen consumption.

cern was expressed about equally prescient experiments involving brain blood flow changes during sciatic nerve stimulation in rodents (Howse et al., 1973; Salford et al., 1975).

However, experiments by Ray Cooper and his colleagues largely circumvented that concern (Cooper et al., 1966, 1975). They demonstrated that oxygen availability measured locally in the cerebral cortex of awake patients undergoing surgery for the treatment of intractable epilepsy increased during changes in behavioral activity (e.g., looking at pictures, manual dexterity, reading). These changes in oxygen availability occurred in the absence of any change in blood pressure and were observed during normal brain function in humans. Surprisingly, these observations were largely ignored until the work of Fox and his colleagues called attention to the phenomenon in normal human subjects with PET (Fox & Raichle, 1986; Fox et al., 1988).

Interpretation of these blood flow-metabolism relationships during changes in functional brain activity are at present controversial. Several schools of thought have emerged. One hypothesis that addresses the role of glycolysis in brain functional activation is most eloquently articulated by Pierre Magistretti and colleagues, based on their work with cultured astrocytes (Tsacopoulos & Magistretti, 1996; Bittar et al., 1996). On this theory, increases in neuronal activity stimulated by the excitatory amino acid transmitter glutamate result in relatively large increases in glycolytic metabolism in astrocytes. The energy supplied through glycolysis in the astrocyte is used to metabolize glutamate to glutamine before it is recycled to neurons. Coupled with estimates that increased firing rates of neurons require little additional energy over and above that required for the normal maintenance of ionic gradients (Creutzfeldt, 1975), this leads to the hypothesis that the primary metabolic change associated with changes (at least increases) in neuronal activity are glycolytic and occur in astrocytes.

In somewhat greater detail, neuronal activation results in sodium ion influx and potassium efflux. This is accompanied by an influx of protons into neurons, initially alkalinizing the extracellular space, which results in alkalinization of the astrocyte (Chesler & Kraig, 1987). Alkalinization of the astrocyte results in stimulation of glycolysis (Hochachka & Mommsen, 1983), the breakdown of glycogen (Swanson et al., 1992), and the production of both pyruvate and lactate in excess of astrocyte metabolic needs and despite normal tissue oxygenation. The lactate can then leave the astrocyte and be taken up by neurons to be oxidatively metabolized (Dringen, Wiesinger, et al., 1993). Because glucose metabolism exceeds oxygen consumption during increases in neuronal activity (Fox et al., 1988), another fate for lactate must be sought. This might possibly occur through enhanced removal from the brain by flowing blood, a hypothesis for which at present we have only indirect evidence (Knudsen et al., 1991; Lear & Kasliwal, 1991), or reincorporation into astrocytic glycogen (Dringen, Schmoll, et al., 1993).

Additional support for this hypothesis comes from in vivo observations that increases in neuronal activity are associated with glycogenolysis in astrocytes (Harley & Bielajew, 1992), a convenient source of readily available energy for such a process that is located in a cell uniquely equipped enzymatically for the process (Bittar et al., 1996; Harley & Bielajew, 1992). Finally, measurements of tissue lactate with magnetic resonance spectroscopy (MRS) in humans (Prichard et al., 1991) and with substrate-induced bioluminescence in laboratory animals (Ueki et al., 1988) has shown localized increases in tissue lactate during physiologically induced increases in neuronal activity.

Not surprisingly, the above hypothesis has been challenged and alternatives have been offered to explain the observed discrepancy between changes in blood flow and glucose utilization, which appear to change in parallel, and oxygen consumption, which changes much less than either. One suggestion is that the observed discrepancy is transient (Frahm et al., 1996). Measuring brain glucose, lactate concentrations, and blood oxygenation with MRI and MRS in normal human volunteers, Frahm and colleagues (1996) observed a rise in visual cortex lactate concentration that peaked after

3 min of visual stimulation and returned to baseline after six min of continuous stimulation. During this same period of time, blood oxygen concentration was initially elevated but also returned to baseline by the end of the stimulation period. In a complementary study Hyder and colleagues (1996) similarly suggest, on the basis of MRS studies of *anesthetized* rats during forepaw stimulation, that "oxidative CMRGlu supplies the majority of energy during *sustained* brain activation." However, in a very careful study of this question in awake humans by Bandettini and associates (1997), they conclude from their own data and a careful analysis of the literature that BOLD signal changes and blood flow remain elevated during prolonged periods of brain activation, provided that there is no *habituation* to the presented stimulus. This conclusion is entirely consistent with the original observations of Fox and Raichle (1986).

Another popular hypothesis is based on optical imaging of physiologically stimulated visual cortex by Grinvald and his associates (Malonek & Grinvald, 1996). In their work they measure changes in reflected light from the surface of visual cortex in *anesthetized* cats. Using wavelengths of light sensitive to deoxyhemoglobin and oxyhemoglobin, they note an almost immediate *increase* in deoxyhemoglobin concentration, followed, after a brief interval, by an increase in oxyhemoglobin that, though centered at the same location as the change in deoxyhemoglobin, is greater in magnitude and extends over a much larger area of the cortex than the changes in deoxyhemoglobin. They interpret these results to mean that increases in neuronal activity are associated with highly localized increases in oxygen consumption which stimulate a vascular response, delayed by several sec, that is large in relation to both the magnitude of the increase in oxygen consumption and the area of cerebral cortex that is active.

In other words, by their theory, increases in neuronal activity in the cerebral cortex are associated with increased oxidative metabolism of glucose. Because the blood flow response to the change in neuronal activity is relatively slow, oxygen reserves in the area of activation are temporarily depleted. When the blood flow response does occur, after a delay of 1–3 sec, it exceeds the needs of the tissue, delivering to the active area of cortex and its surroundings oxygen in excess of metabolic needs. This hypothesis has stimulated interest in the use of high-field-strength MRI systems to detect the initial oxygen depletion predicted by the small increases in deoxyhemoglobin (Menon et al., 1995). The hope would be that both spatial and temporal resolution of fMRI would be improved by focusing on this postulated early and spatially confined event.

Support for the hypothesis of Malonek and Grinvald (1996) comes from theoretical work by Buxton and Frank (1997). In their modeling work they show that in an idealized capillary tissue cylinder in the brain, an increase in blood flow in excess of the increased oxygen metabolic demands of the tissue is needed in order to maintain proper oxygenation of the tissue. This results from the poor diffusivity and solubility of oxygen in brain tissue. On this theory, blood flow remains coupled to oxidative metabolism, but in a nonlinear fashion designed to overcome the diffusion and solubility limitations of oxygen in brain tissue so as to maintain adequate tissue oxygenation.

Although the hypothesis that reactive hyperemia is a normal and necessary consequence of increased neuronal activity merits careful consideration, several observations remain unexplained. *First*, it does not account for the increased glucose utilization that parallels the change in blood flow observed in normal humans (Fox et al., 1988; Blomqvist et al., 1994) and laboratory animals (Ueki et al., 1988; Woolsey et al., 1996; Greenberg et al., 1997). *Second*, it does not agree with the observations of Woolsey and his associates (1996) as well as of others (Greenberg et al., 1997), who have demonstrated a remarkably tight spatial relationship between changes in neuronal activity within a single rat-whisker barrel and the response of the vascular supply, as well as of glucose metabolism, to that barrel. There is little evidence in these studies for spatially diffuse reactive hyperemia surrounding the stimulated area of cortex. *Third*, in the paper by Malonek and Grinvald (1996) the initial rise in deoxyhemoglobin seen with activation is not accompanied by a fall in oxyhemoglobin, as would be expected with a sudden rise in local oxygen consumption that precedes the onset of increased oxygen delivery to the tissue. In the presence of somewhat conflicting evidence on capillary recruitment in brain (Woolsey et al., 1996; Greenberg, Sohn, & Hand, 1997; Powers, Hirsch, & Cryer, 1996) that could explain this observation, we should exercise caution in accepting uncritically the data of Malonek and Grinvald until an explanation for this particular discrepancy is found and better concordance is achieved with other experiments. Clearly, more information is needed on the exact nature of the microvascular events surrounding functional brain activation. *Finally*, we are left without an explanation for the observation that when blood flow decreases below a resting baseline during changes in the functional activity of a region of the brain (see figure 1.2), a negative BOLD signal arises because blood flow decreases more than the oxygen consumption.

One final caveat should be mentioned. From the perspective of this review, it would be easy to assume that because blood flow and glucose utilization appear to increase together, and more than oxygen utilization, during increases in neuronal activity, the increase in blood flow serves to deliver needed glucose. Recent data from Powers and his colleagues (1996) suggest otherwise. They noted no change in the magnitude of the normalized regional blood flow response to physiological stimulation of the human brain during stepped hypoglycemia. They concluded that the increase in blood flow associated with physiological brain activation was not regulated by a mechanism which matched local cerebral glucose supply to local cerebral glucose demand (Powers et al., 1996).

So what are we to conclude? Any theory designed to explain functional brain imaging signals must accommodate three observations. *First*, local increases *and* decreases in brain activity are reliably accompanied by changes in blood flow. *Second*, these blood flow changes exceed any accompanying change in the oxygen consumption. If this were not the case, fMRI based on the BOLD signal changes could not exist. *Third*, though paired data on glucose metabolism and blood flow are limited, they suggest that blood flow changes are accompanied by changes in glucose metabolism of approximately equal magnitude and spatial extent.

Several additional factors must be kept in mind in the evaluation of extant data and the design of future experiments. *Anesthesia*, a factor present in many of the *animal* experiments discussed in this review, may well have a significant effect on the relationships among blood flow, metabolism, and cellular activity during brain activation. Also, *habituation* of cellular activity to certain types of stimuli (Frahm et al., 1996; Bandettini et al., 1997), as well as rapid, practice-induced *shifts in the neuronal circuitry* used for the performance of a task (see figure 1.3), may complicate the interpretation of resulting data if overlooked in experiments designed to investigate these relationships.

At present we do not know why blood flow changes so dramatically and reliably during changes in brain activity or how these vascular responses are so beautifully orchestrated. These questions have confronted us for more than a century and remain incompletely answered. At no time have answers been more important or intriguing than now, because of the immense interest focused on them by the use of functional brain imaging with PET and fMRI. We have at hand tools with the potential to provide unparalleled insights into some of the most important scientific, medical, and social questions facing mankind. Understanding those tools is clearly a high priority.

ISSUES

Since about 1970 members of the medical and scientific communities have witnessed a truly remarkable transformation in the way we are able to examine the human brain through imaging. The results of this work provide a strong incentive for continued development of new imaging methods. Because of the dramatic nature of much of this imaging work and its intuitive appeal, highly creative people from a wide variety of disciplines are increasingly involved. Such people have a choice of many questions on which they can fruitfully spend their time. It remains important to detect subatomic particles, to probe the cosmos, and to sequence the human genome, but to this list we can now add the goal of observing and understanding the human brain at work.

In such a rapidly evolving field it is difficult to make long-range predictions about advances in imaging over the next decade. Functional MRI will likely play an increasingly dominant role in the day-to-day mapping of the brain. The ability to track single cognitive events in individual subjects (see above) is just one of a number of innovations that make fMRI such a powerful and appealing tool for this work. Combining fMRI with ERPs, recorded with either EEG or MEG, will likely provide the spatial and temporal information necessary to understand information processing in the human brain. Whether fMRI has any chance to accomplish all of this alone remains an open question.

PET was obviously a pivotal technique in establishing functional brain imaging. Some might consider its role now only of historical interest. That is unlikely to be the case. PET remains our gold standard for the measurement of many critical variables of physiological interest in the brain, such as blood flow, oxygen consumption, and glucose utilization (to name the most obvious). We have much left to learn about the signals that give rise to fMRI. With so much at stake, understanding these signals must be a high priority item on our agenda. PET will play a significant role in this work.

Functional imaging of the future will undoubtedly involve more than measurements directly related to moment-to-moment changes in neuronal activity (e.g., changes in BOLD contrast). Also of importance will be *changes* in neurotransmitter and neuromodulator release (e.g., diffuse projecting systems involving dopamine, norepinephrine, and serotonin). Such changes are probably involved in learning, reinforcement of behavior, attention, and sensorimotor integration. Here PET is at present in almost sole possession of the agenda. A recent behavioral study with PET demonstrating the release of dopamine in the human brain during the performance of a goal-directed motor task illustrates what is in store (Koepp et al., 1998).

With all of this dramatic recent progress we must never forget our debt to those whose vision and determination laid the necessary groundwork.

ACKNOWLEDGMENTS

I would like to acknowledge many years of generous support from National Institute of Neurological Disorders and Stroke (NINDS), National Heart, Lung, and Blood Institute (NHLBI), and the McDonnell Center for Studies of Higher Brain Function at Washington University, as well as from the John D. and Katherine T. MacArthur Foundation and the Charles A. Dana Foundation.

NOTES

1. Some have wondered whether these reductions in blood flow are merely the hemodynamic consequence of increases elsewhere (i.e., an *intracerebral steal phenomenon*). Such a hypothesis is very unlikely to be correct because of the tremendous hemodynamic reserve of the brain (Heistad and Kontos, 1983) and also because there is no one-to-one spatial or temporal correlation between increases and decreases (e.g., see figures 1.1 and 1.2).

2. Wilder Penfield is frequently given credit for the observation that venous oxygenation increases during a seizure discharge (i.e., "red veins on the cortex"). Careful reading of his many descriptions of the cortical surface of the human brain during a seizure fail to disclose such a description. Rather, he describes quite clearly the *infrequent* appearance of arterial blood locally in pial veins *after* a focal cortical seizure, "... the almost invariable objective alteration in the exposed hemisphere coincident with the onset of the fit is a cessation of pulsation in the brain" (Penfield, 1937, p. 607).

REFERENCES

Ackerman, R. F., Finch, D. M., Babb, T. L., & Engel, J., Jr. (1984). Increased glucose metabolism during long-duration recurrent inhibition of hippocampal cells. *Journal of Neuroscience* 4, 251–264.

Altman, D. I., Lich, L. L., & Powers, W. J. (1991). Brief inhalation method to measure cerebral oxygen extraction fraction with PET: Accuracy determination under pathological conditions. *Journal of Nuclear Medicine* 32, 1738–1741.

Bandettini, P. A., Kwong, K. K., Davis, T. L., Tootell, R. B. H., Wong, E. C., Fox, P. T., Belliveau, J. W., Weisskoff, R. M., & Rosen, B. R. (1997). Characterization of cerebral blood oxygenation and flow changes during prolonged brain activation. *Human Brain Mapping* 5, 93–109.

Bandettini, P. A., Wong, E. C., Hinks, R. S., Tikofsky, R. S., & Hyde, J. S. (1992). Time course EPI of human brain function during task activation. *Magnetic Resonance in Medicine* 25, 390–397.

Berger, H. (1901). *Zur Lehre von der Blutzirkulation in der Schandelhohle des Menschen*. Jena: Verlag Gustav Fischer.

Bittar, P. G., Charnay, Y., Pellerin, L., Bouras, C., & Magistretti, P. (1996). Selective distribution of lactate dehydrogenase isoenzymes in neurons and astrocytes of human brain. *Journal of Cerebral Blood Flow and Metabolism* 16, 1079–1089.

Block, F. (1946). Nuclear induction. *Physiology Review* 70, 460–474.

Blomqvist, G., Seitz, R. J., Sjogren, I., Halldin, C., Stone-Elander, S., Widen, L., Solin, O., & Haaparanta, M. (1994). Regional cerebral oxidative and total glucose consumption during rest and activation studied with positron emission tomography. *Acta Physiologica Scandinavica* 151, 29–43.

Broca, P. (1861). Remarques sur le siège de la faculté du langage articulé; suivies d'une observation d'aphémie (perte de la parole). *Bulletin de la Société Anatomique de Paris* 6, 330–357, 398–407.

Broca, P. (1879). Sur les temperatures morbides locales. *Bulletin de l'Académie de Médecine* (Paris) 2S, 1331–1347.

Brodmann, K. (1909). *Vergleichende lokalisationlehre der grosshirnrinde in inren prinzipien dargestellt auf grand des zellenbaues*. J. A. Barth: Leipzig.

Buckner, R. L., Petersen, S. E., Ojemann, J. G., Miezin, F. M., Squire, L. R., & Raichle, M. E. (1995). Functional anatomical studies of explicit and implicit memory retrieval tasks. *Journal of Neuroscience* 15, 12–29.

Buxton, R. B., & Frank, L. R. (1997). A model for the coupling between cerebral blood flow and oxygen metabolism during neural stimulation. *Journal of Cerebral Blood Flow and Metabolism* 17, 64–72.

Chesler, M., & Kraig, R. P. (1987). Intracellular pH of astrocytes increases rapidly with cortical stimulation. *American Journal of Psychology* 253, R666–R670.

Cooper, R., Crow, H. J., Walter, W. G., & Winter, A. L. (1966). Regional control of cerebral vascular reactivity and oxygen supply in man. *Brain Research* 3, 174–191.

Cooper, R., Papakostopoulos, D., & Crow, H. J. (1975). Rapid changes of cortical oxygen associated with motor and cognitive function in man. In *Blood Flow and Metabolism in the Brain*, A. M. Harper, W. B. Jennett, J. D. Miller, & J. O. Rowan, eds., 14.8–14.9. New York: Churchill Livingstone.

Cormack, A. M. (1963). Representation of a function by its line intergrals, with some radiological physics. *Journal of Applied Physics* 34, 2722–2727.

Cormack, A. M. (1973). Reconstruction of densities from their projections, with applications in radiological physics. *Physics in Medicine & Biology* 18(2), 195–207.

Creutzfeldt, O. D. (1975). Neurophysiological correlates of different functional states of the brain. In *Brain Work: The Coupling of Function, Metabolism and Blood Flow in the Brain*, D. H. Ingvar & N. A. Lassen, eds., 21–46. Copenhagen: Munksgaard.

Creutzfeldt, O., Ojemann, G., & Lettich, E. (1989). Neuronal activity in the human temporal lobe. I. Responses to speech. *Experimental Brain Research* 77, 451–475.

Donders, F. C. (1868; 1969). On the speed of mental processes. *Acta Psychologica* 30, 412–431.

Dringen, R., Schmoll, D., Cesar, M., & Hamprecht, B. (1993). Incorporation of radioactivity from [^{14}C]lactate into the glycogen of cultured mouse astroglial cells. Evidence for gluconeogenesis in brain cells. *Biological Chemistry Hoppe-Seyler* 374(5), 343–347.

Dringen, R., Wiesinger, H., & Hamprecht, B. (1993). Uptake of L-lactate by cultured rat brain neurons. *Neuroscience Letters* 163, 5–7.

Fox, P. T., & Raichle, M. E. (1986). Focal physiological uncoupling of cerebral blood flow and oxydative metabolism during somatosensory stimulation in human subjects. *Proceedings of the National Academy of Sciences USA* 83(4), 1140–1144.

Fox, P. T., Raichle, M. E., Mintun, M. A., & Dence, C. (1988). Nonoxidative glucose consumption during focal physiologic neural activity. *Science* 241, 462–464.

Frackowiak, R. S., Lenzi, G. L., Jones, T., & Heather, J. D. (1980). Quantitative measurement of regional cerebral blood flow and oxygen metabolism in man using 15O and positron emission tomography: Theory, procedure, and normal values. *Journal of Assisted Computed Tomography* 4(6), 727–736.

Frahm, J., Bruhn, H., Merboldt, K. D., & Hanicke, W. (1992). Dynamic MR imaging of human brain oxygenation during rest and photic stimulation. *Journal of Magnetic Resonance Imaging* 2(5), 501–505.

Frahm, J., Kruger, G., Merboldt, K.-D., & Kleinschmidt, A. (1996). Dynamic uncoupling and recoupling of perfusion and oxidative metabolism during focal brain activation in man. *Magnetic Resonance in Medicine* 35, 143–148.

Fulton, J. F. (1928). Observations upon the vascularity of the human occipital lobe during visual activity. *Brain* 51, 310–320.

Garey, L. J. (1994). *Brodmann's "Localization in the Cerebral Cortex."* Smith-Gordon, London.

Georgopoulos, A. P., Kalaska, J. F., Caminiti, R., & Massey, J. T. (1982). On the relations between the direction of two-dimensional arm movements and cell discharge in primate motor cortex. *Journal of Neuroscience* 2, 1527–1537.

Greenberg, J. H., Sohn, N. W., & Hand, P. J. (1997). Vibrissae-deafferentation produces plasticity in cerebral blood flow in response to somatosensory activation. *Journal of Cerebral Blood Flow and Metabolism* 17, S561.

Harley, C. A., & Bielajew, C. H. (1992). A comparison of glycogen phosphorylase a and cytochrome oxidase histochemical staining in rat brain. *Journal of Comparative Neurology* 322, 377–389.

Heistad, D. D., & Kontos, H. A. (1983). Cerebral circulation. In *Handbook of Physiology: The Cardiovascular System*, J. T. Sheppard & F. M. Abboud, eds., vol. 3, 137–182. Bethesda, Md.: American Physiological Society.

Hill, L. (1896). *The Physiology and Pathology of the Cerebral Circulation: An Experimental Research.* London: J. & A. Churchill.

Hochachka, P. W., & Mommsen, T. P. (1983). Protons and anaerobiosis. *Science* 219, 1391–1397.

Hoffman, E. J., Phelps, M. E., Mullani, N. A., Higgins, C. S., & Ter-Pogossian, M. M. (1976). Design and performance characteristics of a whole-body positron transaxial tomography. *Journal of Nuclear Medicine* 17, 493–502.

Hounsfield, G. N. (1973). Computerized transverse axial scanning (tomography): Part I. Description of system. *British Journal of Radiology* 46, 1016–1022.

Howse, D. C., Plum, F., Duffy, T. E., & Salford, L. G. (1973). Cerebral energy metabolism and the regulation of cerebral blood flow. *Transactions of the American Neurological Association* 98, 153–155.

Hyder, F., Chase, J. R., Behar, K. L., Mason, G. F., Rothman, D. L., & Shulman, R. G. (1996). Increased tricarboxylic acid cycle flux in rat brain during forepaw stimulation detected with 1H[13C]NMR. *Proceedings of the National Academy of Sciences USA* 93, 7612–7617.

Ingvar, G. H., & Risberg, J. (1965). Influence of mental activity upon regional cerebral blood flow in man. *Acta Neurologica Scandinavica* suppl. 14, 183–186.

James, W. (1890). *Principles of Psychology.* 2 vols. New York: Holt.

Kety, S. (1960). Measurement of local blood flow by the exchange on an inert diffusible substance. *Methods of Medical Research* 8, 228–236.

Kety, S. (1965). Closing comments. *Acta Neurologica Scandinavica* suppl. 14, 197.

Kim, S. G., & Ugurbil, K. (1997). Comparison of blood oxygenation and cerebral blood flow effects in fMRI: Estimation of relative oxygen consumption change. *Magnetic Resonance in Medicine* 38, 59–65.

Knudsen, G. M., Paulson, O. B., & Hertz, M. M. (1991). Kinetic analysis of the human blood-brain barrier transport of lactate and its influence by hypercapnia. *Journal of Cerebral Blood Flow and Metabolism* 11, 581–586.

Koepp, M. J., Gunn, R. N., Lawrence, A. D., Cunningham, V. J., Dagher, A., Jones, T., Brooks, D. J., Bench, C. J., & Grasby, P. M. (1998). Evidence for striatal dopamine release during a video game. *Nature* 393(6682), 266–268.

Kwong, K. K., Belliveau, J. W., Chesler, D. A., Goldberg, I. E., Weisskoff, R. M., Poncelet, B. P., Kennedy, D. N., Hoppel, B. E., Cohen, M. S., Turner, R., Cheng, H. M., Brady, T. J., & Rosen, B. R. (1992). Dynamic magnetic resonance imaging of human brain activity during primary sensory stimulation. *Proceedings of the National Academy of Sciences USA* 89, 5675–5679.

Landau, W. M., Freygang, W. H. J., Roland, L. P., Sokoloff, L., & Kety, S. S. (1955). The local circulation of the living brain: values in the unanesthetized and anesthetized cat. *Transactions of the American Neurology Association* 80, 125–129.

Lassen, N. A., Hoedt-Rasmussen, K., Sorensen, S. C., Skinhoj, E., Cronquist, B., Bodforss, E., & Ingvar, D. H. (1963). Regional cerebral blood flow in man determined by Krypton-85. *Neurology* 13, 719–727.

Lassen, N. A., Ingvar, D. H., & Skinhoj, E. (1978). Brain function and blood flow. *Scientific American* 239, 62–71.

Lauterbur, P. (1973). Image formation by induced local interactions: Examples employing nuclear magnetic resonance. *Nature* 242, 190–191.

Lear, J. L., & Kasliwal, R. K. (1991). Autoradiographic measurement of cerebral lactate transport rate constants in normal and activated conditions. *Journal of Cerebral Blood Flow and Metabolism* 11, 576–589.

Malonek, D., & Grinvald, A. (1996). Interactions between electrical activity and cortical microcirculation revealed by imaging spectroscopy: Implications for functional brain mapping. *Science* 272, 551–554.

Martin, W. R., & Raichle, M. E. (1983). Cerebellar blood flow and metabolism in cerebral hemisphere infarction. *Annals of Neurology* 14, 168–176.

Menon, R. S., Ogawa, S., Hu, X., Strupp, J. P., Anderson, P., & Ugurbil, K. (1995). BOLD based function MRI at 4 Tesla includes a capillary bed contribution: Echo-planar imaging correlates with previous optical imaging using intrinsic signals. *Magnetic Resonance in Medicine* 33, 453–459.

Mintun, M. A., Raichle, M. E., Martin, W. R. W., & Herscovitch, P. (1984). Brain oxygen utilization measured with O-15 radiotracers and positron emission tomography. *Journal of Nuclear Medicine* 25, 177–187.

Mosso, A. (1881). *Ueber den Kreislauf des Blutes im menschlichen Gehirn*. Leipzig: Verlag von Veit.

Mosso, A. (1894). *La temperatura del cervèllo*. Milan.

Ogawa, S., Lee, T. M., Kay, A. R., & Tank, D. W. (1990). Brain magnetic resonance imaging with contrast depedent on blood oxygenation. *Proceedings of the National Academy of Sciences USA* 87, 9868–9872.

Ogawa, S., Tank, D. W., Menon, R., Ellermann, J. M., Kim, S. G., Merkle, H., & Ugurbil, K. (1992). Intrinsic signal changes accompanying sensory stimulation: Functional brain mapping with magnetic resonance imaging. *Proceedings of the National Academy of Sciences USA* 89, 5951–5955.

Pauling, L., & Coryell, C. D. (1936). The magnetic properties and structure of hemoglobin, oxyghemoglobin and caronmonoxyhemoglobin. *Proceedings of the National Academy of Sciences USA* 22, 210–216.

Penfield, W. (1937). The circulation of the epileptic brain. *Research Publication Association Research Nervous Mental Disorder* 18, 605–637.

Petersen, S. E., Fox, P. T., Posner, M. I., Mintun, M., & Raichle, M. E. (1988). Positron emission tomographic studies of the cortical anatomy of single-word processing. *Nature* 331, 585–589.

Petersen, S. E., Fox, P. T., Posner, M. I., Mintun, M., & Raichle, M. E. (1989). Positron emission tomographic studies of the processing of single words. *Journal of Cognitive Neuroscience* 1, 153–170.

Plum, F., Posner, J. B., & Troy, B. (1968). Cerebral metabolic and circulatory responses to induced convulsions in animals. *Archives of Neurology* 18, 1–3.

Posner, M. I., & Raichle, M. E. (1994). *Images of Mind*. New York: Scientific American Library, c1994.

Powers, W. J., Hirsch, I. B., & Cryer, P. E. (1996). Effect of stepped hypoglycemia on regional cerebral blood flow response to physiological brain activation. *American Journal of Physiology* 270(2 Pt 2), H554–H559.

Prichard, J. W., Rothman, D. L., Novotny, E., Hanstock, C. C., & Shulman, R. G. (1991). Lactate rise detected by II NMR in human visual cortex during physiological stimulation. *Proceedings of the National Academy of Sciences USA* 88, 5829–5831.

Purcell, E. M., Torry, H. C., & Pound, R. V. (1946). Resonance absorption by nuclear magnetic moments in a solid. *Physiological Review* 69, 37.

Raichle, M. E. (1987). Circulatory and metabolic correlates of brain function in normal humans. In *Handbook of Physiology: The Nervous System*. Vol. 5, *Higher Functions of the Brain*, F. Plum, ed., 643–674. Bethesda, Md.: American Physiological Society.

Raichle, M. E., Fiez, J. A., Videen, T. O., MacLeod, A. M., Pardo, J. V., Fox, P. T., & Petersen, S. E. (1994). Practice-related changes in human brain functional anatomy during nonmotor learning. *Cerebral Cortex* 4, 8–26.

Raichle, M. E., Martin, W. R. W., Herscovitch, P., Mintun, M. A., & Markham, J. (1983). Brain blood flow measured with intravenous $H_2^{15}O$. II. Implementation and validation. *Journal of Nuclear Medicine* 24, 790–798.

Reivich, M., Kuhl, D., Wolf, A., Greenberg, J., Phelps, M., Ido, T., Casella, V., Hoffman, E., Alavi, A., & Sokoloff, L. (1979). The [18F] fluorodeoxyglucose method for the measurement of local cerebral glucose utilization in man. *Circulation Research* 44, 127–137.

Roy, C. S., & Sherrington, C. S. (1890). On the regulation of the blood supply of the brain. *Journal of Physiology* London 11, 85–108.

Salford, L. G., Duffy, T. E., & Plum, F. (1975). Association of blood flow and acid-base change in brain during afferent stimulation. In *Cerebral Circulation and Metabolism*, T. W. Langfitt, L. C. McHenry, M. Reivich, & H. Wollman, eds., 380–382. New York: Springer-Verlag.

Shulman, G. L., Corbetta, M., Buckner, R. L., Raichle, M. E., Fiez, J. A., Miezin, F. M., & Petersen, S. E. (1997). Top-down modulation of early sensory cortex. *Cerebral Cortex* 7, 193–206.

Shulman, G. L., Fiez, J. A., Corbetta, M., Buckner, R. L., Miezin, F. M., Raichle, M. E., & Petersen, S. E. (1997). Common blood flow changes across visual tasks: II. Decreases in cerebral cortex. *Journal of Cognitive Neuroscience* 9, 648–663.

Siesjo, B. K. (1978). *Brain Energy Metabolism*. New York: John Wiley & Sons.

Sokoloff, L., Reivich, M., Kennedy, C., Des Rosiers, M. H., Patlak, C. S., Pettigrew, K. D., Sakurada, O., & Shinohara, M. (1977). The [^{14}C]deoxyglucose method for the measurement of local glucose utilization: Theory, procedure and normal values in the conscious and anesthetized albino rat. *Journal of Neurochemistry* 28, 897–916.

Swanson, R. A., Morton, M. M., Sagar, S. M., & Sharp, F. R. (1992). Sensory stimulation induces local cerebral glycogenolysis: Demonstration by autoradiography. *Neuroscience* 51, 451–461.

Ter-Pogossian, M. M., Phelps, M. E., Hoffman, E. J., & Mullani, N. A. (1975). A positron-emission tomography for nuclear imaging (PET). *Radiology* 114, 89–98.

Thulborn, K. R., Waterton, J. C., Matthews, P. M., & Radda, G. K. (1982). Oxygenation dependence of the transverse relaxation time of water protons in whole blood at high field. *Biochimica et Biophysica Acta* 714, 265–270.

Tsacopoulos, M., & Magistretti, P. J. (1996). Metabolic coupling between glia and neurons. *Journal of Neuroscience* 16, 877–885.

Ueki, M., Linn, F., & Hossmann, K.-A. (1988). Functional activation of cerebral blood flow and metabolism before and after global ischemia of rat brain. *Journal of Cerebral Blood Flow and Metabolism* 8, 486–494.

Woolsey, T. A., Rovainen, C. M., Cox, S. B., Henegar, M. H., Liang, G. E., Liu, D., Moskalenko, Y. E., Sui, J., & Wei, L. (1996). Neuronal units linked to microvascular modules in cerebral cortex: Response elements for imaging the brain. *Cerebral Cortex* 6, 647–660.

Yamauchi, H., Fukuyama, H., & Kimura, J. (1992). Hemodynamic and metabolic changes in crossed cerebellar hypoperfusion. *Stroke* 23, 855–860.

Yarowsky, P., Kadekaro, M., & Sokoloff, L. (1983). Frequency-dependent activation of glucose utilization in the superior cervical ganglion by electrical stimulation of cervical sympathetic trunk. *Proceedings of the National Academy of Sciences USA* 80, 4179–4183.

2 Functional Neuroimaging Methods: PET and fMRI

Randy L. Buckner and Jessica M. Logan

INTRODUCTION

An ongoing challenge in the exploration of human cognition is developing and applying methods that can link underlying neuronal activity with cognitive operations.
A complete understanding of the functional anatomy of cognition will ideally encom-
pass knowledge of how cognitive operations arise at the level of individual neurons
and up to the level of distributed systems of brain areas, and how the functional
properties at one level give rise to functional properties at another. This level of
understanding, of course, is a distant target. As a field, functional neuroimaging is
beginning modestly and entering into explorations at a few select points where current experimental methods give glimpses of the functional anatomy of human cognition. Several methods are widely available and discussed throughout this book,
including those based on electrophysiological and related methods (e.g., EEG and
MEG), those based on studying brain injury, and, most recently, those based on
hemodynamic measures (e.g., PET and fMRI). The focus of this chapter is on these
latter two methods—PET and fMRI, which are referred to as functional neuroimaging methods.

Functional neuroimaging methods provide a means of measuring local changes in
brain activity (Frackowiak & Friston, 1995; Posner & Raichle, 1994; Roland, 1993).
In less than an hour or two, a healthy young subject can be led through a noninvasive battery of imaging procedures that yields a picture of active brain areas across
a number of conditions. Imaging can be done on normal as well as compromised
brains. However, current neuroimaging methods are not without their limitations and
challenges. For example, current methods depend on indirect measurements of brain
activity (hemodynamics) that are both sluggish in timing and poorly understood.
Nonetheless, careful application of neuroimaging techniques can provide a window
through which to view the neural basis of cognitive functions.

In this chapter, the basis of each method (PET and fMRI) and how the two relate
to one another are briefly described. Particular focus is placed on a set of methods
referred to as event-related fMRI (ER-fMRI). These methods allow functional neuroimaging procedures to regain the experimental flexibility afforded to traditional
cognitive paradigms, including imaging brain areas active during rapidly presented,
randomly intermixed types of trials and data analysis based on subject performance.
Throughout the chapter, clarifying examples of applications are given that focus on
memory. However, the principles illustrated in such examples apply equally to all
areas of cognition, including attention, language, and emotion.

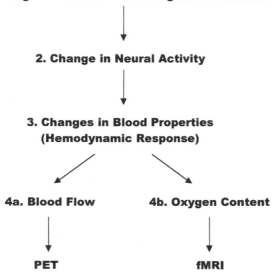

Figure 2.1
Both PET and fMRI functional neuroimaging rely on the observation that (1) changes in behavioral and cognitive task demands lead to (2) changes in neural activity. Through poorly understood mechanisms, changes in neuronal activity correlate closely with (3) changes in blood properties—referred to as hemodynamics. It is these indirect hemodynamic measurements of neuronal activity that both PET and fMRI are based upon. PET measures brain activity through blood property change relating to (4a) blood flow, while fMRI measures a related property involving change in (4b) oxygen content (often referred to as the BOLD-contrast mechanism).

FUNCTIONAL NEUROIMAGING METHODS: PET AND FMRI

Physiological Basis and Limitations of PET and fMRI

Both PET and fMRI measure brain activity indirectly by taking advantage of a for-tuitous physiologic property: when a region of the brain increases activity, both blood flow and the oxygen content of the blood in that region increase (figure 2.1). PET uses radiolabeled tracers to visualize the blood flow changes related to neural activity (Raichle, 1987). fMRI, which has been widely applied only since about 1995, most commonly visualizes neural activity indirectly, through changes in oxygen content of the blood (Kwong et al., 1992; Ogawa et al., 1990, 1992). The signal arises because changes in blood flow bring more oxyhemoglobin into a region than is utilized by local regions of increased neural activity. The net result is a decrease in deoxhemo-globin concentration in the blood, which conveys a signal that can be detected with

MRI. This signal is commonly referred to as the Blood Oxygenation Level Dependent (BOLD) contrast mechanism. Other metabolic and hemodynamic contrast signals appropriate for both PET and fMRI exist but are much less commonly used.

Several sources of data suggest that signals detected by PET and fMRI are valid measurements of local changes in neuronal activity. First, studies of primary visual cortex activation have capitalized on a well-understood retinotopic organization to demonstrate predictable activation patterns (e.g., DeYoe et al., 1996; Engel et al., 1997; Fox et al., 1987; Sereno et al., 1995) and suggest a current practical resolution of about 3 to 6 mm (e.g., Engel et al., 1997; Raichle, 1987). Resolution at this level can be used for mapping within large cortical areas (e.g., V1), as well as to identify smaller cortical areas (e.g., LMT). Subregions of prefrontal cortex can also be separated with this resolution. Imaging at this resolution, however, would not resolve the columnar organization within a functional area (but see Menon et al., 1997). Second, there is evidence that neuroimaging can track and characterize neuronal activity over time. When it has been prolonged or when multiple visual stimuli have been presented to subjects, the hemodynamic signal summates across the separate (Dale & Buckner, 1997; Fox & Raichle, 1985) and continuous (Boynton et al., 1996; Konishi et al., 1996) evoked neuronal events, as would be predicted for a measurement linked to neuronal activity (although deviations from this pattern can be found; Friston et al., 1997; Vazquez & Noll, 1998). Neuroimaging methods have also demonstrated reliability across independent subject groups and even imaging modality (e.g., PET compared to fMRI; Clark et al., 1996; Ojemann et al., 1998).

However, while such findings are indicative of the success of neuroimaging methods in detecting and measuring activity, both techniques come with several limitations that must be considered. A discussion of limitations is important, not to undermine the utility of the techniques discussed here but to understand more critically the types of questions that can successfully be posed, given current technology, and to understand the advances and refinements that must be made before the range of the questions can be expanded. Specifically, it is unlikely that PET or currently applied fMRI will provide much information about local physiologic properties, such as whether a net activity change relies on inhibitory or excitatory synapses, or on the relative combinations of the two. For instance, studies with current functional neuroimaging methods yield only information about net changes in activity (both excitatory and inhibitory) within brain regions spanning several millimeters or more. Furthermore, hemodynamics in response to neuronal activity is revealed on a temporal scale far longer than the neuronal activity itself. For example, for a brief sensory event lasting fractions of a second, hemodynamic changes will take place over 10–12 sec

(Bandettini, 1993; Blamire et al., 1992). Evidence also exists that there may be residual effects that last as long as a minute (Fransson et al., 1999).

While this limitation is less apparent for PET methods, which average data over
time periods of 30 sec to 1 min, this temporal "blurring" of the signal is an acknowledged limitation for fMRI studies, which can potentially detect changes occurring
in well under 1 sec (Cohen & Weisskoff, 1991). Fortunately, the exact restrictions on
measurements are not as severe as one might imagine. In fact, recent developments
in fMRI paradigm design have shown that meaningful signals can be extracted for
events ocurring much more rapidly than once every 10 sec. For example, various
fMRI methods have taken advantage of the reliable timing of the evoked blood flow
signal to demonstrate temporal resolution at the subsecond level (Burock et al., 1998;
Menon et al., 1998; Rosen et al., 1998). In addition, changes in neural activity associated with individual trials or components of a trial in a task can be observed (and
will be discussed more extensively below under "Issues Related to Task Design").

As one illustration of these kinds of paradigms, Richter et al. (1997), in a dramatic
example of the temporal resolution and sensitivity of fMRI, captured brain activity
associated with a *single* momentary cognitive act of mentally rotating a stimulus,
without recourse to averaging over events. O'Craven and Kanwisher (in press) have
demonstrated a similar level of temporal precision and sensitivity by showing that—
on a trial-by-trial basis—brain activity associated with presentation of faces could be
elicited by having an individual simply imagine a single face (without the actual stimulus present). However, despite continued advances in efforts to expand the temporal
resolution capabilities of fMRI and PET, researchers who wish to focus on the fine-
grained analysis of the temporal cascade of brain activity across areas will most likely
continue to rely on techniques more directly coupled to neuronal activity, such as
EEG, MEG, and perhaps even human optical imaging (Gratton & Fabiani, 1998).

Several differences beyond temporal precision exist between PET and fMRI that
are worth mentioning. In contrast to PET, which requires an intravenous injection of
a radioactive isotope, fMRI is completely noninvasive, requiring only that the subject
lie still within the MRI scanner and comply with the behavioral procedures (DeYoe
et al., 1994). In addition, compared to PET, fMRI is relatively inexpensive and can
be performed on scanners already available within most major hospitals, positioning
it as a method available for widespread clinical use. However, fMRI does have disadvantages in regard to PET in that it is is extremely sensitive to a number of artifacts
that can impede examination of brain function, especially brain motion, which poses
one of the most severe challenges to fMRI data collection. Brain motion arising from
many sources, such as subject movement or even motion on the order of millimeters
associated with the respiratory and cardiac cycles, can disrupt the ability to acquire

fMRI data. Motion correction algorithms (e.g., Woods et al., 1998) and head immobilization techniques are routinely used to reduce these difficulties, but motion remains a serious challenge to fMRI studies, especially those concerned with clinical populations. In addition, while overt speech responses are routinely used in the design of PET studies, it is difficult (though not impossible) to image overt speech production during fMRI studies because of the head motion and changes in air volume associated with overt speech (e.g., see Barch et al., 1999; Birn et al., in press; Phelps et al., 1997). With continued technological advances and methodological innovations in research, it seems likely that these limitations due to motion will be overcome in time.

Another limitation of BOLD-contrast fMRI, at least as it is most often applied, is that it does not afford uniform brain sampling. Due to issues surrounding the physics of image acquisition, functional images are insensitive to regions near orbital frontal cortex and in the anterior temporal lobes (Ojemann et al., 1997). In these regions the signal-to-noise ratio is extremely low. Thus, when null results are found in these regions, it is important not to interpret them as a case of no change in brain activity. Rather, a limitation of the the imaging method should be acknowledged by realizing that the method does not sample brain activity in those regions.

While PET has disadvantages in terms of invasiveness and temporal sampling, there is one area in which it has a clear current advantage: quantitation. PET can provide relatively accurate measurements of absolute blood flow (and some other metabolic measures); fMRI currently cannot. Because of this, in addition to images of structural lesions, images of "functional" lesions, such as areas distant from structural lesions that show metabolic abnormalities, can be obtained and can potentially be correlated with behavioral measures, as is often done with structural lesions.

Issues Related to Task Design

Beyond basic technical considerations, one must also confront issues of the practical application of neuroimaging techniques to questions about human cognition. Namely, how can tasks and trials within a task be constructed to disentangle brain-based cognitive operations? This topic presents a number of challenges, and no single answer exists. In fact, many of the authors of chapters in this volume may disagree on specific solutions. Nonetheless, there are a number of constraints and issues that must be faced.

A common goal in conducting neuroimaging studies is to begin to isolate, either by well matched task comparisons or through convergence across multiple studies, the processing roles of specific brain areas. The difficulty in accomplishing this goal is that brain activity changes are revealed as (1) relative changes between pairs of tasks, (2) gradual or nonlinear changes across a series of tasks, or (3) correlations between tasks or measures across subjects. Absolute measures are currently not possible. Relative change between two tasks or a series of tasks must be designed to disentangle cognitive operations based on relative comparisons.

The basic paradigm construct most commonly used is to have subjects engage in a target behavioral task for a period of time and then contrast that task period with periods where subjects perform a reference task. For example, the subject might perform a target task such as a word retrieval task, and the measurement obtained during the performance of that task would be contrasted with a measurement obtained when the subject performed a matched reference task, such as the passive viewing of words with no retrieval demand. The logic of this paradigm construct is that brain activity will change between the two task states and will correlate selectively with the manipulated task demands (e.g., the difference between the word retrieval task and the passive word viewing task will reveal activity associated with retrieval of words and any other task demands that differ between them). When using fMRI, images are taken of the brain repeatedly and in sequence (as rapidly as one set of whole-brain images every 2 sec). Brain areas of activation are identified by examining which specific regions change signal intensity as the task state changes from the reference condition (word viewing or fixation) to the target task (word retrieval). Statistical procedures ranging from simple, direct comparisons between task states to more elaborate assessments of interactions and correlations among task states can then be employed to identify those regions whose activity change is unlikely to occur by chance (Frackowiak & Friston, 1995). Correlation of activity with subjects' behavioral performance is also possible.

One issue associated with task paradigms of this form is that they may cause differences in the processing strategies (or cognitive sets) adopted by subjects during task performance via the blocking of trials, which may result in differential patterns of neural activity that do not have to do with the item-specific processes elicited by the individual trials per se. It is easy to envision such a situation in its extreme form, such as when two task blocks being compared differ markedly in how individual trials (or lack of trials) modulate the arousal level of a subject (for a particularly problematic example of confounding arousal level, see Buckner, Raichle et al., 1996). This issue crops up, however, in considerably more subtle forms in cognitive paradigms where subject strategies may be influenced by the predictability of events.

An illustration of this issue comes from blocked studies of recognition memory (Buckner, Koutstaal, Schachter, Dale, et al., 1998; Buckner, Koutstaal, Schachter, Wagner, et al., 1998; Rugg et al., 1996; Wagner, Desmond, et al., 1998). Debate arose as to the role of certain prefrontal areas in memory retrieval. Rugg et al. (1996), in an influential study, suggested that certain prefrontal areas were most active during trials where subjects successfully retrieved information. The manner in which this conclusion was derived, however, may have influenced the interpretation. In this study and those which preceded it, blocks of trials that had fewer or greater numbers of successfully retrieved items were the basis of exploration. Rugg and colleagues noted that blocks with the most successfully retrieved items activated certain prefrontal areas to the greatest degree.

More recently, paradigms have been developed that avoid the problems of analyzing and interpreting data from blocked designs by isolating individual trials of tasks— "event-related" fMRI (ER-fMRI) procedures (Buckner, Bandettini, et al., 1996; Dale & Buckner, 1997; Josephs et al., 1997; Rosen et al., 1998; Zarahn et al., 1997). These procedures allow experimenters to contrast activity associated with different trial types and even to disentangle activity associated with subcomponents of a trial. In a comparison of an ER-fMRI study and a blocked trial study of memory retrieval similar to that of Rugg et al. (1996), Buckner et al. (Buckner, Bandettini, et al., 1998; Buckner, Koutstaal, Schacter, Dale, et al., 1998) were able to show that modulation of the prefrontal areas in relation to retrieval success was closely tied to the use of a blocked trial procedure; ER-fMRI separation of successfully retrieved and correctly rejected items indicated equal levels of prefrontal signal change. The preliminary conclusion is that the blocked trial paradigm, where item events are predictable, may have encouraged subjects to adjust their strategy (implicitly or explicitly) and influenced prefrontal participation. In other words, set effects specific to an encouraged strategy may have resulted (Düzel et al., 1999; Wagner, Desmond, et al., 1998). ER-fMRI paradigms can circumvent this issue by presenting trials randomly and contrasting different trial types under conditions where the specific upcoming event type cannot be predicted.

More generally, ER-fMRI methods have broadly expanded the spectrum of task designs and analytical techniques that can be used in neuroimaging studies. As illustrated in the example above, ER-fMRI allows paradigms to move from "blocked" testing procedures in which long periods of task performance are integrated, to paradigms that isolate individual trial events or subcomponents of trial events. This provides much greater flexibility in experimental design by allowing for selective averaging of stimulus events or task conditions that may be intermixed on a trial-by-trial basis, as is done in most behavioral studies. Moreover, by focusing on responses to single events rather than to extended blocks, ER-fMRI provides a means of examining questions regarding the dynamics and time course of neural activity under various conditions. Because of its importance to the field and its general relevance to understanding the hemodynamic signal being detected by both PET and fMRI, it is worthwhile to consider the basis of ER-fMRI in more detail.

Event-Related fMRI

The development of ER-fMRI has followed the development of our understanding of the basic principles of the BOLD-contrast hemodynamic response, as elucidated by fMRI and optical imaging studies (e.g., Malonek & Grinvald, 1996). The blood properties contributing to the BOLD signal are most likely similar to blood flow signals measured with PET, although it is difficult to support the link precisely. Specifically, there are two key characteristics of the BOLD hemodynamic response most relevant to cognitive task paradigms: (1) it can be detected following even brief periods of stimulation and (2) it can be characterized by a predictable response function.

The first characteristic of the BOLD hemodynamic response—that it can be elicited by a brief period of neuronal activity—was observed soon after BOLD-contrast became available for functional neuroimaging. Blamire et al. (1992) noted that visual stimuli presented for 2 sec were sufficient to produce detectable hemodynamic responses. Bandettini (1993) demonstrated signal changes in response to even shorter task events, examining responses to finger movements for durations ranging from 0.5 sec to 5 sec. In all situations, including the 0.5 sec finger movement, clear increases in the hemodynamic signal were present. Following these early studies were a number of similar investigations of motor and visual stimulation (Boulanouar et al., 1996; Humberstone et al., 1995; Konishi et al., 1996; Savoy et al., 1995). A bit later this finding was carried over to the realm of cognitive paradigms, where the source of stimulation is not as precisely defined and more subtle responses are elicited.

Buckner, Bandettini, et al. (1996) observed that subtle signal changes in visual and prefrontal brain areas can be detected during isolated trials of a word generation task. Kim et al. (1997) examined responses to tasks involving subject-initiated motor preparation. They detected event-related responses in motor and visual cortex. These and other observations make it clear that fMRI can detect hemodynamic responses to very brief neuronal events, making it possible to be utilized in a truly event-related fashion (Rosen et al., 1998). And, as mentioned, a number of cognitive tasks paradigms have already exploited these methods (e.g., Brewer et al., 1998; Buckner, Goodman, et al., 1998; Carter et al., 1998; Cohen et al., 1997; Courtney et al., 1997; Wagner, Schacter, et al., 1998).

The second characteristic of the BOLD hemodynamic response is the nature and reliability of the shape of the response to a given brief, fixed interval of neuronal activity. Early studies using sustained stimulation paradigms (e.g., Kwong et al., 1992) noted that the hemodynamic response is delayed in onset from the time of presumed neural activity by about 2–6 sec. The work of Blamire et al. (1992) confirmed this finding for brief sensory events, and further demonstrated that the hemodynamic response is prolonged in duration, lasting on the order of 10–12 sec. Certain, more subtle, components of the response may have considerably longer recovery periods (Fransson et al., 1999). From this information, investigators began to incorporate explicit models of the hemodynamic response function into analyses of time-series data, in order to better account for the response lag and delayed offset properties. Analysis methods have been developed to exploit the power and unique characteristics of ER-fMRI paradigms more specifically (Clark et al., 1997; Dale & Buckner, 1997; Friston et al., 1998; Josephs et al., 1997; Zarahn et al., 1997). Several approaches are now being explored that utilize full implementation of the statistical framework of the general linear model (GLM) (e.g., Josephs et al., 1997; Friston et al., 1998; Zarahn et al., 1997). Such methods promise the most flexibility because interactions of event types with time and performance variables can be easily coded.

An important question in the application of ER-fMRI paradigms is the boundary conditions for effectively applying the methods (e.g., how close in time separate trial events can be presented). Extremely rapid presentation rates (less than 2 sec between sequential events) are feasible and provide a powerful means of mapping brain function (Burock et al., 1998). Several distinct issues relate directly to this conclusion. The first issue concerns the linearity of the BOLD response over sequential neuronal events. As mentioned above, recent work in early visual cortex suggests that, on first approximation, changes in intensity or duration have *near* linear and additive effects on the BOLD response (Boynton et al., 1996). These findings appear to hold for higher cognitive processes as well, in that similar results have been observed through manipulations of intensity (load) and duration within working memory paradigms (Cohen et al., 1997). Moreover, data from visual sensory responses suggest that the hemodynamic response of one neural event summates in a *roughly* linear manner on top of preceding events (Dale & Buckner, 1997). Subtle departures from linear summation have been observed in nearly every study that has examined response summation, and in certain studies, the nonlinearities have been quite pronounced (Friston et al., 1997; Vazquez & Noll, 1998). Fortunately, using parameters typical to many studies, the nonlinearities may be subtle enough, in certain situations, to still be considered approximately linear.

These findings suggest that it may be possible to carry out ER-fMRI studies using presentation rates (about 1 event per 2 sec or less) that are much faster than the time course of the BOLD response. Directly relevant to this, Dale and Buckner (1997) showed that individual responses to sensory stimuli can be separated and analyzed by using overlap correction methods. Burock et al. (1998) pushed this limit even farther by randomly intermixing sensory stimuli at a rate of 1 stimulus every 500 msec

(250 msec stimulus duration, 250 msec gap between sequential stimuli). Recent rapid ER-fMRI studies of higher-level cognitive processes, such as repetition priming (Buckner, Goodman, et al., 1998), face memory (Clark et al., 1998), and memory encoding (Wagner, Schacter, et al., 1998), suggest the procedures can be effectively applied to cognitive tasks and higher-order brain regions (e.g., prefrontal cortex).

Example of an Application of Functional Neuroimaging: Episodic Memory Encoding

As an example of how the variety of paradigms and functional neuroimaging methods can be used to study cognition, a series of tasks that examine encoding into episodic memory can be considered. Episodic memory is the form of memory concerned with recollection of specific events from the past (Tulving, 1983). Relevant to this discussion, a number of neuroimaging studies using both PET and fMRI, blocked and event-related paradigms, and both young and older adults have been used to explore episodic encoding, providing an illustration of the many aforementioned principles and the multiple ways in which functional neuroimaging can be effectively applied.

The most basic kind of episodic memory encoding task that can be conducted is an *intentional* memorization task in a blocked task paradigm. During such a task, subjects are presented with a series of items, such as words, and are directly instructed to memorize the words. Alternatively, encoding can be encouraged *incidentally* by having subjects make a meaning-based semantic decision about each word. Meaning-based elaborative processes promote memorization independent of any intent to remember (e.g., Craik & Lockhart, 1972).

Blocked task paradigms have examined intentional and incidental encoding with PET and fMRI (Demb et al., 1995; Fletcher et al., 1995; Kapur et al., 1994, 1996; Kelley et al., 1998). Kapur and colleagues (1994) conducted a study of encoding using a paradigm prototypical of PET studies. In their study, subjects in one task were presented with a series of words and were instructed to decide, for each word, whether it represented a living (e.g., "dog") or nonliving (e.g., "car") entity. Eighty words were presented during the task and a PET image was acquired over a 60-sec period, averaging activity over the brain during that epoch. A second task was examined that was identical in format except the task instruction was to decide whether each word contained the letter "a." One of the two tasks (living/nonliving judgment or letter detection) was presented to the subject about every 10 min—leaving a period of time for the subjects to rest while the level of radiation returned to an acceptable baseline. Memory performance on a later recognition test differed markedly between the two tasks, with the meaning-based processing task showing significantly greater recognition performance. Inferences about brain areas active during encoding were made by directly comparing the images acquired during the living/nonliving task and the letter detection task. They found that several areas within left prefrontal cortex were significantly more active during the meaning-based task, including areas falling along the left inferior frontal gyrus (Brodmann's areas 45, 46, and 47).

Blocked task paradigms can be conducted in a quite similar manner using fMRI, as illustrated by a study of Demb et al. (1995). Much like Kapur et al. (1994), they used a task encouraging incidental encoding. Their meaning-based processing task, however, required subjects to decide whether words were abstract (e.g., "think") or concrete (e.g., "anvil"), and their reference task involved deciding whether words were in uppercase or lowercase letters. Words were presented sequentially in task blocks (similar to PET) and brain activity was temporally integrated over the averaged blocks.

Several subtle differences existed between the two studies owing to the exact constraints of PET and fMRI. In the study of Demb et al. (1995), task blocks involving the meaning-based decision immediately followed those involving the surface-based uppercase/lowercase decision. The tasks alternated every 40 sec for a period of about 5 min. Such a design allows activity to be compared across task blocks that occur close together in time. Thus, while PET requires task blocks to be separated by long periods, fMRI does not. One advantage of this difference in design is that a considerable amount of data can be acquired in an individual subject using fMRI. Consistent with this, Demb et al. (1995) not only were able to generalize the PET findings of Kapur et al. (1994) to fMRI, but also could clearly detect activity in left prefrontal cortex along the inferior frontal gyrus in individual subjects. One further difference to note is that Demb et al. (1995) imaged activity over only a relatively small portion of the brain (within frontal cortex). While this was a limitation at the time, fMRI studies can now sample activity over the whole brain (barring the regions of signal loss). Buckner and Koutstaal (1998), for example, replicated the study of Demb et al. (1995) using whole-brain imaging procedures.

How else might blocked trial encoding studies be conducted? The studies of Kapur et al. (1994) and Demb et al. (1995) compared two task states that each involved similar presentation of words and response selection demands, but differed in terms of task demands related to encoding. The goal was to hold as many processes as possible in common across the tasks and isolate those related to encoding. Both tasks isolated left frontal regions. We refer to this form of task comparison as "tight" because as many variables as possible are held constant between the two tasks being compared. Another approach could have been to make a much broader comparison, without as much control over possibly interacting variables; for instance, a comparison between the meaning-based task promoting encoding and a low-level reference condition involving rest or visual fixation with no word presentation. We refer to this form of task comparison as "loose." Buckner and Koutstaal (1998) made such a loose comparison, using tasks adopted directly from Demb et al. (1995). In their fMRI study, the abstract/concrete meaning-based processing task was compared to a low-level reference condition where subjects simply fixated on a crosshair. The shallow uppercase/lowercase processing task was also compared to the fixation task. This approach might seem odd if the only goal were to isolate areas related to encoding; however, such an approach has several merits.

First and most important, it is not always possible to trust that an experiment has been conducted successfully and that appropriate data have been collected. Imaging methods are noisy, and not all data sets are equal. Some subjects comply, others do not; and, for unknown reasons, there is a belief that some compliant subjects show minimal activation responses due to physiological factors. Whether this belief can be substantiated with data or not, many investigators would agree some subjects repeatedly provide high-quality data while others provide low-quality data. In any individual subject or group of subjects it is often impossible to tell, in advance, what kind of data will result. By making loose task comparisons, activity related to highly predictable regions is not balanced across tasks and can be used to evaluate the quality of data.

For example, in addition to processes related to encoding, the meaning-based decision task required subjects to view words and make motor responses. These demands did not occur in the fixation reference task, where no word stimuli were presented and no responses were made. A strong prediction is that primary visual and motor cortex should be activated for tasks, such as the meaning-based decision task, that involve visual and motor processing (and this activation was in fact evident in the actual study). Observation of activity within these regions does not necessarily tell us about cognitive operations, but it does tell us about the quality of the data. Thus, rather than being dependent solely upon evaluation of activation patterns that are perhaps unknown, as is the case in many tight task comparisons, loose task comparisons can be designed to allow the evaluation of activity changes within predictable locations and, therefore, help to determine the quality of data obtained in a given study.

A second reason to use a loose task comparison is that it is often desirable to survey the entire set of brain areas active during a task and not just the select few that differ in the tight task comparison. For example, left frontal cortex is consistently activated during tasks promoting verbal encoding into episodic memory (Tulving et al., 1994). However, left frontal cortex has been only intermittently reported during episodic *retrieval* of verbal materials. This finding led to the proposal by Tulving and colleagues (1994) that left frontal cortex is preferentially involved in encoding (as compared to right frontal cortex) and right frontal cortex is preferentially involved in retrieval (as compared to left frontal cortex). While we do not disagree that there is some truth to these statements, the latter statement is somewhat misleading, in that the impression is given that left frontal cortex is not robustly activated during episodic retrieval. Quite to the contrary, left frontal cortex is activated robustly during episodic memory retrieval for verbal materials (Buckner et al., 1995), and the impression of strong preferential involvement of right frontal cortex (to the exclusion of left) is partly an artifact of using only a specific form of tight task comparison (Buckner, 1996; Petrides et al., 1995).

Most PET studies of verbal episodic retrieval have compared episodic retrieval of words to a reference task that involves meaning-based elaboration on words. In these studies, left frontal cortex was likely activated to similar degrees across both tasks and was absent in the tight task comparison (consistent with the intent of these tight task comparisons, which sought to control for elaborative verbal processes). In the few instances where additional loose task comparisons were examined, left frontal cortex was clearly present (e.g., Buckner et al., 1995; Petrides et al., 1995). This illustration serves as an example of why it is necessary to determine all of the active areas during a task—both those selective for specific manipulated task demands and those more generally involved in a broad class of tasks.

For these reasons we believe loose task comparisons are important in cognitive functional neuroimaging studies. However, it would be unreasonable to suggest that only loose task comparisons should be included in a study. Loose task comparisons come with their own interpretational challenges (Binder et al., 1999; Shulman et al., 1997). Given the amount of data that can be acquired in fMRI studies, it is often possible to include a variety of task comparisons that involve both loose comparisons, which give information about the entire network of areas active during a task, and tight comparisons, which serve to isolate specific cognitive operations. One can even imagine a parametric design where several tasks are compared that progressively differ in their ability to promote encoding, and all are compared to each other, as well as to a low-level reference task (for such an example in the domain of working memory, see Braver et al., 1997). Interactions within factorial designs are possible as well (Frackowiak & Friston, 1995).

One last point on this issue is worth mentioning. Any single task comparison is likely to be problematic and provide a biased piece of the overall puzzle. Task analyses may be incomplete, and set effects are probably encouraged during blocked testing procedures in ways we have not yet envisioned. Therefore, convergence and multiple approaches to the same cognitive question should be the rule of thumb.

Along these lines, it is possible to consider a second class of studies that can be conducted to isolate encoding processes based on ER-fMRI designs. ER-fMRI paradigms allow one to isolate and extract information associated within individual trials rather than being restricted to temporally averaging over sequential trials. As an example of how ER-fMRI can parallel blocked trial procedures, we consider an ER-fMRI extension of the PET study of Kapur et al. (1994) and the fMRI study of Demb et al. (1995). Rotte et al. (1998) conducted a study in which they randomly intermixed meaning-based and shallowly processed trials. Identical in task construct to Demb et al. (1995), they presented words, one at a time, and randomly cued each trial as to whether the subject should classify the word as abstract or concrete (the meaning-based task), or as uppercase or lowercase. However, the subjects could not anticipate which kind of decision would be required (i.e., set effects were held to a minimum). In addition, randomly interspersed throughout the study were catch trials where no words were presented: subjects simply continued to fixate within these trials as they would normally do between trials. Using ER-fMRI selective averaging procedures (Dale & Buckner, 1997), they were able to show again that meaning-based processing —at the individual item level—was associated with left frontal activation along the inferior frontal gyrus. These words were recognized, on average, more often than words cued for the shallow uppercase/lowercase decision, providing yet another link between left frontal activation and verbal encoding processes.

Another way in which ER-fMRI studies can be conducted has yielded perhaps the strongest link for left frontal involvement in encoding. Trial events can be sorted on the basis of subject performance. Using event-related fMRI, Wagner, Schacter, and colleagues (1998) sorted words by whether they were remembered or forgotten on a later recognition test (similar to many ERP studies; Halgren & Smith, 1987; Paller, 1990; Rugg, 1995). In their study, again extending from Demb et al. (1995), only a single task was used to promote encoding (the abstract/concrete judgment task). Subjects were presented a series of words, one every 2 sec, and instructed to decide whether each word was abstract or concrete. Interspersed throughout the study were catch trials, similar to those mentioned above, where no words were presented. From the subject's point of view, the task appeared as a continuous stream of words with the same goal: meaning-based classification. The catch trials caused the words to appear randomly in time so that subjects experienced gaps between some words and not others, but otherwise, the gaps did not alter the nature of the single meaning-based classification task the subjects were attempting to complete. No reference was made to the fact that a memory test would follow.

After imaging, subjects received a surprise recognition test enabling the experimenter to identify which words were remembered and which were forgotten. The final step involved post hoc sorting of the trials. All trials in which subjects processed words that they later remembered were separated from those that involved forgotten items. Comparing activity associated with words remembered to activity associated with words forgotten showed significantly increased activity in left inferior frontal gyrus in regions similar to those identified by Kapur et al. (1994) and the studies that followed. Brewer et al. (1998) noted similar frontal activation during an ER-fMRI paradigm involving picture processing, but in their study, encoding correlated with right frontal cortex rather than left frontal cortex.

Taken collectively, the studies discussed above show the variety of the kinds of paradigms that can be conducted using functional neuroimaging methods. Different paradigm constructs will be optimal for different cognitive questions. In the study of encoding, convergent results have been suggested by all paradigm constructs ranging from blocked trial PET studies to ER-fMRI paradigms: activity within frontal cortex correlates with episodic memory encoding (Buckner et al., 1999).

Flexibility in the application of functional neuroimaging methods extends beyond the kind of paradigm that can be employed. All of the studies discussed to this point focus on the study of healthy young participants. However, PET and fMRI procedures are not restricted to studies of young adults. For instance, several studies have begun to address effects of aging on brain areas active during memory encoding. Grady et al. (1995), in an influential study, examined brain areas activated during encoding of faces in young and in elderly subjects. Consistent with observations that normal young subjects show prefrontal activation during encoding (as mentioned above), young subjects in their study showed left prefrontal activation during the (nonverbal) encoding task. Elderly subjects, however, did not show significant left prefrontal activation, and the direct comparison between young and old subjects was significant. Medial temporal cortex activity also showed differences between age groups, although the direct comparison was not significant. The relevance of this finding is tied to the behavioral results: elderly subjects recognized significantly fewer of the faces than young subjects. Elderly subjects may have failed to adopt appropriate encoding strategies that would activate left frontal regions and promote encoding (Buckner & Koutstaal, 1998). Thus, as a consequence of misapplied frontally mediated encoding strategies, their recognition performance may have suffered.

Cabeza et al. (1997) noted a complementary finding in a PET study of encoding and retrieval. In their study, young adults showed left frontal activation increases during verbal encoding and additional right-lateralized frontal activation during retrieval. By contrast, older adults showed minimal frontal activity during encoding (similar to Grady et al., 1995) and more bilateral activity during retrieval. Cabeza and colleagues argued that advanced age is associated with two forms of neural change: (1) age-related decreases in local regional activity, indicating less efficient processing, and (2) age-related increases in activity, indicating functional compensation. Thus, the basic kinds of paradigm constructs used with young adults can be applied to older adult populations, and this ability to link neural activity to behavioral performance demonstrates the power of applying these neuroimaging techniques to our basic understanding of cognition.

ISSUES

As we have discussed, a number of issues regarding the limits of the application of functional neuroimaging methods are still in debate and provide an important focus for further research. For instance, Menon et al. (1998) have demonstrated that fMRI procedures can map changes in hemodynamic offsets within regions by as little as a few hundred milliseconds or less (see also Rosen et al., 1998). These data suggest that combining high-speed MRI techniques with event-related task paradigms can be used to map quite rapid hemodynamic changes. Unfortunately, the ultimate limits of temporal resolution with fMRI will most likely be imposed by the underlying changes in physiology that they measure, which are (for BOLD-contrast) fairly indirect, temporally blurred, and affected by differences in regional vasculature (Lee et al., 1995). Across regions of cortex, the hemodynamic response may be systematically offset on the order of seconds in spite of the stable within-region measurements made by Menon et al. (1999).

Transient coordination of neuronal activity known to occur across segments of the cortex on time scales of tens to hundreds of milliseconds will likely remain the domain of techniques capable of resolving more direct correlates of brain activity at such short time scales (e.g., EEG, MEG). These techniques are capable of meaningful, rapid measurements of brain activity but, today, provide relatively coarse spatial resolution. In order to overcome this limitation, methods for combining the temporal resolution of EEG and MEG with the spatial resolution of fMRI are being developed (Dale et al., 1995; Dale & Sereno, 1993; Heinze et al., 1994; Snyder et al., 1995). Using such methods, it may become possible to study the precise spatiotemporal orchestration of neuronal activity associated with cognitive processes. Event-related fMRI allows a refinement of such integration by affording the ability to study the same paradigms in both fMRI settings and during EEG and MEG sessions. Several investigators have suggested that EEG could be conducted simultaneously with fMRI or PET measurements.

Another avenue of future investigation is likely to be in relation to comparisons across populations, in both normal and clinically diagnosed individuals. For example, there has been growing interest in comparisons across age groups. Older adults perform differently than young adults on memory tasks. Why? Functional neuroimaging provides a possible leverage point on this issue, and this can be seen in published studies (e.g., Cabeza & Nyberg, 1997; Grady et al., 1995). Considerably more can be done and will continue to be done. For instance, pathological states of aging, where memory and cognition are most severely impaired, have been investigated minimally to date.

However, conducting functional neuroimaging studies in older adults and across patient groups brings with it a number of challenging technical hurdles. We must progress cautiously, however; basic assumptions about the methods cannot be taken for granted. For example, there is some evidence that the coupling between neural activity and hemodynamics is compromised in older adults. Ross et al. (1997) have suggested that there may be substantial decrements in the amplitude of the hemodynamic response in older as compared to younger adults, even for sensory responses evoked in visual cortex. Taoka et al. (1998) found differences in the timing (shape) of the hemodynamic response that correlated with age. However, a thorough study by D'Esposito and colleagues portrayed a more optimistic picture (D'Esposito et al., 1999). While they showed evidence for differences in the signal-to-noise ratio across age groups and a trend for differences in the between-group variance of the hemodynamic response, the overall shape of hemodynamic response was similar across age groups. Clearly, more work is needed to place constraints on how we are to interpret between-group differences. Moreover, little is known about the behavior of the hemodynamic response in older adults with dementia and other neurological disorders. Nonetheless, the fact that studies are being conducted and are obtaining reliable signal changes in these populations, makes it clear that the methods applied to healthy young adults can be fruitfully applied across other populations (patient groups, different subject groups) as well.

REFERENCES

Bandettini, P. A. (1993). MRI studies of brain activation: Dynamic characteristics. In *Functional MRI of the Brain*. Berkeley, CA: Society of Magnetic Resonance in Medicine.

Barch, D. M., Carter, C. S., Braver, T. S., Sabb, F. W., Noll, D. C., & Cohen, J. D. (1999). Overt verbal responding during fMRI scanning: Empirical investigations of problems and potential solutions. *NeuroImage* 10, 642–657.

Binder, J. R., Frost, J. A., Hammeke, T. A., Bellgowan, P. S. F., Rao, S. M., & Cox, R. W. (1999). Conceptual processing during the conscious resting state. A functional MRI study. *Journal of Cognitive Neuroscience* 11, 80–95.

Birn, R. M., Bandettini, P. A., Cox, R. W., & Shaker, R. (1999). Event-related fMRI of tasks involving brief motion. *Human Brain Mapping* 7, 106–114.

Blamire, A. M., Ogawa, S., Ugurbil, K., Rothman, D., McCarthy, G., Ellerman, J. M., et al. (1992). Dynamic mapping of the human visual cortex by high-speed magnetic resonance imaging. *Proceedings of the National Academy of Sciences USA* 89, 11069–11073.

Boulanouar, K., Demonet, J. F., Berry, I., Chollet, F., Manelfe, C., & Celsis, P. (1996). Study of the spatiotemporal dynamics of the motor system with fMRI using the evoked response of activated pixels: A deconvolutional approach. *Proceedings of the International Society for Magnetic Resonance in Medicine* 3.

Boynton, G. M., Engel, S. A., Glover, G. H., & Heeger, D. J. (1996). Linear systems analysis of functional magnetic resonance imaging in human V1. *Journal of Neuroscience* 16, 4207–4221.

Braver, T. S., Cohen, J. D., Nystrom, L. E., Jonides, J., Smith, E. E., & Noll, D. C. (1997). A parametric study of prefrontal cortex involvement in human working memory. *NeuroImage* 5, 49–62.

Brewer, J. B., Zhao, Z., Glover, G. H., & Gabrieli, J. D. E. (1998). Parahippocampal and frontal responses to single events predict whether those events are remembered or forgotten. *Science* 281, 1185–1187.

Buckner, R. L. (1996). Beyond HERA: Contributions of specific prefrontal brain areas to long-term memory retrieval. *Psychonomic Bulletin & Review* 3, 149–158.

Buckner, R. L., Bandettini, P. A., O'Craven, K. M., Savoy, R. L., Petersen, S. E., Raichle, M. E., et al. (1996). Detection of cortical activation during averaged single trials of a cognitive task using functional magnetic resonance imaging. *Proceedings of the National Academy of Sciences of the United States of America* 93, 14878–14883.

Buckner, R. L., Goodman, J., Burock, M., Rotte, M., Koutstaal, W., Schacter, D. L., et al. (1998). Functional-anatomic correlates of object priming in humans revealed by rapid presentation event-related fMRI. *Neuron* 20, 285–296.

Buckner, R. L., & Koutstaal, W. (1998). Functional neuroimaging studies of encoding, priming, and explicit memory retrieval. *Proceedings of the National Academy of Sciences of the United States of America* 95, 891–898.

Buckner, R. L., Kelley, W. M., & Petersen, S. E. (1999). Frontal cortex contributes to human memory formation. *Nature Neuroscience* 2, 311–314.

Buckner, R. L., Koutstaal, W., Schacter, D. L., Dale, A. M., Rotte, M. R., & Rosen, B. R. (1998). Functional-anatomic study of episodic retrieval: II. Selective averaging of event-related fMRI trials to test the retrieval success hypothesis. *NeuroImage* 7, 163–175.

Buckner, R. L., Koutstaal, W., Schacter, D. L., Wagner, A. D., & Rosen, B. R. (1998). Functional-anatomic study of episodic retrieval using fMRI: I. Retrieval effort versus retrieval success. *NeuroImage* 7, 151–162.

Buckner, R. L., Petersen, S. E., Ojemann, J. G., Miezin, F. M., Squire, L. R., & Raichle, M. E. (1995). Functional anatomical studies of explicit and implicit memory retrieval tasks. *Journal of Neuroscience* 15, 12–29.

Buckner, R. L., Raichle, M. E., Miezin, F. M., & Petersen, S. E. (1996). Functional anatomic studies of memory retrieval for auditory words and visual pictures. *Journal of Neuroscience* 16, 6219–6235.

Burock, M. A., Buckner, R. L., Woldorff, M. G., Rosen, B. R., & Dale, A. M. (1998). Randomized event-related experimental designs allow for extremely rapid presentation rates using functional MRI. *NeuroReport* 9, 3735–3739.

Cabeza, R., Grady, C. L., Nyberg, L., McIntosh, A. R., Tulving, E., Kapur, S., et al. (1997). Age-related differences in neural activity during memory encoding and retrieval: A positron emission tomography study. *Journal of Neuroscience* 17, 391–400.

Cabeza, R., & Nyberg, L. (1997). Imaging cognition: An empirical review of PET studies with normal subjects. *Journal of Cognitive Neuroscience* 9, 1–26.

Carter, C. S., Braver, T. S., Barch, D. M., Botvinick, M. M., Noll, D., & Cohen, J. D. (1998). Anterior cingulate cortex, error detection, and the online monitoring of performance. *Science* 280, 747–749.

Clark, V. P., Keil, K., Maisog, J. M., Courtney, S., Ungerleider, L. G., & Haxby, J. V. (1996). Functional magnetic resonance imaging of human visual cortex during face matching: A comparison with positron emission tomography. *NeuroImage* 4, 1–15.

Clark, V. P., Maisog, J. M., & Haxby, J. V. (1997). fMRI studies of face memory using random stimulus sequences. *NeuroImage* 5, S50.

Clark, V. P., Maisog, J. M., & Haxby, J. V. (1998). fMRI study of face perception and memory using random stimulus sequences. *Journal of Neurophysiology* 79, 3257–3265.

Cohen, J. D., Perlstein, W. M., Braver, T. S., Nystrom, L. E., Noll, D. C., Jonides, J., et al. (1997). Temporal dynamics of brain activation during a working memory task. *Nature* 386, 604–607.

Cohen, M. S., & Weisskoff, R. M. (1991). Ultra-fast imaging. *Magnetic Resonance Imaging* 9, 1–37.

Courtney, S. M., Ungerleider, L. G., Keil, K., & Haxby, J. V. (1997). Transient and sustained activity in a distributed neural system for human working memory. *Nature* 386, 608–611.

Craik, F. I. M., & Lockhart, R. S. (1972). Levels of processing: A framework for memory research. *Journal of Verbal Learning and Verbal Behavior* 11, 671–684.

Dale, A., Ahlfors, S. P., Aronen, H. J., Belliveau, J. W., Houtilainen, M., Ilmoniemi, R. J., et al. (1995). Spatiotemporal imaging of coherent motion selective areas in human cortex. *Society for Neuroscience Abstracts* 21, 1275.

Dale, A. M., & Buckner, R. L. (1997). Selective averaging of rapidly presented individual trials using fMRI. *Human Brain Mapping* 5, 329–340.

Dale, A. M., Halgren, E., Lewine, J. D., Buckner, R. L., Paulson, K., Marinkovic, K., et al. (1997). Spatio-temporal localization of cortical word repetition-effects in a size judgement task using combined fMRI/ MEG. *NeuroImage* S592.

Dale, A. M., & Sereno, M. I. (1993). Improved localization of cortical activity by combining EEG and MEG with cortical surface reconstruction: A linear approach. *Journal of Cognitive Neuroscience* 5, 162–176.

Demb, J. B., Desmond, J. E., Wagner, A. D., Vaidya, C. J., Glover, G. H., & Gabrieli, J. D. E. (1995). Semantic encoding and retrieval in the left inferior prefrontal cortex: A functional MRI study of task difficulty and process specificity. *Journal of Neuroscience* 15, 5870–5878.

D'Esposito, M., Zarahn, E., Aguirre, G. K., & Rypma, B. (1999). The effect of normal aging on the coupling of neural activity to the BOLD hemodynamic response. *NeuroImage* 10, 6–14.

DeYoe, E. A., Bandettini, P., Neitz, J., Miller, D., & Winans, P. (1994). Functional magnetic resonance imaging (fMRI) of the human brain. *Journal of Neuroscience Methods* 54, 171–187.

DeYoe, E. A., Carman, G. J., Bandettini, P., Glickman, S., Wieser, J., Cox, R., et al. (1996). Mapping striate and extrastriate visual areas in human cerebral cortex. *Proceedings of the National Academy of Sciences USA* 93, 2382–2386.

Düzel, E., Cabeza, R., Picton, T. W., Yonelinas, A. P., Scheich, H., Heinze, H. J., et al. (1999). Task-related and item-related brain processes of memory retrieval: A combined PET and ERP study. *Proceedings of the National Academy of Sciences USA* 94, 1794–1799.

Engel, S. A., Glover, G. H., & Wandell, B. A. (1997). Retinotopic organization in human visual cortex and the spatial precision of functional MRI. *Cerebral Cortex* 7, 181–192.

Fletcher, P. C., Frith, C. D., Grasby, P. M., Shallice, T., Frackowiak, R. S. J., & Dolan, R. J. (1995). Brain systems for encoding and retrieval of auditory-verbal memory: An in vivo study in humans. *Brain* 118, 401–416.

Fox, P. T., Miezin, F. M., Allman, J. M., Van Essen, D. C., & Raichle, M. E. (1987). Retinotopic organization of human visual cortex mapped with positron emission tomography. *Journal of Neuroscience* 7, 913–922.

Fox, P. T., & Raichle, M. E. (1985). Stimulus rate determines regional brain blood flow in striate cortex. *Annals of Neurology* 17, 303–305.

Frackowiak, R. S. J., & Friston, K. J. (1995). Methodology of activation paradigms. In *Handbook of Neuropsychology* vol. 10, F. Boller and J. Grafman, eds., 369–382. Amsterdam: Elsevier.

Fransson, P., Kruger, G., Merboldt, K. D., & Frahm, J. (1999). Temporal and spatial MRI responses to subsecond visual activation. *Magnetic Resonance in Medicine* 17, 1–7.

Friston, K. J., Fletcher, P., Josephs, O., Holmes, A., Rugg, M. D., & Turner, R. (1998). Event-related fMRI: Characterizing differential responses. *Neuroimage* 7, 30–40.

Friston, K. J., Josephs, O., Rees, G., & Turner, R. (1997). Nonlinear event-related responses in fMRI. *Magnetic Resonance in Medicine* 39, 41–52.

Grady, C. L., McIntosh, A. R., Horwitz, B., Maisog, J. M., Ungerleider, L. G., Mentis, M. J., et al. (1995). Age-related reductions in human recognition memory due to impaired encoding. *Science* 269, 218–221.

Gratton, G., & Fabiani, F. (1998). Dynamic brain imaging: Event-related optical signal (EROS) measures of the time course and localization of cognitive-related activity. *Psychonomic Bulletin & Review* 5, 535–563.

Halgren, E., & Smith, M. E. (1987). Cognitive evoked potentials as modulatory processes in human memory formation and retrieval. *Human Neurobiology* 6, 129–139.

Heinze, H. J., Mangun, G. R., Burchert, W., Hinrichs, H., Scholtz, M., Münte, T. F., et al. (1994). Combined spatial and temporal imaging of brain activity during visual selective attention in humans. *Nature* 372, 543–546.

Humberstone, M., Barlow, M., Clare, S., Coxon, R., Glover, P., Hykin, J., et al. (1995). Functional magnetic resonance imaging of single motor events with echo planar imaging at 3T, using a signal averaging technique. *Proceedings of the Society of Magnetic Resonance* 2, 858.

Josephs, O., Turner, R., & Friston, K. (1997). Event-related fMRI. *Human Brain Mapping* 5, 243–248.

Kapur, S., Craik, F. I. M., Tulving, E., Wilson, A. A., Houle, S. H., & Brown, G. M. (1994). Neuroanatomical correlates of encoding in episodic memory: Levels of processing effects. *Proceedings of the National Academy of Sciences of the United States of America* 91, 2008–2011.

Kapur, S., Tulving, E., Cabeza, R., McIntosh, A. R., Houle, S., & Craik, F. I. M. (1996). The neural correlates of intentional learning of verbal materials: A PET study in humans. *Cognitive Brain Research* 4, 243–249.

Kelley, W. M., Miezin, F. M., McDermott, K. B., Buckner, R. L., Raichle, M. E., Cohen, N. J., et al. (1998). Hemispheric specialization in human dorsal frontal cortex and medial temporal lobe for verbal and nonverbal encoding. *Neuron* 20, 927–936.

Kim, S. G., Richter, W., & Ugurbil, K. (1997). Limitations of temporal resolution in functional MRI. *Magnetic Resonance in Medicine* 37, 631–636.

Konishi, S., Yoneyama, R., Itagaki, H., Uchida, I., Nakajima, K., Kato, H., et al. (1996). Transient brain activity used in magnetic resonance imaging to detect functional areas. *NeuroReport* 8, 19–23.

Kwong, K. K., Belliveau, J. W., Chesler, D. A., Goldberg, I. E., Weisskoff, R. M., Poncelet, B. P., et al. (1992). Dynamic magnetic resonance imaging of human brain activity during primary sensory stimulation. *Proceedings of the National Academy of Sciences USA* 89, 5675–5679.

Lee, A. T., Glover, G. H., & Meyer, C. H. (1995). Discrimination of large venous vessels in time-course spiral blood-oxygen-level-dependent magnetic-resonance functional neuroimaging. *Magnetic Resonance in Medicine* 33, 745–754.

Malonek, D., & Grinvald, A. (1996). Interactions between electrical activity and cortical microcirculation revealed by imaging spectroscopy: Implications for functional brain mapping. *Science* 272, 551–554.

Menon, R. S., Luknowsky, D. C., & Gati, G. S. (1998). Mental chronometry using latency-resolved functional MRI. *Proceedings of the National Academy of Sciences USA* 95, 10902–10907.

Menon, R. S., Ogawa, S., Strupp, J. P., & Ugurbil, K. (1997). Ocular dominance in human V1 demonstrated by functional magnetic resonance imaging. *Journal of Neurophysiology* 77, 2780–2787.

O'Craven, K., & Kanwisher, N. (in press). Mental imagery of faces and places activates corresponding stimulus-specific brain regions. *Journal of Cognitive Neuroscience*.

Ogawa, S., Lee, T., Nayak, A., & Glynn, P. (1990). Oxygenation-sensitive contrast in magnetic resonance image of rodent brain at high magnetic fields. *Magnetic Resonance in Medicine* 14, 68–78.

Ogawa, S., Tank, D. W., Menon, R., Ellerman, J. M., Kim, S. G., Merkle, H., et al. (1992). Intrinsic signal changes accompanying sensory stimulation: Functional brain mapping with magnetic resonance imaging. *Proceedings of the National Academy of Sciences USA* 89, 5951–5955.

Ojemann, J. G., Akbudak, E., Snyder, A. Z., McKinstry, R. C., Raichle, M. E., & Conturo, T. E. (1997). Anatomic localization and quantitative analysis of gradient refocused echo-planar fMRI susceptibility artifacts. *NeuroImage* 6, 156–167.

Ojemann, J. G., Buckner, R. L., Akbudak, E., Snyder, A. Z., Ollinger, J. M., McKinstry, R. C., et al. (1998). Functional MRI studies of word stem completion: Reliability across laboratories and comparison to blood flow imaging with PET. *Human Brain Mapping* 6, 203–215.

Paller, K. A. (1990). Recall and stem-completion priming have different electrophysiological correlates and are modified differentially by directed forgetting. *Journal of Experimental Psychology: Learning, Memory, and Cognition* 16, 1021–1032.

Petrides, M., Alivisatos, B., & Evans, A. C. (1995). Functional activation of the human ventrolateral frontal cortex during mnemonic retrieval of verbal information. *Proceedings of the National Academy of Sciences of the United States of America* 92, 5803–5807.

Phelps, E. A., Hyder, F., Blamire, A. M., & Shulman, R. G. (1997). fMRI of the prefrontal cortex during overt verbal fluency. *NeuroReport* 8, 561–565.

Posner, M. I., & Raichle, M. E. (1994). *Images of Mind*. New York: Scientific American Books.

Raichle, M. E. (1987). Circulatory and metabolic correlates of brain function in normal humans. In *The Handbook of Physiology: The Nervous System*. vol. 5, *Higher Functions of the Brain*, F. Plum and V. Mountcastle, eds., 643–674. Bethesda, Md.: American Physiological Association.

Richter, W., Georgopoulos, A. P., Ugurbil, K., & Kim, S. G. (1997). Detection of brain activity during mental rotation in a single trial by fMRI. *NeuroImage* 5, S49.

Roland, P. E. (1993). *Brain Activation*. New York: Wiley-Liss.

Rosen, B. R., Buckner, R. L., & Dale, A. M. (1998). Event-related Functional MRI: Past, present, and future. *Proceedings of the National Academy of Sciences USA* 95, 773–780.

Ross, M. H., Yurgelun-Todd, D. A., Renshaw, P. F., Maas, L. C., Mendelson, J. H., Mello, N. K., et al. (1997). Age-related reduction in functional MRI response to photic stimulation. *Neurology* 48, 173–176.

Rotte, M. R., Koutstaal, W., Buckner, R. L., Wagner, A. D., Dale, A. M., Rosen, B. R., et al. (1998). Prefrontal activation during encoding correlates with level of processing using event-related fMRI. *Supplement of the Journal of Cognitive Neuroscience* 5, 114.

Rugg, M. D. (1995). ERP studies of memory. In *Electrophysiology of Mind: Event-Related Brain Potentials and Cognition*, M. D. Rugg and M. G. H. Coles, eds., 132–170. Oxford: Oxford University Press.

Rugg, M. D., Fletcher, P. C., Frith, C. D., Frackowiak, R. S. J., & Dolan, R. J. (1996). Differential activation of the prefrontal cortex in successful and unsuccessful memory retrieval. *Brain* 119, 2073–2083.

Savoy, R. L., Bandettini, P. A., O'Craven, K. M., Kwong, K. K., Davis, T. L., Baker, J. R., et al. (1995). Pushing the temporal resolution of fMRI: Studies of very brief visual stimuli, onset variability and asynchrony, and stimulus-correlated changes in noise. *Proceedings of the Society of Magnetic Resonance* 2, 450.

Sereno, M. I., Dale, A. M., Reppas, J. B., Kwong, K. K., Belliveau, J. W., Brady, T. J., et al. (1995). Borders of multiple visual areas in humans revealed by functional magnetic resonance imaging. *Science* 268, 889–893.

Shulman, G. L., Fiez, J. A., Corbetta, M., Buckner, R. L., Miezin, F. M., Raichle, M. E., et al. (1997). Common blood flow changes across visual tasks: II. Decreases in cerebral cortex. *Journal of Cognitive Neuroscience* 9, 648–663.

Snyder, A. Z., Abdullaev, Y. G., Posner, M. I., & Raichle, M. E. (1995). Scalp electrical potentials reflect regional cerebral blood flow responses during processing of written words. *Proceedings of the National Academy of Sciences USA* 92, 1689–1693.

Taoka, T., Iwasaki, S., Uchida, H., Fukusumi, A., Nakagawa, H., Kichikawa, K., et al. (1998). Age correlation of the time lag in signal change on EPI-fMRI. *Journal of Computer Assisted Tomography* 22, 514–517.

Tulving, E. (1983). *Elements of Episodic Memory*. New York: Oxford University Press.

Tulving, E., Kapur, S., Craik, F. I. M., Moscovitch, M., & Houle, S. (1994). Hemispheric encoding/retrieval asymmetry in episodic memory: Positron emission tomography findings. *Proceedings of the National Academy of Sciences USA* 91, 2016–2020.

Vazquez, A. L., & Noll, D. C. (1998). Nonlinear aspects of the BOLD response in functional MRI. *NeuroImage* 7, 108–118.

Wagner, A. D., Desmond, J. E., Glover, G. H., & Gabrieli, J. D. E. (1998). Prefrontal cortex and recognition memory: fMRI evidence for context-dependent retrieval processes. *Brain* 121, 1985–2002.

Wagner, A. D., Schacter, D. L., Rotte, M., Koutstaal, W., Maril, A., Dale, A. M., et al. (1998). Building memories: Remembering and forgetting of verbal experiences as predicted by brain activity. *Science* 281, 1188–1191.

Woods, R. P., Grafton, S. T., Holmes, C. J., Cherry, S. R., & Mazziotta, J. C. (1998). Automated image registration: I. General methods and intrasubject, intramodality validation. *Journal of Computer Assisted Tomography* 22, 139–152.

Zarahn, E., Aguirre, G. K., & D'Esposito, M. (1997). A trial-based experimental design for fMRI. *NeuroImage* 6, 122–138.

3 Functional Neuroimaging: Network Analyses

L. Nyberg and A. R. McIntosh

INTRODUCTION

This chapter emphasizes how we can understand the neurobiology of cognition from the perspective of interacting neural systems. Part of the emphasis is on analyses of functional neuroimaging data that attempt to identify how the influences which brain regions have on one another change across different cognitive and behavioral operations. Henceforth, such analyses will be referred to as *network analyses.* We will start by outlining the theoretical motivation for network analyses; next, we will discuss various statistical methods that can be used. Examples of results will be provided, with a focus on cognitive domains that have been discussed in the other chapters and that, in our opinion, constitute very clear examples of how network analyses go beyond more traditional univariate data analysis.

Why should you conduct network analyses? The underlying idea that motivates analyses of interactions among brain regions is that cognitive processes result from such interactions. That is, processes such as memory or attentional operations do not result from the workings of single brain areas, but rather from the "collaboration" of several areas. This is not a new perspective unique to the field of functional neuroimaging. It has a long history that arose out of early anatomical, neuropsychological, and physiological studies (Lashley, 1933; Finger, 1994). Importantly, though, by being able to sample whole-brain activity, functional neuroimaging techniques are especially well suited to provide empirical support for the operation of large-scale neurocognitive networks. In order to do so, however, it is necessary to go beyond the standard way of analyzing functional neuroimaging data. This usually involves comparison of the activity pattern associated with the execution of a target task against that associated with a reference task such that a map of differential activity emerges. For example, it may be found that relative to the reference task, the target task is associated with increased activity in regions A, B, and C, and with decreased activity in regions D and E. The outcome of such an analysis of relative changes in regional activity may be interpreted in terms of components of networks (i.e., regions A–E form a functional network), but this outcome alone does not constitute an index of the network operation. Some of the regions that showed differential activity may not be part of a specific functional network. Moreover, regions where activity does not change significantly as a function of the manipulation may be part of the relevant network (as exemplified below). And, most important, the network that serves a particular function must be quantified while those regions are engaged in that function. Therefore, techniques such as those described below must be considered:

How can you conduct network analyses? There are several ways to analyze functional interactions among brain regions. Partly, the selection of data analytic technique may be affected by the type of neuroimaging data to be analyzed. Here, we will for most part be concerned with data generated by measuring brain blood flow with positron emission tomography (PET), but the analytic tools we describe below are just as easily applied to functional MRI (Büchel & Friston, 1997) and serve a purpose similar to that of tools used in electrophysiology (for a discussion of similar analyses of electrophysiological data, see Aertsen et al., 1987; Nunez et al., 1997).

In the context of introducing tools for network analyses, it is useful to consider the distinction between *effective* and *functional* connectivity (e.g., Friston, 1994; Gerstein et al., 1978). Functional connectivity can be defined as the correlation of activity among brain regions—no reference is made to how a correlation is mediated. For example, a strong correlation between the activity in two regions may be driven by a shared functional relation with a third region. In contrast, in the case of effective connectivity, the influence that one region has on another is directly estimated. A measure of effective connectivity requires constraints that are not imposed in estimates of functional connectivity. For example, one constraint may be derived through a combination of anatomical and functional information and allows conclusions of region-to-region influences. Others may be imposed through the use of a multiple regression analysis (McIntosh & Gonzalez-Lima, 1994; Friston, 1994). In what follows, we will describe techniques that address both functional and effective connectivity (see table 3.1), starting with functional techniques. Following the description of techniques, a brief discussion of their relative merits will be presented.

Horwitz (1989) laid the foundation for analyses of interactions among brain regions by presenting results of analyses of pairwise regional interrelations. It is possible to select a region and analyze how the activity in this region correlates, across subjects, with activity in the rest of the brain (a sort of seed-region correlation anal-

Table 3.1
Techniques for Network Analyses

Connectivity	Analytic Technique	Reference Paper
Functional	Pairwise regional interrelations	Horwitz (1989)
	Partial least squares	McIntosh et al. (1997)
	Principal components analysis	Friston (1994), Strother et al. (1995)
Effective	Structural equation modeling	
	Between-subjects model	McIntosh & Gonzalez-Lima (1994)
	Within-subjects model	Büchel & Friston (1997)
	Multiple regression	Friston et al. (1993)

ysis). The specific region may be selected a priori, but the selection can also be guided by results of activation analyses. The result of such a correlational analysis is a map of brain areas that are interrelated with the selected region. To identify task-related changes in correlation patterns, the map can be compared with another map based on data from a second task (see Horwitz et al., 1992).

McIntosh (e.g., McIntosh et al., 1997) has presented a multivariate extension of the procedure proposed by Horwitz, using partial least squares (PLS). By sorting the correlations into what is similar and what is different across tasks, PLS facilitates the comparison of the correlation maps across experimental conditions. It can also be used when it is of interest to use more than one seed region. For example, McIntosh et al. (1997) used the PLS procedure to analyze whole-brain correlation maps formed from a left hippocampal and two right prefrontal brain regions. The results revealed that some of these regions had a similar correlation pattern across all four conditions, but task-specific correlation patterns involving one or more of the three regions were also observed. More recently, McIntosh et al. (1999) showed that the pattern of left prefrontal functional connectivity could distinguish subjects that were aware of stimulus relationships in a sensory learning task from subjects who were not aware of the relationships. Without the aid from PLS, such interrelations would have been impossible to identify.

PLS can also be used to analyze activation data. Here, "task" PLS identifies spatial patterns of brain activity that represent the optimal association between brain images and a block of contrast vectors coding for the experimental design (see McIntosh, Bookstein, et al., 1996). PLS is similar to some other multivariate analytic procedures that attempt to relate brain regions and experimental conditions (e.g., Friston et al., 1993; see McIntosh, Bookstein, et al., 1996, for discussion and Worsley et al., 1997 for an extension to fMRI). As with the seed-region version of PLS, task PLS is a *multivariate* analysis of activation changes that serves to identify distributed systems that *as a whole* relate to some aspect of the experimental design. As such, task PLS can be considered a form of network analysis. An example of results from a task PLS analysis is given in figure 3.1.

Figure 3.1 shows results from a task PLS analysis of data from a PET study of episodic memory encoding and retrieval (Nyberg, McIntosh, et al., 1996). The study had seven conditions, each consisting of a single word presented in the center of a computer screen or to the left or right of fixation. The instructions given to the subject provided a bias to a particular cognitive operation. In reference to the labels on the x-axis of the graph, "Read" refers to a baseline task where subjects simply read the word; "Item-Enc" was a task involving explicit encoding of single words; "Item-Ret" was a task involving yes/no recognition of single words encoded in the previous con-

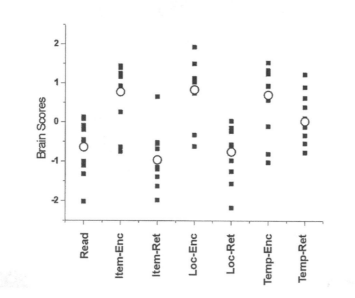

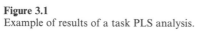

Figure 3.1
Example of results of a task PLS analysis.

dition; "Loc-Enc" involved the encoding of single words as well as the location of the word on the screen (left or right of fixation); "Loc-Ret" was a task that involved remembering whether test words at study had been presented to the left or right of fixation; "Temp-Enc" involved encoding of single words as well as whether the word came from a designated first or second list; "Temp-Ret" involved remembering of whether test words had been part of the first or second study list.

PLS analysis of task differences identified "singular images" representing a task effect and "brain scores" that indicate the variation of the task effect across scans. The brain images identify areas that distinguish between encoding and retrieval conditions; the graph shows the variation in activity in this image across the seven conditions. Peak areas are plotted on axial MRI sections, which run from ventral to dorsal, going from left to right. The numbers beside the rows of images identify the Talairach atlas slice location in mm from the AC–PC line for the slices in the leftmost column. Slices move in increments of 4 mm. The "brain scores" derived from the image are the dot-product of the brain image and each subject's data in the original PET scan. The open circles in the graph represent the average score within each scan, and the black squares are the scores for each individual subject. During encoding scans, subjects showed more activity in black areas (notably left prefrontal cortex and left fusiform gyrus), whereas during retrieval and read scans subject showed more activity in areas white (notably right prefrontal cortex and midbrain). The fact that the reading baseline scan grouped with retrieval scans may suggest that there are retrieval operations occurring during the *read* condition.

The multivariate analyses we have discussed identify systems of brain regions relating to an experimental manipulation and systems that are in some way related to one particular or several brain regions. They do not provide information on region-to-region influences, but can be said to address issues of functional connectivity. By contrast, the final statistical procedure that will be considered, *structural equation modeling* (SEM), can be used to address questions relating to effective connectivity. This procedure relates to analysis of a global neural system as well as to the investigation of interrelations in such a system. It goes beyond these approaches by taking into account existing anatomical connections and the direction of influences (feedforward vs. feedback; direct effects vs. indirect effects). In general, the basic steps are shown below. (For a more complete discussion of SEM analysis of PET data, see McIntosh & Gonzalez-Lima, 1994).

• Selection of regions. Network components can be selected on the basis of theoretical consideration and/or results of different kinds of initial analyses. Initial analyses can, for example, be in the form of PLS analyses of activation data, as described above ("task" PLS). Univariate activation analyses can also be used at this stage, and both kinds of activation analyses can be complemented by analyses of interrelations (i.e., not only regions showing differential activation can be included in the model).

• Specifying the model. When the network components have been selected, the primate neuroanatomy literature is consulted to specify anatomic connections between the included regions. Some simplifying steps may be required, such as reducing the number of connections or regions, but such omissions should be explicitly stated. The decision of which connections to include/exclude has to be made by the investigator, and such a decision should, if possible, be guided by previous findings/theory. Fortunately, from simulation work it appears that omissions from the model may not impact on the portions of the network that are modeled, but rather on the residual influences on the model (McIntosh & Gonzalez-Lima, 1994).

• Computation of interregional covariances. The next step involves calculation of the interregional covariances. This is generally done within conditions and across subjects. With functional MRI, where more scans per subject can be done, the single-subject covariances can be computed using trial variance (Büchel & Friston, 1997). To ensure generalizability, however, both within-subject and between-subjects models need to be compared.

• Computation of path coefficients and model comparison. On the basis of the covariance matrix, SEM is used to compute path coefficients for the existing connections (figure 3.2). These coefficients represent the strength of the influence of one region upon another. Such influences can be direct as well as indirect, and coefficients can be computed for both kinds of connections. It should also be noted that, unlike interregional correlations, in the case of reciprocal connections the path coefficients can show that the influence of region A upon region B is stronger than that of B upon A (this holds only in cases where A and B also have unique influences). When path coefficients have been computed for all connections within conditions, it is possible to statistically compare models for different tasks to find out whether there are task-related changes in functional interactions. If the results suggest that there are, one can do further post hoc analyses to specify the source(s) of the effect.

We have described techniques for addressing functional connectivity, notably PLS, as well as effective connectivity, notably SEM. Although powerful, each of these approaches has its limitations. As noted above, when evaluating findings of functional connectivity, it is crucial to keep in mind that the data cannot speak to the direction of functional interactions. Therefore, inferences regarding the modulation of one area by another are not warranted. Such inferences can be made based on use of SEM, but

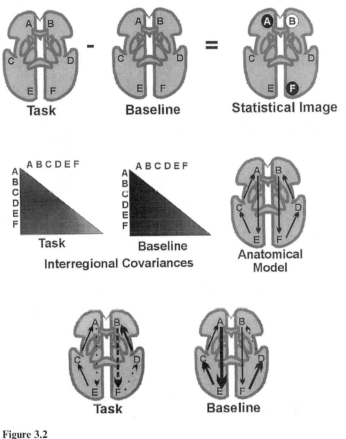

Figure 3.2
Graphic representation of essential steps in structural equation modeling for imaging data. In the top row, regions for the model are selected partly on the basis of the statistical differences between task and baseline (regions A and F showing deactivation and B showing activation), and partly on theoretical considerations, such as anatomical completeness or a theoretical model (regions C, D, and E). In the middle row, the activity correlations between areas are computed within task, and the anatomical model is constructed on the basis of published neuroanatomical work. Finally, in the bottom row, the correlations are used to derive path coefficients for each anatomical connection within task, yielding two functional models. Positive weights are solid, and negative are dashed, with the thickness of the line indicating the size of the weight. The "deactivations" identified from the subtraction image in region A correspond to a reduced involvement of region A, whereas the deactivation of F is because of strong negative feedback from region B. The activation in region B corresponds to its increased (suppressive) influence on F plus the stronger afferent influence from D.

it must be taken into account that the models used in such analyses leave out much anatomical detail. Indeed, if a key region has been left out of the model, the conclusions may not hold. It can also be noted that, generally, neither technique will capture nonlinear relationships between brain areas, although SEM can be extended to capture such relations (for an example, see Büchel & Friston, 1997).

NETWORK ANALYSES: EMPIRICAL EXAMPLES

Perception—Attention—Language

Numerous studies have examined activity changes related to perception, attention, and language (for a review, see Cabeza & Nyberg, 1997). The results point to a highly complex pattern of activations for each process, with specific regions being activated depending on the specific task demands. While several of these studies discuss their results in terms of network operations, we focus on studies where these network operations were the point of investigation.

We start by describing a study that bears on all three processes (McLaughlin et al., 1992). In this study, blood flow was measured in three conditions: (1) diotic presentation of a narrative with instruction to try to memorize the content; (2) dichotic presentation of single words with instruction to try to remember as many words as possible; and (3) presentation of white noise with instruction to pay attention to how many times the intensity of the noise changed. A principal components analysis on data from 28 a priori determined regions were conducted to identify three independent factors. These components were interpreted as statistical analogues of neural networks. Based on various statistical and theoretical considerations, different functions were ascribed to the different factors. The first factor was suggested to serve auditory/linguistic functions; and regions associated with auditory and language stimulation, including Broca's and Wernicke's areas, had high loadings on this factor. The second factor was seen as serving attentional processes; and regions loading high on this factor, including the frontal eye fields and cingulate gyrus, have been associated with attentional functions. The third factor was suggested as serving visual imaging activities; and visual association areas loaded high on this factor. Based on these findings, the authors concluded that the auditory tasks activated three separate neural networks, and multivariate factor analysis was held to have a central role in identifying these networks.

A study by McIntosh et al. (1994) used network analysis to examine visual perception in spatial and object-identification domains. SEM was applied to data from a PET study of an object vision (face matching) and spatial vision (dot-location matching) task. The anatomic model included dorsal and ventral visual regions in occipital, temporal, and parietal cortices and a frontal region near area 46. The analyses of functional networks revealed significant differences between the spatial and object tasks in the right hemisphere. During object vision, interactions among ventral occipital and temporal regions were strong, whereas during spatial vision, interactions among dorsal occipitoparietal regions were stronger. A further difference had to do with feedback influences from the frontal region to occipital cortex, which were strong for the spatial task but absent during the object task. This task-related difference relating to the frontal area was not obvious on the basis of analysis of activation changes. Prefrontal and anterior temporal regions did not show a net change in activity, despite these remarkable changes in functional interactions. Additional information that was provided by the network analyses included findings of strong interactions between the dorsal and ventral pathways. This final result suggests that although one pathway is especially challenged during processing of a particular kind of information, interactions with regions in the nondominant pathways are important as well. Such interdependencies are difficult to appreciate in activation analysis, but are likely critical to the normal operations of parallel systems. The functional networks for the two tasks are shown in figure 3.3.

Turning now to attention, a study by Büchel and Friston (1997) explored attentional modulation of visual processing through SEM analysis of data obtained by functional magnetic resonance imaging (fMRI). One condition involved looking at moving dots that were presented on a screen (no-attention condition). Another con-

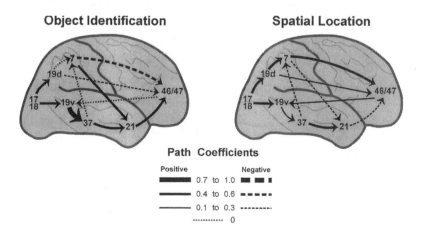

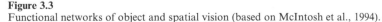

Figure 3.3
Functional networks of object and spatial vision (based on McIntosh et al., 1994).

dition involved identical visual presentation, but subjects were instructed to attend to changes in the speed of the moving dots (attention condition). An anatomical model was constructed that involved primary visual cortex (V1), a middle temporal region (V5), and a posterior parietal cortex region (PPC). The model included only uni-directional connections from V1 and onward. The SEM analyses indicated stronger influences of V1 on V5 and of V5 on PPC in the attention condition, suggesting that attending to changes in speed of moving objects is mediated by changes in functional influences among regions in the dorsal visual pathway. In a second step, the question of which brain region(s) can modulate these influences was addressed. Based on empirical and theoretical considerations, the dorsolateral prefrontal cortex (DLPFC) and/or the anterior cingulate (AC) were seen as likely candidates. Of these regions, only the right DLPFC region showed activation changes relating to the manipulation of attentional demands, and this region was included in the model as a possible moderator of functional interactions in the dorsal pathway. Specifically, by including an interaction term in the analysis, the possibility that DLPFC might modulate the influence of V5 upon PPC was tested. The results provided support for this possibility, and hence suggested that interactions between frontal and posterior visual pathway regions underlie this form of attentional processing.

Further examples of multivariate analyses of imaging data related to components of language processing have been reported by Friston and colleagues (Friston et al., 1991) and Bullmore and colleagues (Bullmore et al., 1996). In the section "Cognitive Dysfunction and Aging," an example of language processing in normal and dyslexic readers will be discussed in some detail.

Working Memory–Long-Term Memory

There is some consensus that human memory is not a unitary system, but is composed of several independent and interacting systems. A very broad division is the traditional time-based distinction, which can be conceptualized as working memory ("active" temporary remembering of various kinds of information) versus long-term memory ("passive" remembering of information over long periods of time). In turn, working memory and long-term memory can be further subdivided. Baddeley (e.g., Baddeley & Hitch, 1974) has proposed a model of working memory in which a central executive controls the operation of "slave systems" devoted to verbal or visuospatial information. Functional neuroimaging studies have been based on this model, and separate analyses of the central executive (D'Esposito et al., 1995), as well as the verbal (e.g., Paulesu et al., 1993) and visuospatial (e.g., Jonides et al., 1993) components, have been presented.

With regard to long-term memory, a broad classification in terms of declarative versus nondeclarative memory has been proposed by Squire (e.g., 1992). Declarative memory can be separated into episodic and semantic memory (Tulving, 1983), and functional neuroimaging studies suggest that different neural systems are engaged by episodic and semantic memory retrieval (e.g., Fletcher et al., 1995; Nyberg et al., 1998; Tulving et al., 1994). Nondeclarative memory refers to a very broad class of memory functions, each associated with a specific neural signature (for a recent review, see Gabrieli, 1998). Many nondeclarative memory functions have been studied with functional neuroimaging techniques, including priming (for a review, see Schacter & Buckner, 1998), motor (e.g., Karni et al., 1995) and nonmotor (Raichle et al., 1994) learning, and nonaversive (Molchan et al., 1994) and aversive (Fredriksson et al., 1995) conditioning. The empirical examples of network analyses include one example from the domain of working memory, one example of a declarative long-term memory function, and one example of a nondeclarative long-term memory function.

Building on a working memory study by Haxby et al. (1995), McIntosh, Grady, et al. (1996) conducted a SEM analysis of data from a delayed match-to-sample test of faces. The delays varied systematically, ranging between 1 and 21 sec. It was found that the functional interactions changed as a function of the length of the delay. At short delays (1–6 sec), the SEM analysis revealed strong functional interactions in the right hemisphere between ventral temporal, hippocampal, anterior cingulate, and inferior frontal regions. At the long delay (21 sec), both hemispheres were involved and strong functional interactions involved bilateral frontal and frontocingulate interactions. As suggested by the authors, these findings may reflect the use of a specific strategy at short delays that involved maintaining iconlike mental images of the faces. This strategy was mediated by right hemisphere corticolimbic interactions. Over longer delays, maintaining icons of the faces may be an inefficient strategy, and the involvement of frontal regions, notably in the left hemisphere, becomes more prominent. The increased left prefrontal involvement may reflect expanded encoding strategies.

Turning now to long-term memory, and more specifically to declarative long-term memory, we will discuss a network analysis of episodic memory retrieval. Episodic memory refers to encoding and retrieval of personally experienced events. Hippocampus, in the medial temporal lobe (MTL), has been held to play a central role in episodic memory functioning. Regarding its specific functional role, many different accounts have been proposed (see Tulving et al., 1999), and a rather intense current debate has to do with the possibility that different MTL structures are involved during episodic encoding and retrieval (Gabrieli et al., 1997; LePage et al., 1998; Schacter & Wagner, 1999). The study to be discussed here explored the possibility that MTL structures interact with specific posterior neocortical brain regions, depending on what type of information is retrieved (Köhler et al., 1998).

SEM was conducted on data from a PET study of episodic recognition memory for spatial location and object identity. Based on a PLS analysis, six right-hemisphere regions were selected for inclusion in the anatomical model. These were located in middle frontal gyrus, parieto-occipital sulcus, superior temporal sulcus, supramarginal gyrus, fusiform gyrus, and cuneus. In addition, on theoretical grounds, a right MTL region was included in the model.

The examination of the functional retrieval networks revealed significant task-related effects. The right MTL region was found to interact with posterior cortical regions in a task-dependent manner. During retrieval of spatial information, positive interactions between MTL and dorsal cortical regions were observed. During retrieval of information about object identity, these interactions were negative. By contrast, interactions between MTL and ventral regions were positive during object retrieval and negative during spatial retrieval. The networks showing these functional interactions are presented in figure 3.4.

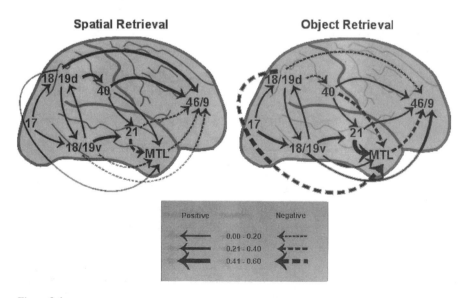

Figure 3.4
Functional networks of retrieval of object and of spatial information (based on Köhler et al., 1998).

The results of the network analyses indicated that the nature of interactions between MTL and posterior neocortical regions depends on the type of information to be retrieved, and it was proposed that such interactions may support recovery of information that is represented in posterior neocortex. It is noteworthy that these results were obtained despite the fact that there were no signs of task-related changes in activity in the MTL regions. This shows that analyses of regional interactions can generate significant information beyond what can be gained from analyses of activation changes. A further important observation in both of these declarative memory studies was the replicability of the basic posterior cortical networks for object and spatial vision. The object vision network showed similar basic interactions in the two memory studies and the original visual perception study mentioned above, and the spatial vision network in the retrieval study showed strong similarities with the spatial vision network in the perceptual study. Such replication of the basic perceptual network across studies using different subjects, different materials, and somewhat different processes attests to the robustness of the network analytic approach.

Our final network example in this section concerns nondeclarative long-term memory, and more specifically sensory-sensory associative learning (McIntosh et al., 1998). In this study, subjects were presented with two visual stimuli (circles), one designated target and one designated distractor, and instructed to respond by pressing a key when the target stimulus was presented. In addition to the visual stimuli, an auditory stimulus (a tone) was presented through headphones. In one phase, the low-probability phase, the tone predicted the presentation of either of the two visual stimuli with a probability of 0.12. In another phase, the high-probability phase, the same probability was 0.80. Using this design, two hypotheses were tested. The first was that once the association between the tone and the circles had been learned (as indicated by faster reaction times on trials where the tone preceeded the circle), presentation of the tone alone would activate visual brain regions. A univariate activation analysis confirmed the first hypothesis by showing that, by the end of training (four blocks of 50 trials), activity in a left dorsal occipital region was as high when the tone was presented alone as when a visual stimulus was presented.

The second hypothesis had to do with examination of which brain regions could have mediated this increase in visual cortex activity. The seed PLS analysis, using the visual cortex region, was used to identify candidate regions, and it was found that four regions showed a covariance pattern with the left occipital region that changed from strongly negative to strongly positive as learning progressed. These were right occipital cortex (area 18), right auditory cortex (area 41/42), right motor cortex (area 6), and right anterior prefrontal cortex (area 10). The identified regions formed the

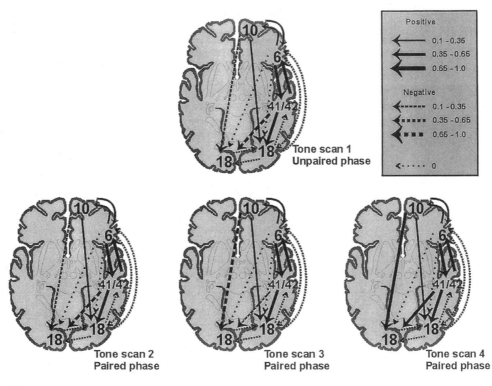

Figure 3.5
Functional networks of sensory-sensory associative learning (based on McIntosh et al., 1998). Unpaired phase denotes the point of the experiment where a tone and visual stimulus had a low probability of a joint occurrence, whereas in the paired phase, there was a high probability that a tone would signal a visual stimulus. Four successive PET scans were taken of the tone presented in isolation to measure the change in the learned response to the tone as it acquired behavioral relevance.

anatomical model for a subsequent SEM analysis, and the model included feedback effects from each of these four regions upon the left occipital region.

The results of the SEM analysis showed that as learning progressed, feedback influences of area 10 and area 41/42 on left area 18 changed from initially being negative to being moderately positive by the end of training (figure 3.5). The change in functional influences from negative to positive was interpreted as a switch from inhibitory to excitatory influences at the level of neural populations. It was proposed that the change from inhibitory to excitatory influences of the prefrontal cortex may have facilitated integration between activity in the auditory and visual systems, resulting in the formation of the association between the tone and the visual stimuli.

Cognitive Dysfunction and Aging

It has been argued that network analyses should be useful in the examination of clinical populations, since they allow examination of how interactions in brain networks are affected by damage or disease (McIntosh et al., 1994). One syndrome associated with cognitive dysfunction is schizophrenia. Structural (e.g., Andreasen et al., 1994) and functional (e.g., Andreasen et al., 1996; Friston et al., 1992) abnormalities associated with this syndrome have been explored using brain imaging, even under conditions of hallucinations that accompany the disease (Silbersweig et al., 1995). Frith and Friston (e.g., Friston & Frith, 1995) have suggested that a core feature of the schizophrenic syndrome is disruption of prefrontotemporal integration. Prefrontal and temporal (including hippocampus) regions have been associated with normal episodic memory functioning (Cabeza & Nyberg, 1997; Fletcher et al., 1997), pointing to the possibility that abnormal functioning/integration of these regions underlies impaired episodic memory processes in schizophrenia. Some more recent results provide support for this view (Heckers et al., 1998; see also Fletcher, 1998). Moreover, a network analysis of prefrontal interactions provides clear support for the fronto-temporal dysconnection (Jennings et al., 1998).

A group of patients with schizophrenia was compared against age-matched controls in a task where subjects indicated whether a visually presented noun was a living or nonliving thing (semantic processing task). One highlight of the functional network for controls was strong positive interactions between left inferior prefrontal, superior temporal, and anterior cingulate cortices. In the patient group, the fronto-temporal interactions were weaker, with negative prefrontal feedback, and the fronto-cingulate interactions were also negative. Interestingly, response latencies in this task were equal between groups and there was only a slight difference in accuracy between groups. These data are consistent not only with the proposed frontotemporal dis-connection in schizophrenia, but also with a more general idea that cognitive dys-functions may be appreciated in terms of the disorganization of large-scale neural cognitive networks.

The network analysis presented above demonstrates the important information that can be derived from the between-groups examination of functional interactions on cognitive tasks where performance is relatively equal. Historically, imaging and behavioral work have used tasks where controls and the patient groups differ, which leads to an interpretive difficulty because group differences may not reflect the pathology per se, but rather the performance difference. When performance is matched, and the functional interactions differ, then one can be reasonably confident that the difference reflects some aspect of the pathology. Clearly, an ideal experimental protocol

would be one where cognitive load varied from easy to difficult and the performances of the patient groups similarly go from relatively spared to deficient. This
would provide a more comprehensive assessment of the consequences of the different
functional networks underlying equivalent performance as the functional network is
tasked by increasing cognitive demands.

A further demonstration of different functional networks supporting equivalent
performance comes from studies of normal aging. Cabeza and colleagues (1997)
tested the hypothesis that age-related changes in activation during memory tasks
are due to an age-related reorganization of neural systems underlying the tasks. PET
scans were obtained from a group of young (mean age = 26 years) and older (mean
age = 70 years) adults during encoding of word pairs and during subsequent cued
recall (the first word of each pair served as cue). Based on analyses of activation
changes, 13 regions were selected for the construction of the anatomical model. These
were located in bilateral lateral frontal regions, in midline frontal and posterior
regions, in bilateral temporal regions, and in thalamus. Based on known neuroanatomy, some 25 reciprocal connections were specified between the regions. On the
assumption that feedback effects depend on feedforward influences, feedforward connections were computed in a first step, followed by computation of feedback effects.

The SEM analyses showed significant differences in functional networks underlying encoding versus recall for both age groups. However, the nature of these differences tended to differ as a function of age group. In keeping with the activation
results, and with numerous findings showing that left prefrontal regions tend to be differentially active during encoding, whereas right prefrontal regions tend to be differentially activated during retrieval (Nyberg, Cabeza, et al., 1996; Tulving et al., 1994),
in the young group, functional interactions involving left prefrontal area 47 were positive during encoding and negative during recall, whereas interactions involving right
prefrontal area 47 tended to be negative during encoding and positive during recall.
In the old group, such an asymmetric pattern of functional interactions during encoding and recall was not observed, and the activation data showed minimal activation
of the left frontal region during encoding and a bilateral activation pattern during
recall. There were other group differences in functional interactions as well, but these
will not be detailed here.

The network analyses helped to understand the age-differences in frontal activation
patterns during encoding and recall. It was suggested that the involvement of left prefrontal cortex in recall for the old adults, partly mediated by stronger interhemispheric fronto-frontal interactions, may reflect some sort of functional compensation,
since the recall task can be hypothesized as being more difficult to perform in old age.
(Performance was equal between groups, but it is not unlikely that the cognitive effort

associated with achieving this level of performance was greater for the older adults.) This view is in line with findings from younger adults, suggesting that the frontal involvement in episodic memory retrieval tends to be bilateral during more complex retrieval tasks (Nolde et al., 1998). In the study by Cabeza et al. (1997), the retrieval task was held constant, but one might see the manipulation of age as an alternative way of varying complexity. More generally, the network analyses helped to understand age differences in activation levels and suggested that such differences may be the result of more global alterations of network operations rather than local regional changes.

Turning now to a study of Alzheimer dementia (AD) patients (Horwitz et al., 1995), patients and age- and sex-matched controls were PET-scanned while they performed a face-matching task and a sensorimotor control task. An anatomical model based on the right hemisphere ventral model presented by McIntosh et al. (1994; discussed above) was used to test for differences in functional interactions between patients and controls. This model included feedforward connections from area 17 to area 18, from area 18 to area 37, from area 37 to area 21, and from area 21 to frontal area 47. In addition, a feedback projection from area 47 to area 18 was included. The functional network for the controls resembled that previously obtained for young subjects (McIntosh et al., 1994), but with more prefrontal feedback. It is noteworthy that accuracy for the old subjects in this task was not distinguishable from accuracy in young subjects, in spite of the difference in interactions (and activity; Grady et al., 1992). The functional network of the AD patients was significantly different from that of the controls (figure 3.6). In particular, the functional linkage between anterior temporal area 21 and frontal area 47 changed from moderately positive for the controls to weakly negative for the AD patients. These results were interpreted as reflecting an inability of the AD patients to fully and automatically activate the neural circuit that young and healthy old persons use to perform the face-matching task, possibly because of impaired cortico-cortical connections. In addition, regions in the frontal lobes showed stronger functional interactions for the AD patients than for the controls (as indicated by stronger interregional correlations among frontal regions for patients than for controls), which may reflect a compensatory function of frontal subsystems. Such compensatory brain functional interactions may enable the AD pathology to develop over many years without being accompanied by behavioral dysfunction.

Our third example of dysfunctional cognitive processing comes from a PET study of language processing, and more specifically, single-word reading (Horwitz et al., 1998). A region in the superior part of the left temporal lobe, the angular gyrus, has traditionally been held to play a central role in reading. It has been suggested that the angular gyrus functionally interacts with extrastriate regions associated with visual

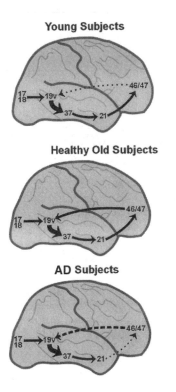

Figure 3.6
Functional networks of object and spatial vision for AD patients and controls (based on Horwitz et al., 1995).

processing of letterlike and wordlike stimuli, and also with posterior language regions such as Wernicke's area. The latter interaction is thought to be crucial for the transformation of visual input into lingusitic representations. To explore functional interactions between angular gyrus and other brain regions, interregional correlations between blood flow in the angular gyrus and blood flow in all other brain areas were examined while subjects were engaged in two reading tasks. Two groups of subjects were studied: normal readers and dyslexic readers (developmental dyslexia).

We will focus here on data from a task involving reading of pseudo words. This task was predicted to engage the interaction of the angular gyrus with other network elements more fully. In the normal readers, activity in left angular gyrus was strongly functionally linked to activity in areas of left visual association cortex. Moreover, angular gyrus was also functionally linked to Wernicke's and Broca's areas. The results of a similar analysis for right angular gyrus suggested that functional interactions were more pronounced in the left hemisphere. These findings agree well with predictions based on brain-damaged individuals, and serve to outline a normal reading network. The pattern observed for dyslexic readers (developmental dyslexia) differed significantly from that observed for the normal readers, and suggested a functional disconnection of angular gyrus from other reading-related regions. This observation is in agreement with observations of acquired alexia in which there is an anatomical disconnection of the angular gyrus from other language regions, thus pointing to similarities between acquired alexia and developmental dyslexia (for a network analysis with SEM of data from literate and illiterate subjects, see Petersson et al., 2000).

Finally, SEM has been used to study functional interactions between cortical and subcortical areas in Parkinson's disease patients and controls while they performed a motor task (Grafton et al., 1994). The patients were scanned before and after left globus pallidotomy. It was found that following surgery there were significant reductions in the strength of interactions between globus pallidus and thalamus and between thalamus and mesial frontal areas. It was concluded that SEM can identify regional interactions not apparent from between-condition comparisons of activation changes.

ISSUES

The purpose of this chapter was to introduce covariance-based analyses of functional brain-imaging data, and to show how such analytic techniques have been used to explore functional networks underlying several different cognitive processes. The network perspective should by no means be seen as being in conflict with categorical analyses of brain-imaging data. Rather, the two types of analyses complement one another, and, as was shown in several of the examples, analysis of activation changes is often an important first step in network analyses. At the same time it is important to stress that network analyses can support conclusions not apparent from activation analyses. Examples of this are the findings by McIntosh et al. (1994) and Köhler et al. (1998), demonstrating that a region can show task-related changes in functional interactions without showing task-related changes in activity.

Aside from the possibility of pulling additional information from the data, an important theoretical reason for conducting network analyses is the notion that examination of functional interactions is necessary for a full appreciation of the functional role of regional activation changes (cf. McIntosh et al., 1997). Based on the assumption that interregional interactions constitute the basis for most of brain function, increased activity of a region may mean one thing in the context of certain kinds of functional interactions and something other under conditions of different functional interactions (e.g., D'Esposito et al., 1998).

Several of the specific examples presented here combined anatomical and functional (task-related interregional covariances) information (SEM) to evaluate functional interactions, although a few studies simply looked at interregional correlations. The specification of connections in the anatomical model is generally done on the basis of information from studies of neural connectivity in the brains of non-human primates. Before discussing further issues relating to network analyses of brain-imaging data, we will briefly describe an innovative approach to determining connectivity in the human brain. Paus and colleagues have combined PET and transcranial magnetic stimulation (TMS) to assess neural connectivity (Paus et al., 1997). While PET was used to monitor brain blood flow, TMS was used to stimulate the left frontal eye field (FEF). Across six separate PET scans, the number of TMS pulse trains was varied (5, 10, 15, 20, 25, 30). Thereafter the effect of number of pulse trains on regional blood flow responses was estimated. Significant correlations were observed between TMS pulse trains and blood flow in regions remote from left FEF, including left cuneus and bilateral superior parietal regions. Thus, activity in these remote regions increased when left FEF was activated by TMS, suggesting the existence of neural connections between FEF and these regions. This pattern is consistent with findings based on studies of anatomic connectivity of monkey FEF, and more generally the study by Paus and colleagues points to the possibility of in vivo studies of neural connectivity in the human brain by the combined TMS/PET technique (for further discussion of this approach, see Wassermann & Grafman, 1997).

A further point relating to interpretation that is important to consider is that PET data represent time-integrated information. Although analyses of effective connectivity provide suggestive evidence on the temporal ordering of effects (for example, by distinguishing between feedforward and feedback effects), it is desirable to constrain the modeling by temporal information. By considering data from techniques that provide temporal information, such as event-related potential and perhaps fMRI (see chapter 2), this can be solved. Also, network analyses of data based on measurement of electrical brain activity have been presented (e.g., Gevins, 1996), and analyses of data from studies combining measurement of blood flow and electrical activity (e.g., Düzel et al., 1999) have great potential.

In conclusion, the use of modern brain-imaging techniques allow simultaneous measures of activity in the whole brain. In turn, this advancement in measuring whole-brain activity while participants perform various cognitive tasks points to the possibility (and necessity) of integrating the multitude of observations in a way which acknowledges that the brain is a truly multivariate dynamic system. The analytical approaches we have discussed here represent a step in this direction.

REFERENCES

Aertsen, A., Bonhoeffer, T. and Kruger, J. (1987). Coherent activity in neuronal populations: analysis and interpretation. In E. R. Caianiello (Ed.), Physics of Cognitive Processes, World Scientific Publishing, Singapore, pp. 1–34.

Andreasen, N. C., Arndt, S., Swayze, V., II, Cizadlo, T., Flaum, M., O'Leary, D., Ehrhardt, J. C., & Yuh, W. T. C. (1994). Thalamic abnormalities in schizophrenia visualized through magnetic resonance image averaging. *Science* 266, 294–298.

Andreasen, N. C., O'Leary, D. S., Cizadlo, T., Arndt, S., Rezai, K., Boles Ponto, L. L., Watkins, G. L., & Hichwa, R. D. (1996). Schizophrenia and cognitive dysmetria: A positron-emission tomography study of dysfunctional prefrontal-thalamic-cerebellar circuitry. *Proceedings of the National Academy of Sciences USA* 93, 9985–9990.

Baddeley, A. D., & Hitch, G. J. (1974). Working memory. In *The Psychology of Learning and Motivation*, G. Bower, ed., 47–90. San Diego: Academic Press.

Bullmore, E. T., Rabe-Hesketh, S., Morris, R. G., Williams, S. C. R., Gregory, L., Gray, J. A., & Brammer, M. J. (1996). Functional magnetic resonance image analysis of a large-scale neurocognitive network. *NeuroImage* 4, 16–33.

Büchel, C., & Friston, K. J. (1997). Modulation of connectivity in visual pathways by attention: Cortical interactions evaluated with structural equation modelling and fMRI. *Cerebral Cortex* 7, 1047–3211.

Cabeza, R., McIntosh, A. R., Tulving, E., Nyberg, L., & Grady, C. L. (1997). Age-related differences in effective neural connectivity during encoding and recall. *NeuroReport* 8, 3479–3483.

Cabeza, R., & Nyberg, L. (1997). Imaging cognition: An empirical review of PET studies with normal subjects. *Journal of Cognitive Neuroscience* 9, 1–26.

D'Esposito, M., Ballard, D., Aguirre, G. K., & Zarahn, E. (1998). Human prefrontal cortex is not specific for working memory: A functional MRI study. *NeuroImage* 8, 274–282.

D'Esposito, M., Detre, J. A., Alsop, D. C., Shin, R. K., Atlas, S., & Grossman, M. (1995). The neural basis of the central executive system of working memory. *Nature* 378, 279–281.

Düzel, E., Cabeza, R., Picton, T. W., Yonelinas, A. P., Scheich, H., Heinze, H. J., & Tulving, E. (1999). "Task- and item-related processes in memory retrieval: A combined PET and ERP study." *Proceedings of the National Academy of Sciences USA* 96, 1794–1799.

Finger, S. (1994). Origins of neuroscience: A history of explorations into brain function, Oxford University Press, New York, 462 pp.

Fletcher, P. (1998). The missing link: A failure of fronto-hippocampal integration in schizophrenia. *Nature Neuroscience* 1, 266–267.

Fletcher, P. C., Frith, C. D., Grasby, P. M., Shallice, T., Frackowiak, R. S. J., & Dolan, R. J. (1995). Brain systems for encoding and retrieval of auditory-verbal memory: An in vivo study in humans. *Brain* 118, 401–416.

Fletcher, P. C., Frith, C. D., & Rugg, M. D. (1997). The functional neuroanatomy of episodic memory. *Trends in Neurosciences* 20, 213–218.

Fredriksson, M., Wik, G., Fischer, H., & Anderson, J. (1995). Affective and attentive neural networks in humans: A PET study of Pavlovian conditioning. *NeuroReport* 7, 97–101.

Friston, K. J. (1994). Functional and effective connectivity: A synthesis. *Human Brain Mapping* 2, 56–78.

Friston, K. J., & Frith, C. D. (1995). Schizophrenia: A disconnection syndrome? *Clinical Neuroscience* 3, 89–97.

Friston, K. J., Frith, C. D., Liddle, P. F., & Frackowiak, R. S. J. (1991). Investigating a network model of word generation with positron emission tomography. *Proceedings of the Royal Society of London* B244, 101–106.

Friston, K. J., Frith, C. D., Liddle, P. F., & Frackowiak, R. S. J. (1993). Functional connectivity: The principal-component analysis of large (PET) data sets. *Journal of Cerebral Blood Flow and Metabolism* 13, 5–14.

Friston, K. J., Liddle, P. F., Frith, C. D., Hirsch, S. R., & Frackowiak, R. S. J. (1992). The left medial temporal region and schizophrenia. A PET study. *Brain* 115, 367–382.

Gabrieli, J. D. E. (1998). Cognitive neuroscience of human memory. *Annual Review of Psychology* 49, 87–115.

Gabrieli, J. D. E., Brewer, J. B., Desmond, J. E., & Glover, G. H. (1997). Separate neural bases of two fundamental memory processes in the human medial temporal lobe. *Science* 276, 264–266.

Gerstein, G. L., Perkel, D. H., & Subramanian, K. N. (1978). Identification of functionally related neural assemblies. *Brain Research* 140, 43–62.

Gevins, A. (1996). High resolution evoked potentials of cognition. *Brain Topography* 8, 189–199.

Grady, C. L., Haxby, J. V., Horwitz, B., Ungerleider, L. G., Schapiro, M. B., Carson, R. E., Herscovitch, P., Mishkin, M., & Rapoport, S. I. (1992). Dissociation of object and spatial vision in human extrastriate cortex: Age-related changes in activation of regional cerebral blood flow measured with [15O] water and positron emission tomography. *Journal of Cognitive Neuroscience* 4, 23–34.

Grafton, S. T., Sutton, J., Couldwell, W., Lew, M., & Waters, C. (1994). Network analysis of motor system connectivity in Parkinson's disease: Modulation of thalamocortical interactions after pallidotomy. *Human Brain Mapping* 2, 45–55.

Haxby, J. V., Ungerleider, L. G., Horwitz, B., Rapoport, S. I., & Grady, C. L. (1995). Hemispheric differences in neural systems for face working memory: A PET–rCBF study. *Human Brain Mapping* 3, 68–82.

Heckers, S., Rauch, S. L., Goff, D., Savage, C. R., Schacter, D. L., Fischman, A. J., & Alpert, N. M. (1998). Impaired recruitment of the hippocampus during conscious recollection in schizophrenia. *Nature Neuroscience* 1, 318–323.

Horwitz, B. (1989). Functional neural systems analyzed by use of interregional correlations of glucose metabolism. In *Visuomotor Coordination*, J.-P. Ewert & M. A. Arbib, eds., 873–892. New York: Plenum Press.

Horwitz, B., Grady, C. L., Haxby, J. V., Schapiro, M. B., Rapoport, S. I., Ungerleider, L. G., & Mishkin, M. (1992). Functional associations among human extrastriate brain regions during object and spatial vision. *Journal of Cognitive Neuroscience* 4, 311–322.

Horwitz, B., McIntosh, A. R., Haxby, J. V., Furey, M., Salerno, J. A., Schapiro, M. B., Rapoport, S. I., & Grady, C. L. (1995). Network analysis of PET-mapped visual pathways in Alzheimer type dementia. *NeuroReport* 6, 2287–2292.

Horwitz, B., Rumsey, J. M., & Donohue, B. C. (1998). Functional connectivity of the angular gyrus in normal reading and dyslexia. *Proceedings of the National Academy of Sciences USA* 95, 8939–8944.

Jennings, J. M., McIntosh, A. R., Kapur, S., Zipursky, R. B., & Houle, S. (1998). Functional network differences in schizophrenia: A rCBF study of semantic processing. *NeuroReport* 9, 1697–1700.

Jonides, J., Smith, E. E., Koeppe, R. A., Awh, E., Minoshima, S., & Mintun, M. A. (1993). Spatial working memory in humans as revealed by PET. *Nature* 363, 623–625.

Karni, A., Meyer, G., Jezzard, P., Adams, M. M., Turner, R., & Ungerleider, L. G. (1995). Functional MRI evidence for adult motor cortex plasticity during motor skill learning. *Nature* 377, 155–158.

Köhler, S., McIntosh, A. R., Moscovitch, M., & Winocur, G. (1998). Functional interactions between the medial temporal lobes and posterior neocortex related to episodic memory retrieval. *Cerebral Cortex* 8, 451–461.

Lashley, K. S. (1933). Integrative functions of the cerebral cortex. *Physiological Review* 13(1), 1–42.

LePage, M., Habib, R., & Tulving, E. (1998). Hippocampal PET activations of memory encoding and retrieval: The HIPER model. *Hippocampus* 8, 313–322.

McIntosh, A. R., Bookstein, F. L., Haxby, J. V., & Grady, C. L. (1996). Spatial pattern analysis of functional brain images using partial least squares. *NeuroImage* 3, 143–157.

McIntosh, A. R., Cabeza, R. E., & Lobaugh, N. J. (1998). Analysis of neural interactions explains the activation of occipital cortex by an auditory stimulus. *Journal of Neurophysiology* 80, 2790–2796.

McIntosh, A. R., & Gonzalez-Lima, F. (1994). Structural equation modelling and its application to network analysis in functional brain imaging. *Human Brain Mapping* 2, 2–22.

McIntosh, A. R., Grady, C. L., Haxby, J. V., Ungerleider, L. G., & Horwitz, B. (1996). Changes in limbic and prefrontal functional interactions in a working memory task for faces. *Cerebral Cortex* 6, 571–584.

McIntosh, A. R., Grady, C. L., Ungerleider, L. G., Haxby, J. V., Rapoport, S. I., & Horwitz, B. (1994). Network analysis of cortical visual pathways mapped with PET. *Journal of Neuroscience* 14, 655–666.

McIntosh, A. R., Nyberg, L., Bookstein, F. L., & Tulving, E. (1997). Differential functional connectivity of prefrontal and medial temporal cortices during episodic memory retrieval. *Human Brain Mapping* 5, 323–327.

McIntosh, A. R., Rajah, M. N., & Lobaugh, N. J. (1999). Interactions of prefrontal cortex related to awareness in sensory learning. *Science* 284, 1531–1533.

McLaughlin, T., Steinberg, B., Christensen, B., Law, I., Parving, A., & Friberg, L. (1992). Potential language and attentional networks revealed through factor analysis of rCBF data measured by SPECT. *Journal of Cerebral Blood Flow and Metabolism* 12, 535–545.

Mesulam, M. M. (1990). Large-scale neurocognitive networks and distributed processing for attention, language, and memory. *Annals of Neurology* 28, 597–613.

Molchan, S. E., Sunderland, T., McIntosh, A. R., Herscovitch, P., & Schreurs, B. G. (1994). A functional anatomic study of associative learning in humans. *Proceedings of the National Academy of Sciences USA* 91, 8122–8126.

Nolde, S. F., Johnson, M. K., & Raye, C. L. (1998). The role of the prefrontal cortex during tests of episodic memory. *Trends in Cognitive Sciences* 2, 399–406.

Nyberg, L., Cabeza, R., & Tulving, E. (1996). PET studies of encoding and retrieval: The HERA model. *Psychonomic Bulletin & Review* 3, 135–148.

Nyberg, L., McIntosh, A. R., Cabeza, R., Habib, R., Houle, S., & Tulving, E. (1996). General and specific brain regions involved in encoding and retrieval of events: What, where, and when. *Proceedings of the National Academy of Sciences USA* 93, 11280–11285.

Nyberg, L., McIntosh, A. R., & Tulving, E. (1998). Functional brain imaging of episodic and semantic memory with positron emission tomography. *Journal of Molecular Medicine* 76, 48–53.

Paulesu, E., Frith, C. D., & Frackowiak, R. S. J. (1993). The neural correlates of the verbal component of working memory. *Nature* 362, 342–345.

Paus, T., Jech, R., Thompson, C. J., Comeau, R., Peters, T., & Evans, A. C. (1997). Transcranial magnetic stimulation during positron emission tomography: A new method for studying connectivity of the human cerebral cortex. *Journal of Neuroscience* 17, 3178–3184.

Petersson, K. M., Reis, A., Askelöf, S., Castro-Caldas, A., and Ingvar, M. (2000). Language processing modulated by literacy: A network-analysis of verbal repetition in literate and illiterate subjects. Journal of Cognitive Neuroscience, 12, 1–19.

Raichle, M. E., Fiez, J. A., Videen, T. O., MacLeod, A. M., Pardo, J. V., Fox, P. T., & Petersen, S. E. (1994). Practice-related changes in the human brain functional anatomy during nonmotor learning. *Cerebral Cortex* 4, 8–26.

Schacter, D. L., & Buckner, R. L. (1998). Priming and the brain. *Neuron* 20, 185–195.

Schacter, D. L., & Wagner, A. D. (1999). Medial temporal lobe activations in fMRI and PET studies of episodic encoding and retrieval. *Hippocampus* 9, 7–24.

Silbersweig, D. A., Stern, E., Frith, C. D., Holmes, A., Grootoonk, Sylke, Seaward, J., McKenna, P., Chua, S. E., Schnorr, L., Jones, T., & Frackowiak, R. S. J. (1995). A functional neuroanatomy of hallucinations in schizophrenia. *Nature* 378, 176–179.

Squire, L. R. (1992). Memory and the hippocampus: A synthesis from findings with rats, monkeys, and humans. *Psychological Review* 99, 195–231.

Strother, S. C., Anderson, J. R., Schaper, K. A., Sidtis, J. J., Liow, J.-S., Woods, R. P., & Rottenberg, D. A. (1995). Principal components analysis and the scaled subprofile model compared to intersubject averaged and statistical parametric mapping: I. "Functional connectivity" of the human motor system studied with [15O] water PET. *Journal of Cerebral Blood Flow and Metabolism* 15, 738–753.

Tulving, E. (1983). *Elements of Episodic Memory*. New York: Oxford University Press.

Tulving, E., Kapur, S., Craik, F. I. M., Moscovitch, M., & Houle, S. (1994). Hemispheric encoding/retrieval asymmetry in episodic memory: Positron emission tomography findings. *Proceedings of the National Academy of Sciences USA* 91, 2016–2020.

Tulving, E., Habib, R., Nyberg, L., LePage, M., & McIntosh, A. R. (1999). Position emission tomography correlations in and beyond medial temporal lobes. *Hippocampus* 9, 71–82.

Wasserman, E. M., & Grafman, J. (1997). Combining transcranial magnetic stimulation and neuroimaging to map the brain. *Trends in Cognitive Sciences* 1, 199–200.

Worsley, K. J., Poline, J. B., Friston, K. J., & Evans, A. C. (1997). Characterizing the response of PET and fMRI data using multivariate linear models. *NeuroImage* 6, 305–319.

II COGNITIVE DOMAINS

4 Functional Neuroimaging of Attention

Todd C. Handy, Joseph B. Hopfinger, and George R. Mangun

INTRODUCTION

The empirical study of human cortical function advanced dramatically during the 1990s due to the advent of hemodynamic neuroimaging (Posner & Raichle, 1994). Methods such as positron emission tomography (PET) and functional magnetic resonance imaging (fMRI) allow the volumetric variations in regional cerebral blood flow that are correlated with cognitive activity to be indexed with millimeter-level spatial resolution. In this chapter, we examine the use of these neuroimaging methods in relation to one of the central components of human cognition: *selective attention*.

We begin by introducing one form of selective visual attention, spatial attention, and then detail the role neuroimaging has played in furthering our understanding of both how attention functions at the cognitive level and how it is implemented at the neural level. In the second section of the chapter, we discuss the ongoing efforts in spatial attention research to combine neuroimaging with other, electrophysiologically based measures of neural activity. The central goal here is to cultivate an appreciation of how the main weakness of PET and fMRI measures, low temporal resolution, can be offset by integrating nonhemodynamic measures into a common experimental paradigm. In the conclusion of the chapter, we turn from looking at how neuroimaging has illuminated our understanding of spatial attention to discussing how more general views of selective attention can illuminate critical aspects of neuroimaging. In particular, we argue that resource-based theories of selective attention provide an effective—and ultimately necessary—cognitive model for describing and predicting the complex patterns of multivariate neural activity that are the characteristic outcome of most neuroimaging experiments.

FUNCTIONAL NEUROIMAGING OF ATTENTION

At the most basic level, selective attention can be characterized as the "filtering" of sensory information, a process that is central to normal human function in that it allows us to rapidly isolate important input from the sensory environment for the highest levels of cognitive analysis. The empirical study of visual selective attention has stemmed from three general questions regarding such filtering: (1) Where in the afferent visual processing stream does selection occur? (2) What neural mechanisms control or mediate these selective effects? (3) What are the functional consequences of the selection process? While the ultimate goal of this chapter is to outline the different ways in which neuroimaging techniques have been applied to the study of selective attention, we must begin by reviewing the cognitive foundations of this elementary process.

From a cognitive perspective, selective attention can take many forms in visual processing, involving both "early" perceptual (e.g., Egly et al., 1994; Treisman & Gelade, 1980) and "later" postperceptual (e.g., Pashler, 1998; Shiu & Pashler, 1994; Sperling, 1984) processing operations. This suggests that selection has no unitary locus in the visual system. Rather, selection of visual input can occur on the basis of a variety of stimulus criteria (e.g., color, shape, or spatial location), with the locus of selection varying as a function of the processing operations performed on the sensory input (e.g., Johnston et al., 1995, 1996). In terms of attentional control, a general distinction is made at the cognitive level between stimulus-driven or *bottom-up* effects on attentional selection, and goal-driven or *top-down* influences (e.g., Desimone & Duncan, 1995; Yantis, 1998). For example, the physical features of visual stimulation, such as the spatial arrangement of objects in an array or whether any objects within an array are moving, will affect what information is selected (e.g., Driver, 1996; Folk et al., 1994; Prinzmetal, 1995). In turn, these bottom-up factors qualitatively differ from top-down effects, which involve actively choosing a specific stimulus criterion on which to base selection, as described above.

Given the range of factors affecting visual selective attention, when considering the neural substrates of the selection process, both the form of selection and the manner of its control must be made explicit. In this section and the next, we will limit the scope of discussion to one widely studied form of selection in vision: spatial attention and its top-down modulation.

Spatial Attention

As studied in the visual domain, spatial attention refers to the act of covertly attending to nonfoveal locations within the visual field. Although descriptions of spatial attention and its functional consequences can be traced back to James (1890), contemporary research in spatial attention has its roots in two seminal, behavioral-based studies. First, Eriksen and Hoffman (1972) measured vocal reaction times (RTs) to the onset of nonfoveal target letters that subjects were required to discriminate. Importantly, Eriksen and Hoffman found that if a target letter was presented simultaneously with a set of task-irrelevant noise letters, the effect of the noise letters on target RTs depended on their proximity to the target. When the noise letters were presented within a degree of visual angle from the target, target RTs were delayed relative to when no noise letters were present. However, this effect was eliminated when the noise letters were presented a degree or more from the target. This finding suggested that when attending to a nonfoveal location, the spatial extent of the attended region is restricted to about 1° of visual angle.

Second, Posner (1980) reported a number of experiments that measured manual RTs to nonfoveal targets as a function of whether the targets were presented in attended or unattended spatial locations. The critical manipulation in these studies was to cue the subjects prior to target onset—via an arrow or letter at fixation—as to the most likely location of the impending target. Independent of whether the task involved detection or discrimination, Posner found that RTs were consistently faster when the targets were presented at the cued (or attended) location, relative to when the targets were presented at the uncued (or unattended) location. Whereas Eriksen and Hoffman (1972) had demonstrated the focal nature of spatial attention within the visual field, Posner's (1980) results indicated that focused spatial attention can directly alter the processing of stimulus inputs.

The Cognitive Model The research inspired by Eriksen and Hoffman (1972) and Posner (1980) has led to the suggestion that spatial attention is analogous to a mental spotlight or zoom lens that facilitates the processing of all stimuli falling within its focus (e.g., Eriksen & St. James, 1986; Posner, 1980; for a review, see Klein et al., 1992). In this manner, covertly orienting spatial attention to a discrete location within the visual field operates as a mechanism of selective attention by conferring a processing "benefit" for attended stimuli, and a processing "cost" for unattended stimuli, relative to conditions where attention is uniformly distributed across all spatial locations (Posner, 1980). The general cognitive model thus posits that the attentional focus can be moved from location to location (e.g., Tsal, 1983), and—independent of their physical properties—any stimuli falling within this focus will receive measurable benefits in visual processing relative to stimuli falling outside of the focus. Within this framework, the "spotlight" model has been further refined by data indicating that spatial attention can affect perceptual sensitivity (or d'; e.g., Downing, 1988; Müller & Humphreys, 1991; Hawkins et al., 1990), that both the size of the focus (e.g., Eriksen & Yeh, 1985) and the rate at which processing benefits drop off from the focus (e.g., Handy et al., 1996) are dependent on the specific parameters of the task being performed, and that the attentional focus can be split, at least under certain stimulus conditions (e.g., Kramer & Hahn, 1995).

The Neural Correlates When considering the neural correlates of spatial attention, a distinction must be made between those brain areas which serve as the *source* of the attention effect and those which are the *site* of the attention effect (Posner, 1995; Posner & Petersen, 1990). In relation to the spotlight model, the attentional source involves those neural structures which are devoted exclusively to the operation of the spotlight per se, such as moving the spotlight from location to location. The source also includes those neural structures mediating the top-down *or executive* control of the spotlight, such as deciding where in the visual field the spotlight should be moved and when the movement should be initiated. In contrast, the attentional site involves those visuocortical areas which are primarily involved in stimulus processing, but whose functional activity can be modulated by spatial attention. For example, although spatial attention can affect perceptual sensitivity (e.g., Downing, 1988; Handy et al., 1996; Müller & Humphreys, 1991; Hawkins et al., 1990), these effects are manifest in processing operations that can proceed independent of any attention-related modulation.

However, before considering the contributions that neuroimaging has made in elucidating the neural correlates of spatial attention, we must consider the wider context provided by research methodologies that predate the advent of hemodynamic measures. In particular, electrophysiological and neuropsychological studies have revealed many critical insights into the neural implementation of spatial attention, and these contributions must be detailed prior to introducing the evidence from neuroimaging. Here we examine these nonneuroimaging data in relation to the three general questions driving spatial attention research: identifying the locus, the control mechanisms, and the functional consequences of spatial selection.

LOCUS OF SELECTION   Identifying the neural loci of spatial-based attentional selection has been an issue especially amenable to studies using electrophysiological measures. In particular, owing to their millisecond-level temporal resolution, event-related potentials (ERPs)—signal-averaged voltage fluctuations recorded from the scalp that are time-locked to sensory, motor, or cognitive events (see Hillyard & Picton, 1987)—have been used with much success in investigating how early in the afferent visuocortical pathway spatial attention can modulate stimulus processing. Applied to the issue of localizing the site of attentional modulation, the critical assumption regarding ERPs is that the time course of spatial attention effects (relative to stimulus onset) can be correlated with the progression of visuocortical processing areas activated by the given stimulus. The earlier in time an attention effect is observed, the earlier in visuocortical processing the site of the attention effect is assumed to be (see Mangun & Hillyard, 1995).

Using ERPs, researchers have shown that spatial attention can modulate the lateral occipital P1 and N1 ERP components, which peak at about 120 and 170 msec post stimulus, respectively. In particular, the amplitudes of the P1 and N1 are larger for stimuli in attended spatial locations, relative to physically identical stimuli presented outside of the attentional focus (e.g., Eason, 1981; Mangun & Hillyard, 1991; Van Voorhis & Hillyard, 1977). Given the time course of the sensory-evoked P1 and N1, these ERP data indicate that spatial attention can affect visual processing within the first 120 msec after the onset of a visual stimulus. In contrast, efforts to show similar attention-related modulations in the C1 ERP component, which peaks at about 70 msec post stimulus, have produced negative results (e.g., Clark & Hillyard, 1996; Mangun et al., 1993). On the basis of the relative time windows of the P1, N1, and C1 (and their characteristic scalp topography), the ERP data thus suggest that the initial site of spatial attention effects in visual processing lies within extrastriate visual cortex, encompassing areas V2–V4 (e.g., Clark et al., 1995; Gomez Gonzalez et al., 1994).

Although spatial attention can selectively modulate processing in extrastriate cortex, further ERP research has now indicated that these effects of attention depend directly on the perceptual load of the given task. In particular, Handy and Mangun (2000) found that the magnitude of attentional modulation in the P1 and N1 ERP components increased positively with the perceptual load of target items in an endogenous spatial cuing paradigm (figure 4.1). These results suggest that the effects of attention within extrastriate cortex can be described via resource allocation, where a greater proportion of limited-capacity attentional resources are allocated to the cued location under high versus low perceptual load. This positive relationship between

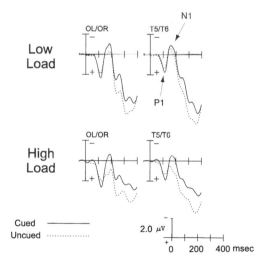

Figure 4.1
The effect of perceptual load on the magnitude of the spatial attention effect in the P1 and N1 ERP components reported by Handy and Mangun (2000). Under the high load condition, there is greater difference in amplitude between the cued and uncued conditions, relative to the low load condition. From a resource perspective, such data are consistent with the view that attention acts to selectively amplify the magnitude of neural responses. These ERPs were recorded from lateral occipital electrode sites contralateral to the visual field of the ERP-evoking stimulus.

neuronal response and attentional resource allocation is critical for understanding selective attention in relation to multivariate neural activity, and will be discussed in greater detail below.

CONTROL OF SELECTION   The neuropsychological study of brain-lesioned patients has been a particularly effective technique for identifying the neural structures involved in attentional control (e.g., Driver, 1998; Mesulam, 1981; Rafal, 1996; Rafal & Henik, 1994). Much of the research in this domain has been premised on defining the act of attentional orienting as a three-step process (e.g., Posner et al., 1984; see Posner, 1995, for a review). According to this view, when a subject is cued to move her spatial attention to a new location, attention must first be *disengaged* from its current location within the visual field. Following disengagement, attention must be *moved* from its initial location to the new location. Finally, once the attentional spotlight has been moved to the new location, attention must be *engaged* with whatever stimuli are in the new location. Each of these three steps—disengage, move, and engage—involves an attention-specific operation associated with spotlight function, and the evidence from lesion studies has strongly suggested that these operations are performed by different neural structures.

For example, Posner et al. (1984) reported that when patients with unilateral damage to the parietal lobe oriented their attention to their ipsilesional visual field, they were greatly impaired in their ability to respond to targets presented in the contralesional visual field. Because patients showed no such impairments for contralesional targets when attention was precued to the contralesional visual field, this was taken as evidence that the parietal lobe is involved in mediating the act of disengaging attention from its current focus (see also Baynes et al., 1986; Morrow & Ratcliff, 1988; Posner et al., 1987).

In contrast, studies of patients with progressive supranuclear palsy—which results in degeneration of the superior colliculus and other midbrain structures involved in the control of saccadic eye movements—have shown that these patients are slowed in their ability to move their attentional focus (e.g., Posner et al., 1982; Posner et al., 1985). Specifically, if subjects had difficulty making saccades in a specific direction, their responses to nonfoveated targets were consistently delayed whenever they had to move their attention in the impaired direction in order to make the target response. These data thus suggest that the superior colliculus and related midbrain areas are responsible for the act of moving the attentional spotlight (see also Rafal, 1996).

Finally, the third component of attentional orienting—engaging stimuli at a new location—appears to be mediated by the pulvinar nucleus of the thalamus. Specifically, given sufficient time to orient their attention to a nonfoveal location, patients with unilateral damage to the pulvinar nevertheless showed selective delays in responding when the targets were in the contralesional visual field (see Posner, 1988). Because there were no similar delays in responding to targets in the ipsilesional visual field, and that targets were occurring after attention had been moved, the delay in responding to targets in the contralesional field could be attributed to a selective impairment of the engagement operation—an effect on stimulus processing similar to that seen in patients with parietal-based visual neglect (e.g., Rafal, 1996; Rafal & Henik, 1994).

The question of what neural areas mediate the executive control of these orienting operations has brought lesion and ERP techniques into a single empirical paradigm (see Swick & Knight, 1998). In particular, recent data suggest that prefrontal cortex (Brodmann's areas 9 and 46) modulates processing in posterior cortical areas via parallel excitatory and inhibitory reafferent projections (see Knight et al., in press), pathways critical for spatial attention as well as for oculomotor function (e.g., Corbetta, 1998). When ERPs were recorded for visual stimuli in patients with lesions of dorsolateral prefrontal cortex, there was a selective decrease in the N1 amplitude for stimuli in the ipsilesional visual field (Knight, 1997), indicating that these patients had an impaired ability to modulate processing in extrastriate visual cortex via spatial attention. Such data provide compelling evidence that top-down inputs from prefrontal cortex are intimately involved in mediating sensory processing in extrastriate cortex, although it remains to be determined exactly how these effects are implemented. One possibility is that these top-down effects on early visual processing are subserved by a corticothalamic network involving the pulvinar nucleus, which may act to provide an amplification signal to those posterior visuocortical areas which are processing inputs from attended spatial locations (LaBerge, 1995).

CONSEQUENCES OF SELECTION   ERPs have been used to investigate two different aspects of how spatial attention may affect the processing of stimulus inputs. First, studies have shown that when spatial selection is combined with a second form of selection, such as attending to both the location and the color of a stimulus, selection for the nonspatial attribute is hierarchically dependent on whether or not the stimulus was in an attended spatial location. For example, Hillyard and Münte (1984) required subjects to detect target items of a specific color (either red or blue) at a specific (i.e., attended) location. Independent of color, they found that the P1 and N1 for items at the attended location were larger in amplitude, relative to items presented in an unattended location. Critically, however, the later-latency ERP components associated with attending to color showed selective enhancements only for items of the target color that were at the attended location. These data suggest that stimuli are first selected on the basis of their spatial location, and that selection for color could thus occur only for stimuli presented in the attended location (see also Eimer, 1995).

Similar findings have been reported for combined spatial and motion selection, where selection for attended motion attributes occurred only for moving stimuli in attended locations (Anllo-Vento & Hillyard, 1996). Taken together, the data thus indicate that spatial selection precedes other forms of selection, and directly limits the processing of stimuli at higher stages within the afferent visual pathways (see also Green et al., 1998).

Second, the modulatory effects of spatial attention on the amplitudes of the P1 and N1 ERP components have long been taken as evidence that spatial attention acts as a mechanism of sensory facilitation *or gain* (e.g., Mangun et al., 1987). The sensory gain hypothesis has been further refined by the proposal that the P1 and N1 reflect that activity of qualitatively distinct and dissociable selection-based operations within extrastriate cortex. In particular, it has been suggested that the amplitude of the P1 covaries positively with the *suppression* of stimulus information falling *outside* the focus of attention, while the N1 amplitude covaries positively with the *amplification* of information *within* the attentional focus (e.g., Hillyard et al., 1998; Luck, 1995; Mangun & Hillyard, 1991). This proposal for the P1 and N1 would indicate that spatial attention can enhance the contrast between attended and unattended sensory signals by the combined system of boosting the signals from attended locations and dampening the signals from unattended locations.

In sum, neuropsychological and electrophysiological studies have provided a wealth of important information about the neural underpinnings of spatial attention and its effects on early processing in vision. However, like all methods of empirical analysis, the lesion and ERP techniques described above have their inherent limitations, limitations that transcend the study of visual attention. In lesion studies, for example, a deficit in a specific cognitive process (e.g., attentional disengagement) can be linked to a specific neural structure, but this method tells us little about what other structures may be involved—that is, there might not be one-to-one mapping of the impaired operation onto the impaired structure. Further, it can be difficult to determine whether a cognitive deficit in a lesion patient is caused by damage to the neural structure per se, or whether it is caused by damage to pathways extending through the lesioned area. Similarly, ERPs are well known to have limited spatial resolution, making it difficult to reliably identify the cortical loci of different ERP generators. Only with the advent of hemodynamic neuroimaging has an empirical tool been found that can overcome these methodological limitations.

PET and fMRI Evidence

Neuroimaging studies of spatial attention have closely paralleled the general issues addressed using neuropsychological and electrophysiolgical methodologies: Where does selection take place, what areas control the selection process, and what are the functional consequences of selection? However, relative to what has been learned via lesion and ERP studies, the nature of PET and fMRI methods has led to a variety of new and unique approaches to these basic questions. As a consequence, not only has neuroimaging confirmed many of the central findings from lesion and ERP research but, more important, it has provided an invaluable resource for building upon this already vast knowledge base. What follows is a nonexhaustive review of the imaging literature that highlights the different and essential ways in which neuroimaging has been applied to the empirical study of visuospatial attention.

Locus of Selection At least two different approaches have been used in neuroimaging for localizing the site of spatial attention effects in the afferent visual pathway. The first approach, which is based on comparing sensory-evoked visuocortical responses as a function of different attention conditions, is not unique to neuroimaging. For example, the ERP studies reviewed have been based in large part on comparing the amplitude of sensory-evoked responses in visual cortex for stimuli in attended versus unattended spatial locations (e.g., Mangun & Hillyard, 1991). In contrast, the second approach we discuss—which is premised on exploiting the retinotopic organization of striate and extrastriate visuocortical areas—is unique to neuroimaging, since it depends directly on the finegrained spatial resolution provided by hemodynamic measures of neural activity. Importantly, however, the results obtained via both approaches remain consistent with the corpus of evidence from human electrophysiology, which strongly suggests that spatial attention can affect processing in extrastriate but not in striate visual cortex.

MODULATION OF SENSORY RESPONSES A number of spatial attention studies using ERPs have been premised on comparing the sensory-evoked responses to nonfoveal stimuli as a function of whether or not the stimuli were in a covertly attended spatial location. The same technique can be applied in neuroimaging, where the critical measure is to compare changes in PET or fMRI signal strength for attended versus unattended stimuli. The site(s) of attentional modulation in visuocortical processing can then be localized by identifying those cortical areas showing a significant increase in signal intensity under focused spatial attention conditions, relative to conditions where the activity-evoking stimuli are physically identical but presented in unattended spatial locations.

Adopting this approach, Kastner et al. (1998: experiment 2) used fMRI to examine the effects of spatial attention under two different stimulus conditions: either four stimuli were presented simultaneously within the upper right visual field quadrant, or the stimuli were presented sequentially over time, with only one stimulus appearing in the upper right quadrant at any moment. Within this design, Kastner et al. also manipulated attention such that subjects either covertly attended to the stimulus location nearest fixation, or attention was maintained at fixation. Although this experiment was included in a study that was ultimately designed to explore the suppressive interactions that arise in cortical processing between multiple stimulus representations—and the role spatial attention may play in mediating these interactions (see below)—the results of this experiment speak directly to localizing the site of attentional modulation in visual cortex. Specifically, Kastner et al. reported that, independent of the simultaneous versus sequential stimulus condition, spatial attention increased stimulus-driven activity in ventral extrastriate visual areas V2, V4, and TEO, but not in striate area V1.

RETINOTOPIC MAPPING   In order to more precisely localize where in the afferent visual pathway spatial attention can modulate sensory-evoked processing, mapping techniques have been developed that rely on the retinotopic organization of extrastriate cortical regions. Specifically, for visual areas such as V2, VP, and V4, the location of stimulus-driven activity within each area systematically varies with the visual field location of the stimulus. Further, the borders between adjacent visual regions have a characteristic "mirror image," such that if the topographic representations in one area move from lower to upper visual field, when the boundary is reached with the next visual area, its topographic representations will move from upper to lower visual field. As a result, if neuroimaging is used to track activations in visual cortex as a function of the visual field location of a stimulus, the borders between visual areas can be identified as the point where these visuotopic mappings reverse their direction along the cortical ribbon (e.g., Sereno et al., 1995).

The use of retinotopic mapping to localize spatial attention-related modulations in visual cortex was first reported by Jha et al. (1997). In this study, the borders of V1, V2, VP, and V4 were first mapped in each subject by stimulating the vertical and horizontal meridians of each visual field with a reversing checkerboard pattern, and these activations were spatially coregistered with high-resolution anatomical "template" images. Subjects then performed a spatial attention task where stimuli were presented bilaterally, while attention was oriented to either the left or the right visual field in alternating 16 sec blocks throughout the approximately 4 min scanning period. With two letterlike stimuli presented in each hemifield, the task required subjects to make a manual response whenever the two symbols in the attended hemifield matched. For upper visual field stimuli, attention-related activations were found in the posterior lingual and fusiform gyri contralateral to the attended visual field. When these activations were coregistered to the anatomical templates defining the different ventral occipital visual areas, the data indicated that attention was modulating activity only in areas V2, VP, and V4.

Retinotopic mapping has also been utilized by other research groups. In parallel studies, Brefczynski and DeYoe (1999) and Tootell et al. (1998) had subjects attend to discrete spatial locations and required them to respond to any targets presented at the currently attended location. Presented concurrently during the spatial attention task were stimuli in other, nonattended locations. The critical manipulation in each of these studies was to vary the attended location while holding the physical stimulation parameters constant. In this manner, the cortical areas selectively activated by spatial attention could be isolated by subtracting the images from each attention condition (i.e., attending to a particular spatial location) from a condition where the same stimuli were passively viewed. The results from these experiments indicated that spatial attention modulates processing in extrastriate cortex in a highly retinotopic pattern. As spatial attention was moved from location to location in the visual field, the cortical area selectively modulated by spatial attention moved in a systematic fashion through dorsomedial and ventral occipital cortex, including areas V2, V3, and V3a. Importantly, both Brefczynski and DeYoe and Tootell et al. showed that this retinotopic pattern of attention-driven activity directly matched the pattern of activity obtained in a control condition, where each spatial location was selectively stimulated without stimuli elsewhere in the visual field.

Control of Selection As reviewed above, neuropsychological data have implicated parietal, prefrontal, and subcortical structures in the control of spatial attention. In the following section, we first review the neuroimaging evidence that supports this view of the attentional network. We then look at a number of studies that have compared the operation of the spatial attention network with other forms of attentional orienting, in order to distinguish between those control operations which are unique to spatial attention and those operations which can be shared with other systems. Finally, we examine how knowledge of the neural structures involved in the orienting of spatial attention can lead to direct and testable predictions of cognitive-based theories.

THE ATTENTIONAL NETWORK In a seminal PET study, Corbetta et al. (1993) compared sensory-evoked cortical activations as a function of whether attention was shifting to nonfoveal locations in the visual field or remained focused on fixation. In the shifting attention condition, subjects made voluntary attentional movements to the left or right of fixation throughout the scanning period while engaged in a target detection task. In the fixation condition, subjects were required to detect the onset of a target at fixation while ignoring nonfoveal probe stimuli that matched the shifting attention condition in total peripheral stimulation. Corbetta et al. found activations in the superior parietal lobule (approximating BA 7) and superior frontal cortex (within BA 6) during the shifting attention condition, activations that were absent during the attention at fixation. That activity in both parietal and frontal regions was selective for movements of the attentional spotlight confirmed the findings from neuropsychological studies reviewed in the section "The Neural Correlates" (above).

However, comparing the parietal and frontal activations against a third condition —where subjects passively viewed the peripheral probes while maintaining gaze at fixation—revealed that the parietal and frontal areas were involved in different aspects of the attention movement. In this third condition, the peripheral stimulation due to the probes was assumed to cause involuntary *or reflexive* shifts of spatial attention (see Posner & Cohen, 1984), shifts that did not occur during the fixation condition because attention was actively maintained at fixation. As a result, while the parietal areas were active during both voluntary and reflexive attentional movements, the frontal areas were active only during the voluntary movements. Consistent with the lesion data reviewed above, Corbetta et al. (1993) concluded that the parietal activations reflected processes associated with attentional movements, while the frontal activations selectively reflected the top-down executive control of voluntary movement.

COMPARISONS WITH NONVISUOSPATIAL ATTENTION   Given that the results of Corbetta et al. (1993) confirm parietal and frontal involvement in the control of spatial attention, might either of these areas control other forms of selective attention as well, such as attention to visual motion or auditory space? A number of PET and fMRI studies have addressed this question by comparing activations associated with spatial attention against activations arising during other forms of selective attention, in both the visual and the nonvisual domains.

For example, Coull and Nobre (1998) used PET and fMRI measures to examine whether the same cortical systems are involved in orienting attention to visual space and orienting attention to discrete time intervals, such as when an event is expected to occur at a predictable moment in time. Subjects attended a central fixation point, where a cue was presented on each trial that indicated with .80 probability either the most likely location (left or right of fixation) of an impending target, the most likely time interval during which it would occur (300 or 1500 msec post cue), or the most likely location *and* time interval. The simple detection task required a rapid manual response to the onset of the nonfoveal target while maintaining gaze at fixation. Coull and Nobre found that both forms of attentional orienting produced frontal activations that included bilateral activation of the dorsolateral prefrontal cortex (BA 46).

However, whereas spatial attention selectively activated the *right* intraparietal sulcus, temporal orienting selectively activated the *left* intraparietal sulcus. Further, when both spatial and temporal attention were concurrent, bilateral activations were seen in the intraparietal sulcus. These results strongly suggest that while the frontal control mechanisms overlap between spatial and temporal orienting, the posterior cortical areas mediating these different forms of attentional orienting are domain-specific.

In another study, Nobre et al. (1997) used PET to compare the cortical network activated by the top-down *or voluntary* orienting of spatial attention with the cortical network activated when spatial attention is *reflexively* oriented to a nonfoveal location by the rapid onset of a peripheral visual stimulus. Subjects maintained fixation on a central diamond that was flanked by two peripheral squares, one in each visual hemifield, 7° to the left and right of fixation. In the reflexive attention condition, a brief brightening of one of the two boxes indicated with .80 probability that the impending target stimulus would occur in the flashed box. In the voluntary attention condition, the same box brightening indicated with .80 probability that the target would occur in the nonflashed box. The task required subjects to discriminate whether the target item was an " × " or a " + ." Interestingly, Nobre et al. found few differences in the cortical areas activated by the two visuospatial attention tasks—both produced activations that included bilateral premotor cortex in the frontal lobe—again suggesting a common frontal control mechanism for attentional orienting.

PARIETAL ACTIVATIONS AND THEORY TESTING   According to cognitive theory, serial searches of multielement displays involve successive movements of the attentional spotlight to the location of each display element, an iterative process that continues until the target item has been detected (e.g., Treisman & Gelade, 1980). As a result, if target detection time is plotted as a function of the number of elements in the display, detection time increases with display set size under conditions requiring serial searches. In contrast, conditions conducive to parallel visual searches, which yield a perceptual "pop-out" phenomenon for the target against the background of non-target elements, produce target detection times that remain constant as set size is increased. The assumption is that because the target perceptually pops out from the background elements, parallel visual searches do not require or induce any movements of the attentional spotlight.

Testing this prediction, Corbetta et al. (1995) used PET to examine cortical activations produced during conditions of serial versus parallel visual search. Based on the results of Corbetta et al. (1993), which showed that the superior parietal lobule is active during covert shifts of spatial attention, Corbetta et al. predicted that if attentional movements occur only during serial visual searches, parietal activations should be observed only in that condition. Subjects viewed moving, nonfoveal dots that were in all four visual quadrants, with the task requiring them to signal the presence within a subset of dots of a target color, a target speed of motion, or a target conjunction of color *and* speed of motion. Corbetta et al. found that when task conditions produced behavioral evidence of serial visual search (the conjunction condition), activations were found in the superior parietal lobule—activations that were absent under the other two conditions, which produced behavioral evidence of parallel visual search. These results thus provided direct neural evidence implicating the role of spatial attention in guiding the serial scanning of cluttered visual scenes.

Taking a similar approach, Culham et al. (1998) examined the role of spatial attention within the visual tracking system. Subjects were required to covertly track the motion of a subset of "bouncing balls" within a visual display. Comparing fMRI images taken during this tracking task with images obtained during passive viewing of the bouncing ball display revealed bilateral activations in both parietal and frontal cortex, and, albeit to a lesser degree, within motion-sensitive area MT as well. These activations were then compared against activations observed during a variant of the tracking task that was specifically designed to induce the shifting of visuospatial attention. This second comparison showed that both the tracking and the shifting attention tasks produced comparable parietal and frontal activations. Based on this similarity in activation patterns, Culham et al. concluded that attentional tracking engages the network of cortical areas involved in the control of spatial attention.

Consequences of Selection   A number of neuroimaging studies have shown that selective attention to different stimulus classes or attributes can lead to selective enhancement (or amplification) of neural activity in the specialized cortical areas where the attended attributes are processed (e.g., Haxby et al., 1994). For example, O'Craven et al. (1997) demonstrated that when subjects viewed a screen containing an overlapping mixture of moving and stationary dots, activity in motion-sensitive areas MT and MST was greater when subjects were selectively attending to the moving dots, in comparison to when subjects were selectively attending to the stationary dots. In relation to the functional consequences of *spatial* attention, the central question is whether these sorts of attentional effects on cortical processing can be selective for stimuli in attended spatial locations. Here we examine this issue in relation to two closely related phenomena that have been associated with the effects of spatial attention: sensory gain and perceptual salience.

INCREASED SENSORY GAIN   As discussed above, ERP evidence has led to the suggestion that spatial attention can act as a mechanism of sensory gain, where stimulus information arising in attended locations is perceptually enhanced and stimulus information arising in unattended locations is perceptually dampened (e.g., Luck, 1995; Mangun, 1995). However, based on data from both single-unit recordings in nonhuman primates and on human neuropsychology, it has also been suggested that when multiple objects are presented in the visual field, the object representations in cortex "compete" for access to the limited-capacity visual processing system (Desimone & Duncan, 1995). This competition between objects has been character-ized as a mutually suppressive interaction, such that each object representation sup-presses to a degree the processing of other, concurrent object representations. It now appears that these suppressive interactions may be closely linked to the sensory gain that is associated with spatial attention.

In particular, Kastner et al. (1998) used fMRI to examine the processing of unitary versus multiple visual stimuli, on the hypothesis that if stimuli engage in mutually suppressive interactions, greater activations should arise for a stimulus presented in isolation versus a stimulus presented with other stimuli. In the first experiment, sub-jects passively viewed stimuli in the upper right visual field quadrant under two con-ditions: when four stimuli were presented sequentially (i.e., one after the other) and when four stimuli were presented simultaneously. Consistent with their hypothesis, Kastner et al. found that weaker activations occurred in visuocortical areas V1, V2, VP, V4, and TEO under the simultaneous versus sequential stimulus conditions. Following this finding up in a second experiment, Kastner et al. repeated the design used in the first experiment while adding a second condition: varying whether or not spatial attention was covertly oriented to one of the stimulus locations. They found that, in comparison to when the stimuli were unattended, spatial attention led to a bigger increase in the fMRI signal in the simultaneous versus the sequential condition. These results strongly suggest that the sensory gain properties associated with spatial attention may be subserved, at least in part, by biasing the suppressive interactions between multiple stimuli such that the sensory signal associated with an attended stimulus will be enhanced relative to stimuli in unattended locations.

DECREASED PERCEPTUAL SALIENCE   Similar to the notion of sensory gain, several studies have examined the effects of spatial attention on the perceptual salience of stimuli in attended versus unattended visual field locations. In terms of neuroimaging, such studies have relied on the strength of PET or fMRI signals as an indicator of the degree to which a given stimulus is perceived—the weaker the hemodynamic signal, the less perceptually salient the stimulus. For example, Rees, Frith, et al. (1997) exam-ined the processing of nonfoveal moving stimuli as a function of the perceptual load of a task at fixation, on the assumption that spatial attention is withdrawn from non-foveal locations as the load of a foveal task increases (see Lavie & Tsal, 1994). In the low-load task, subjects discriminated whether or not single words presented at fixation were in uppercase letters, and in the high-load task they were instructed to discriminate the number of syllables in each word. Throughout each task condition, task-irrelevant moving stimuli were presented parafoveally. Importantly, Rees, Frith, et al. found that activation in motion-sensitive area MT was reduced in the high-load versus the low-load condition, suggesting that the withdrawal of spatial attention from parafoveal locations had reduced the perceptual salience of the moving stimuli.

In a similar study, Wojciulik et al. (1998) compared the processing of faces in the human fusiform face area (FFA) as a function of whether or not the facial stimuli were in an attended spatial location. Subjects viewed displays that had four stimuli presented in different parafoveal locations—two houses and two faces—and were required to discriminate (in different conditions) whether the faces or houses matched. As a result, while spatial attention was oriented to the locations of the faces in the face-matching condition, the faces were in unattended locations during the house-matching condition. Given this manipulation of spatial attention, Wojciulik et al. found that fMRI activations in bilateral FFA were larger when subjects were attending to the location of the faces versus the houses, suggesting that there was reduced perceptual salience of the faces when they were in unattended locations.

ISSUES

Current Issues: Combined Methodologies

As the above review indicates, PET and fMRI have been invaluable tools in examining the neural basis of selective spatial attention. However, like lesion and ERP methodologies, neuroimaging has its inherent limitations. The hemodynamic responses that form the basis of both PET and fMRI signals are on the order of hundreds of milliseconds at best (e.g., Kim et al., 1997), a time scale that is relatively sluggish when compared to the millisecond-level speed of neural processing. Compounding this concern, neuroimaging typically relies on scanning functional activity over several seconds at the shortest, further blurring the temporal resolution these measures allow. While coarse temporal resolution is a negligible concern for many important questions that have been—and can be—effectively addressed using hemodynamic measures, efforts are being made to offset this limitation by combining hemodynamic and electrophysiological measures within the same experimental paradigm.

The resulting "hybrid" studies can thus integrate the high spatial resolution of PET or fMRI with the high temporal resolution of ERPs, a strategy that can be used to address questions for which neither method would be appropriate alone. This approach has been particularly effective in spatial attention research, which has relied heavily on ERPs in relation to issues of site localization, and which can greatly benefit from using neuroimaging to improve the localization of attention-sensitive ERP generators in early visual cortex. We discuss combined paradigms by first introducing the theoretical issues guiding the design of such studies—issues that transcend attention research—and then by examining the specific ways in which these paradigms have been employed in the study of spatial attention.

Theoretical Framework   To properly correlate hemodynamic and electrophsyiological measures of neural activity, two primary issues must be taken into consideration: What are the experimental conditions under which each measure will be obtained, and how might function-related hemodynamic and electrophysiological activity mirror the same underlying processes—if at all—at the physiological level? While the answer to the former is under experimenter control, the latter remains a somewhat open question.

EXPERIMENTAL DESIGN   Mangun, Hopfinger, et al. (1998) presented a theoretical account of how the high spatial resolution of neuroimaging can be combined with the high temporal resolution of ERPs in order to provide a more complete account of cortical processing, relative to using either method in isolation. The combined approach advocated by Mangun, Hopfinger, et al. rests on a *frames of reference* logic, which details the necessary paradigm structures that must be in place in order to confidently correlate hemodynamic and electrophysiologically based measures of neural activity. Although this chapter focuses on the study of visual attention in relation to neuroimaging, the theoretical issues discussed here are applicable to all domains of perceptual, cognitive, and motor study that utilize neuroimaging techniques.

First, given that imaging and ERP recording do not take place at the same time, the combined study must have a common *sensory* reference frame, indicating that identical stimuli are used in each testing session. This will ensure that each measure of neural activity is obtained under the same sensory-evoked conditions. Second, to minimize issues of between-session variability, it is imperative to have a common *biological* reference frame, where the same subjects are used in all testing sessions. If this condition is not met, potential differences in the outcomes of the electrophsyiological and hemodynamic measures will be confounded with differences that may arise due to intersubject variation. Third, the study must have a common *experimental* frame of reference, where the comparisons of imaging and ERP data are based on the same conditions—for example, using the same subtraction conditions to isolate task-specific hemodynamic and electrophysiological activity. Finally, to maximize the likelihood of correlating the proper foci of hemodynamic and electrophysiological activity, the study requires an appropriate *spatial* frame of reference. This issue involves using dipole modeling of ERP scalp topography in order to establish an approximate cortical location of the ERP-generating dipole of interest—a location that should have a strong spatial correspondence with the foci of hemodynamic activity.

PHYSIOLOGICAL CORRELATES Although combining hemodynamic and electrophysiological measures can be a powerful tool for examining the neural substrates of cognition, one must carefully consider how electrical scalp recordings may relate to regional cerebral blood flow (rCBF). ERPs reflect electrical current generated by postsynaptic neural activity, whereas neuroimaging indexes changes in rCBF that are coupled to neural activity. Although incorporating appropriate frames of reference within a paradigm can minimize the likelihood of measuring qualitatively different neural activities, ERPs may nevertheless map onto rCBF in at least three different ways. Specifically, task-dependent ERP and rCBF measures may be reflections of the same underlying neural activity and its unitary function; they may manifest different functional aspects of neuronal activity, but in the same population of neurons; or they may reflect the activity of entirely different populations of neurons. Further, in relation to attentional manipulations, one must differentiate within each of these scenarios whether the measured responses reflect stimulus-evoked activity modulated by attention, or an attention-driven change in cortical excitability (or tonic state) that is not time-locked to any particular stimulus input (see, e.g., Rees, Frackowiak, et al., 1997). Most likely, each of these possibilities is equally viable, depending on the specific cognitive operations and neural structures under study (for a more detailed discussion, see Mangun, Hopfinger, et al., 1998).

Imaging and Electrophysiology Directly applying the theoretical structures outlined by Mangun, Hopfinger, et al. (1998), a number of spatial attention studies have adopted combined neuroimaging and electrophysiological paradigms. These efforts have taken two basic forms, with a focus on using either PET or fMRI to localize the visuocortical generators of electrophysiological activity, or using ERPs to help delineate the likely time course of processing events reflected in PET and fMRI images.

ERP LOCALIZATION In human-based studies of visuocortical processing, attention-related modulations in the P1 ERP component remain the primary evidence indicating the initial point in visual processing where attention can influence stimulus-evoked activity (see above). In order to precisely localize the cortical generator of the P1 ERP component, which has a maximal scalp distribution overlying lateral occipital cortex, Heinze et al. (1994) integrated PET and ERP measures within the same experimental paradigm. Specifically, they had each subject perform the same task—symbol matching—in separate PET and ERP testing sessions. While subjects maintained gaze on a central fixation point, letterlike symbols were presented bilaterally in a rapid and random sequence, with two symbols in the upper left visual field quadrant and two symbols in the upper right quadrant. The subjects were instructed to attend exclusively to either the left or the right visual field, and to make a rapid, manual response whenever the two symbols in the attended visual field matched.

When comparing PET images of the attention conditions against images taken during passive viewing of the stimuli, Heinze et al. (1994) found that attending to either the left or the right visual field produced significant activation in contralateral fusiform gyrus. Critically, making this same comparison in the ERP data revealed attention-related modulations of the contralateral P1 ERP component (see color plate 2, figure 4.2A). In order to ensure that these data patterns were not an artifact of comparing passive and active task conditions, Heinze et al. subtracted the attend-right condition from the attend-left condition in both the PET and the ERP data, which revealed data patterns parallel to the initial subtractions (figure 4.2B). The focus of the PET activation in the fusiform gyrus was then used to help model the scalp topography of the P1 data shown in figure 4.2B, with the PET data serving to constrain the anatomical location of the P1-generating dipole. Two different dipole modeling conditions were used: a "seeded forward" solution, where the location of the dipole was held constant but the orientation (relative to the scalp surface) was allowed to vary in order to minimize the difference between predicted and recorded P1 topography, and a "best fit" inverse solution, where both the orientation and the location of the dipole were allowed to vary (figure 4.2C). Importantly, when examining the amount of variance accounted for by the modeled dipole source, the seeded solution—which kept the dipole located in the center of the fusiform PET activations—accounted for 96.2% of the variance within the 110–130 msec time window of the P1. Allowing the dipole to move from the fusiform location in the "best fit" solution improved the amount of variance accounted for by only 2.2% (figure 4.3).

The results of Heinze et al. (1994), which suggest that the P1 is generated in extrastriate cortex, have now been extended in two important ways. First, Heinze et al. used upper visual field stimuli, which produced activations in ventral occipital cortex below the calcarine fissure. Given the retinotopic organization of early visual cortex, Woldorff et al. (1997) predicted that if the P1 is generated in extrastriate cortex, activations should be observed in dorsal occipital cortex if *lower* visual field stimuli were used instead. Bilateral stimuli were presented in the lower visual field in a rapid sequence, and PET and ERP measures were recorded (in separate sessions) as subjects selectively attended to stimuli on the left or the right. Consistent with their prediction, Woldorff et al. found a focus of activation in dorsal occipital cortex that was contralateral to the attended visual field. During iterative dipole modeling, the best fit for the ERP data occurred when the dipole was located in this dorsal area, above the cal-

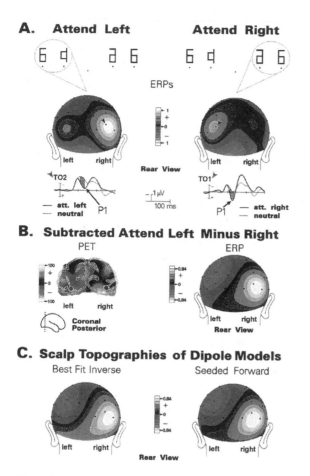

Figure 4.2
Comparing PET and ERP attention effects from the combined study of Heinze et al. (1994). (*A*) Topographic isovoltage maps showing the lateral occipital focus of the P1 attention effect for both attend-left minus passive and attend-right minus passive conditions. The corresponding ERP waveforms, showing the associated attention effects, are below each map, along with the time window of the shown scalp topography (shaded). (*B*) The attend-left minus attend-right ERP data are shown on the right, and a coronal section through the posterior occipital region in the PET data is shown on the left, for the same subtraction condition as the ERP data. The PET data reveal foci of activations in both the left and right fusiform gyrus (indicated by the dots), although the left activation appears as a decrease due to the subtraction condition. These data show that the attention effects in the PET and ERP data have similar spatial frames of reference. (*C*) Two different scalp topographies obtained using dipole modeling procedures. In the "seeded forward" solution (right) the dipole was held constant in the center of the fusiform PET activation, whereas in the "best fit" solution (left) the dipole was allowed to vary in position. The comparison demonstrates that the PET fusiform activation provides a good predictor of the actual dipole location. (Reprinted with permission from *Nature*, copyright 1994, Macmillan Magazines, Ltd.) (See color plate 2.)

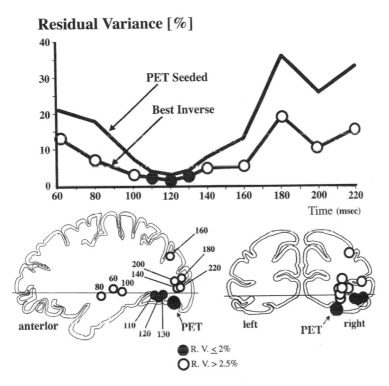

Figure 4.3
Comparing the amount of residual variance (RV) accounted for in modeling the scalp topography of the ERP data, as a function of the seeded and best-fit solutions, across 20 msec time windows. Lower values of RV indicate a closer correspondence between ERP attention effects and the modeled data. (*Top*) RV is minimized in both solutions in the 110–130 msec time window associated with the P1 attention effect (see figure 4.2). (*Bottom*) The location of the "best fit" dipole solution most closely converges with the location of the fusiform PET activation (black circles) during the time window of the P1 attention effect (shaded circles), shown in both saggital (left) and coronal (right) slices. The figure shows a Talairach section through the fusiform gyrus. (Reprinted with permission from *Nature*, copyright 1994, Macmillan Magazines, Ltd.)

carine fissure. Second, Mangun, Bounocore, et al. (1998) have shown, using fMRI and ERP measures, that the prior group-averaged data patterns reported by Heinze et al. and Woldorff et al. are consistent within individual subjects, where on an individual basis attentional modulations of the P1 were found to co-occur with enhanced contralateral activations in the posterior fusiform and middle occipital gyri.

STEADY-STATE VISUAL EVOKED POTENTIALS   Another measure of electrophysiological activity is the steady-state visual evoked potential (SSVEP), a surface-recorded electrical potential that is elicited in response to an oscillating and continuously present visual stimulus, such as a flickering light. The waveform of the SSVEP is typically sinusoidal, and takes on the fundamental frequency of the oscillating stimulus. Like the P1 ERP component, the amplitude of the SSVEP can be modulated by spatial attention, with the amplitude being larger when the evoking stimulus is an attended versus an unattended visual field location (e.g., Morgan et al., 1996). To localize the cortical generator of the SSVEP, Hillyard et al. (1997) recorded fMRI and SSVEP measures in separate sessions as subjects attended to letter sequences in either the left or the right visual field. Importantly, the letters in each visual field were superimposed over square backgrounds that were flickering at either 12 Hz (in the left visual field) or 8.6 Hz (in the right visual field). This difference in flickering rate between locations produced SSVEPs with a unique fundamental frequency for each location, allowing Hillyard et al. to compare the amplitudes of the SSVEPs as a function of both attention and location. Consistent with Morgan et al., the amplitudes of the SSVEPs were larger when the evoking stimuli were attended. When dipole modeling was used to examine the scalp topography of the attention-related modulations of the SSVEPs, the best-fit dipole locations coincided with foci of fMRI activations that were found in ventrolateral occipital cortex. Taken with the above data from combined imaging and ERP studies, the results of Hillyard et al. lend further support to the position that spatial attention first modulates afferent visual processing in extrastriate cortex.

ATTENTION AND STRIATE MODULATION   Although combined neuroimaging and ERP methods have strongly suggested that spatial attention can selectively modulate sensory-evoked processing in extrastriate cortex, neuroimaging studies of spatial attention have found attention-related activations in primary visual cortex (e.g., Watanabe et al., 1998). Such findings are at odds with the data from ERP studies, which have failed to show attention-related modulations in the C1 ERP component, a component that has been localized—based on electrophysiological evidence alone —to primary *or striate* visual cortex (e.g., Clark et al., 1995; Clark & Hillyard, 1996; Gomez Gonzalez et al., 1994; Mangun et al., 1993). One hypothesis for these apparently contradictory findings has been that whether or not attentional effects are seen in striate cortex may depend on the type of visual display used. Whereas both neuroimaging in humans (e.g., Schneider et al., 1995) and single-unit studies in nonhuman primates (e.g., Motter, 1993) have shown attention-related modulations in striate cortex under conditions of cluttered or multielement visual scenes, the ERP studies showing no comparable modulations in the C1 have used single-element displays. This discrepancy suggests that spatial attention may affect striate processing, but only when the subject must selectively isolate a target from a background of nontarget distractor elements.

This hypothesis was examined in a combined fMRI and ERP study by Martinez et al. (1999). In separate fMRI and ERP sessions, they had subjects discriminate unilateral stimuli that were randomly flashed to the left and right of fixation, and that were surrounded by an array of task-irrelevant distractors such that the visual field was "cluttered." Under these conditions, Martinez et al. found fMRI activations in both striate (i.e., the calcarine fissure) and extrastriate visual cortex, a data pattern consistent with Schneider et al. and Tootell et al. (1998). However, attention-related modulations were found only in the P1 ERP component—the C1 showed no such comparable effect. Following analytic procedures comparable to those of Heinze et al. (1994; see above), Martinez et al. localized the C1 generator to the site of the calcarine activation. These results thus strongly suggest that while attention may be capable of modulating stimulus processing in striate cortex, these effects may be the result of later, reafferent input from higher cortical areas that follows the initial, sensory-evoked response indexed by the C1.

SYSTEMATIC COVARIATION   One final approach for combining imaging and electrophysiological measures relies on making parametric variations in a given cognitive operation, and then correlating this manipulation with quantitative changes in signal strength in each dependent measure. This method rests on the assumption that cognitive operations have an "intensity vector" (i.e., they can be engaged in graded amounts; see Just & Carpenter, 1992), and that a change in processing intensity or *load* for a given operation will produce a quantitative change in activation level at the neural locus (or loci) where the operation is implemented (e.g., Handy, in press). For example, the cortical areas mediating working memory have been identified in neuroimaging studies by showing a positive relationship between activation level and memory load, where load was manipulated by varying the number of digits that subjects were required to hold in storage (e.g., Jonides et al., 1997; Manoach et al., 1997).

Applying parametric load manipulations to combined neuroimaging and ERP paradigms, if both measures reflect the same underlying neural and computational processes, then the measures should covary positively as a systematic change is made in processing load. Using this logic, Mangun et al. (1997) replicated the basic symbol-matching experiment performed by Heinze et al. (1994), but varied the perceptual load of the task. In the high-load condition, the stimuli and task were identical to Heinze et al., as described above. However, in the low-load condition a small but visually salient dot was added to a small percentage of the symbols, and the subjects' task was to detect any symbols with dots in the attended visual field. Although an attention effect was found in the P1 ERP component in both load conditions, there was an interaction between attention and load as well, indicating that the attention effects were greater in the P1 in the high-load condition. Importantly, the PET images showed load-related increases in signal intensity in both the posterior fusiform and

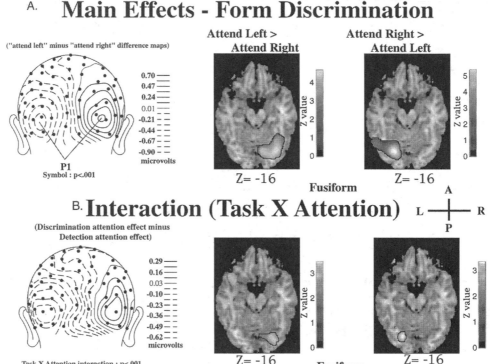

Figure 4.4
The PET and ERP data from the covariation study by Mangun et al. (1997). (*A*) On the left is the topographic isovoltage map of the P1 attention effect, in an attend-left minus attend-right subtraction that reveals the lateral occipital locus of the P1 generators in each hemisphere. On the right are the PET data showing similar activations in the fusiform gyrus, under the same stimulus and subtraction conditions as the ERP data. (*B*) The significant interaction between attention and load in both the ERP (left) and the PET (right) data, showing that the interaction in the fusiform gyrus is consistent with the scalp topography of the interaction in the P1.

the middle occipital gyri (figure 4.4), providing strong converging evidence with prior combined imaging and ERP data suggesting that the P1 is generated in extrastriate cortex (e.g., Heinze et al., 1994; Woldorff et al., 1997).

Future Issues: Selection and Multivariate Activations

So far, discussion has focused primarily on qualitative issues of *what happens where* in relation to the site and source of spatial attention effects in visual processing. However, the data reported by Mangun et al. (1997), which show covariations in PET and ERP measures as a function of perceptual load, demonstrate that function-related neural behavior has important *quantitative* properties as well. Indeed, it has been argued that the answers to qualitative questions of neural function directly depend on the quantitative properties of the given task parameters (Carpenter et al., 1999)—if a cognitive operation of interest is not sufficiently engaged by the task a subject is performing, neuroimaging may fail to reveal any significant activation clusters associated with that cognitive operation. In closing, we address two central questions regarding the quantitative relationship between processing load and neural activation: What theoretical principles link parametric variations in cognitive states to quantitative changes in neural activity, and what implications do these principles have for the imaging of cortical function? The answers to these questions lie in understanding the role selective attention can play in describing and predicting the complex patterns of multivariate neural activity typically observed in functional neuroimaging studies. Below we first briefly review the general model of selective attention that applies to the relationship between load and neural activation—attentional resource theory— and then we detail the specific implications that arise from applying resource theory to neuroimaging data.

Attentional Resources Borrowing terms germane to economics, capacity theories of selective attention have likened attention to a limited-capacity resource that is in demand during cognitive processing (for reviews, see Kramer & Spinks, 1991; Näätänen, 1992). The concept of processing load—which can take various operational forms, such as perceptual or memory load—directly follows from this resource view of attention. The load a task places on a given cognitive stage is positively correlated with the task-related demand for attentional resources at that stage (e.g., Lavie & Tsal, 1994). In turn, both imaging and ERP studies have shown that activation levels in discrete cortical processing areas increase with the load a task places on the cognitive operations performed in those loci (e.g., Alho et al., 1992; Carpenter et al., 1999; Handy & Mangun, 2000; Jonides et al., 1997; Mangun et al., 1997; Manoach et al., 1997). These results suggest that, as argued by Just and Carpenter (1992), attentional resources at the cognitive level can be correlated with activation intensity at the neural level (see also Posner & Dehaene, 1994; Posner & Driver, 1992). However, selection implies a limited capacity to perform cognitive operations, and from a resource perspective, these capacity limits are incorporated into the general model by assuming that there is a fixed amount *or pool* of attentional resources upon which cognitive processes can draw. As one operation consumes a greater amount of resources in response to an increase in load, there will be fewer residual resources available for allocation to other ongoing operations.

Implications The implications of applying attentional resource theory to the analysis of neuroimaging data stem from considering how multivariate neural activity may relate to the concept of resource pools. In dual task situations, the level of performance on a primary task is gauged as a function of performance on a secondary task (e.g., Navon & Gopher, 1980; Pashler, 1993). If both tasks share a common resource pool, and the primary task demands sufficient resources such that resource demand exceeds available supply for the secondary task, performance on the secondary task will be relatively degraded in direct proportion to the size of the resource deficit. Applying these concepts to the function-related activity of two neural loci, the activation level at one locus can be compared against changes in intensity at the second locus as a function of load. If the two loci subserve different cognitive operations but share a common resource pool, increasing the resource demand at one locus will increase activation at that locus, and reduce activation in the second locus due to the drop in resource availability. That is, the two loci will manifest a negative covariance in response to the load manipulation. For example, Rees et al. (1997) showed decreased fMRI activations in motion-sensitive cortical area V5 with increases in linguistic load (see above). From a trade-off perspective, the effect on V5 may have been the result of an increase in resource allocation to linguistic processing areas, on the assumption that motion and linguistic processing draw on a common resource pool.

This "trade-off" relationship applies to distributed neural systems as well. As used here, a "distributed neural system" refers to an elementary cognitive operation that is implemented at the neural level across multiple, discrete loci. For example, a study of visual working memory showed functional dissociations between a group of activations in occipitotemporal cortex that were correlated with the initial perceptual encoding of information, and a group of activations in prefrontal cortex that were correlated with the maintenance of that information in memory (Courtney et al., 1997). While this *functional integration* across multiple neural loci is presumably supported at the neuroanatomical level by relatively dense intrinsic connections between integrated loci (e.g., Friston, 1998), at the functional level these loci should manifest comparable task-dependent activation profiles. As a result, if the load on a given cognitive stage is varied, the distributed neural loci implementing this stage should show a strong *positive* activation covariance (e.g., Carpenter et al., 1999).

However, manipulations of processing load may also lead to *negative* covariances. As discussed above, negative covariance is indicative of a trade-off in resource allocation between two functionally *segregated* loci, and these principles apply to distributed neural systems as well. For example, Raichle (2000) has identified two neural regions—the posterior cingulate cortex and adjacent precuneus—that are most metabolically active when the brain is in a resting state. Interestingly, these areas decrease in activity if subjects are performing a novel task, but maintain relatively high activation levels if subjects are performing a familiar task. Raichle suggested that this dynamic pattern of activity reflects an activation trade-off between different distributed neural systems; the system associated with activity in the posterior cingulate and adjacent precuneus becomes active only when other systems are not placing a demand on limited "brain" resources. Similar evidence has been found in other meta-analyses of imaging data, where changes in various task parameters (e.g., from passive to active viewing of stimuli) have been shown to produce systematic activations *and* deactivations in different neural structures (e.g., Petersen et al., 1998; Shulman et al., 1997). From the processing load perspective, as one distributed system draws resources away from a second, the loci in the different distributed systems should manifest negative activation covariance, while the loci within each system should manifest positive covariance.

While selective attention theory provides a viable framework for making direct and testable predictions regarding the functional relationships between multiple neural processing loci, data from neuroimaging may also provide crucial means by which to advance extant cognitive theory. In particular, one of the central debates in attentional resource theory has been over whether there is a single, unitary pool of attentional resources upon which all cognitive operations must draw, or whether multiple resource pools exist, such that not all operations utilize the same resource pool (e.g., Pashler & Johnston, 1998; Shah & Miyake, 1996). One argument in favor of the multiple resource view has been that operations implemented in different cortical regions (e.g., the left and right hemispheres) may rely on different resource pools (e.g., Boles & Law, 1998; Polson & Friedman, 1988; Wickens, 1992). If multiple resource pools exist, orthogonal cognitive processes utilizing different resource pools would be expected to show no trade-offs in activation levels—in the neural loci where those operations are implemented—as the load on one process is varied (figure 4.5). If found, such evidence from neuroimaging would lend strong support to the multiple resource view.

Conclusions   Hemodynamic neuroimaging has provided researchers with an invaluable tool for studying the neural correlates of cognitive processing, and here we have reviewed how these techniques have been used to detail the cortical and subcortical structures involved in selective visuospatial attention. However, research in selective attention has produced several important advances for imaging neuroscience as well. First, neuroimaging represents an approach that directly complements other investigative methodologies, and the study of spatial attention has given rise to effective paradigms for integrating PET and fMRI with electrophysiological measures of cortical function. These resulting "combined" paradigms have been developed so that the relative weakness of hemodynamic neuroimages—low temporal resolution—is offset by the high temporal resolution of ERPs. Second, it has been argued that to advance

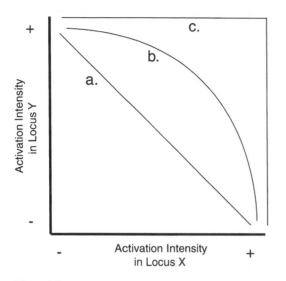

Figure 4.5
Three idealized curves representing the potential trade-offs in activation levels that may arise between two different neural loci as processing load is manipulated. (*a*) The two loci show a perfect trade-off; as the given task increases activation in locus X, activation decreases in equal proportion in locus Y. (*b*) The two loci show a less than 1 : 1 trade-off in activation. (*c*) The two loci show no trade-off in activation levels; a load-mediated change in activation in one locus has no effect on activation in the other locus. In terms of resource pools, the relationships in a and b suggest whole (a) or partial (b) sharing of resources between two loci, whereas c suggests that the processing operations implemented in the two loci draw on separate resource pools. The principles embodied in this graph would also apply to distributed neural systems, where each axis would represent the group of neural loci where a given function is implemented.

our understanding of mind–brain relations, we need to move beyond making topographic maps of human brain function to uncovering the emergent properties underlying multivariate neural behavior (Friston, 1998). Central to this process will be the incorporation of attentional resource theory as a means by which to predict and describe such multivariate activity.

For example, cortical areas mediating a common cognitive operation should be expected to covary positively (in terms of activation intensity) with a parametric variation in that operation, while cortical areas mediating different operations—but sharing a common resource pool—should be expected to covary negatively. Likewise, Friston (1997: 213) has proposed the hypothesis that within distributed neural systems, functional integration is subserved by *neural transients*, defined as "the mutual expression and induction of reproducible, stereotyped spatiotemporal patterns of activity that endure over extended periods of time." Taken within a processing load framework, does the induction and maintenance of neural transients require the consumption of attentional resources, and if so, does this limit the induction and maintenance of other, concurrent transient states? These represent the next generation of questions to be addressed by imaging neuroscience, and the tenets of selective attention theory will likely be integral in the search for definitive answers.

ACKNOWLEDGMENTS

We would like to thank the many individuals whose work contributed to the content of this chapter. We are grateful to Hajo Heinze, Steve Hillyard, Massimo Girelli, Amishi Jha, Wayne Khoe, Maryam Soltani, Erinrose Matheney, Alan Kingstone, Ray Klein, Steve Luck, and Michael Gazzaniga for numerous helpful discussions of the issues and topics presented here.

REFERENCES

Alho, K., Woods, D. L., Algazi, A., & Näätänen, R. (1992). Intermodal selective attention. II. Effects of attentional load on processing of auditory and visual stimuli in central space. *Electroencephalography and Clinical Neurophysiology* 82, 356–368.

Anllo-Vento, L., & Hillyard, S. A. (1996). Selective attention to the color and direction of moving stimuli: Electrophysiological correlates of hierarchical feature selection. *Perception & Psychophysics* 58, 191–206.

Baynes, K., Holtzman, J. D., & Volpe, B. T. (1986). Components of visual attention: Alterations in response pattern to visual stimuli following parietal lobe infarction. *Brain* 109, 99 114.

Boles, D. B., & Law, M. B. (1998). A simultaneous task comparison of differentiated and undifferentiated hemispheric resource theories. *Journal of Experimental Psychology: Human Perception and Performance* 24, 204–215.

Brefczynski, J. A., & DeYoe, E. A. (1999). A physiological correlate of the "spotlight" of visual attention. *Nature Neuroscience* 2, 370–374.

Carpenter, P. A., Just, M. A., Keller, T. A., Eddy, W., & Thulborn, K. (1999). Graded functional activation in the visuospatial system with the amount of task demand. *Journal of Cognitive Neuroscience* 11, 9–24.

Clark, V. P., Fan, S., & Hillyard, S. A. (1995). Identification of early visual evoked potential generators by retinotopic and topographic analyses. *Human Brain Mapping* 2, 170–187.

Clark, V. P., & Hillyard, S. A. (1996). Spatial selective attention affects early extrastriate but not striate components of the visual evoked potential. *Journal of Cognitive Neuroscience* 8, 387–402.

Corbetta, M. (1998). Frontoparietal cortical networks for directing attention and the eye to visual locations: Identical, independent, or overlapping neural systems? *Proceedings of the National Academy of Sciences USA* 15, 831–838.

Corbetta, M., Miezin, F. M., Shulman, G. L., & Petersen, S. E. (1993). A PET study of visuospatial attention. *Journal of Neuroscience* 13, 1202–1226.

Corbetta, M., Shulman, G. L., Miezin, F. M., & Petersen, S. E. (1995). Superior parietal cortex activation during spatial attention shifts and visual feature conjunction. *Science* 270, 802–805.

Coull, J. T., & Nobre, A. C. (1998). Where and when to pay attention: The neural systems for directing attention to spatial locations and to the time intervals as revealed by both PET and fMRI. *Journal of Neuroscience* 18, 7426–7435.

Culham, J. C., Brandt, S. A., Cavanagh, P., Kanwisher, N. G., Dale, A. M., & Tootell, R. B. H. (1998). Cortical fMRI activation produced by attentive tracking of moving targets. *Journal of Neurophysiology* 80, 2657–2670.

Desimone, R., & Duncan, J. (1995). Neural mechanisms of selective visual attention. *Annual Review of Neuroscience* 18, 193–222.

Downing, C. J. (1988). Expectancy and visuo-spatial attention: Effects on perceptual quality. *Journal of Experimental Psychology: Human Perception and Performance* 13, 228–241.

Driver, J. (1996). Attention and segmentation. *The Psychologist* 9, 119–123.

Driver, J. (1998). The neuropsychology of spatial attention. In *Attention*, H. Pashler, ed., 297–340. Hove, UK: Psychology Press.

Eason, R. G. (1981). Visual evoked potential correlates of early neural filtering during selective attention. *Bulletin of the Psychonomic Society* 18, 203–206.

Egly, R., Driver, J., & Rafal, R. D. (1994). Shifting visual attention between objects and locations: Evidence from normal and parietal lesion patients. *Journal of Experimental Psychology: General* 123, 161–177.

Eimer, M. (1995). Event-related potential correlates of transient attention shifts to color and location. *Biological Psychology* 41, 167–182.

Eriksen, C. W., & Hoffman, J. E. (1972). Temporal and spatial characteristics of selective encoding from visual displays. *Perception & Psychophysics* 12, 201–204.

Eriksen, C. W., & St. James, J. D. (1986). Visual attention within and around the field of focal attention: A zoom lens model. *Perception & Psychophysics* 40, 225–240.

Eriksen, C. W., & Yeh, Y.-Y. (1985). Allocation of attention in the visual field. *Journal of Experimental Psychology: Human Perception and Performance* 11, 583–597.

Folk, C. L., Remington, R. W., & Wright, J. H. (1994). The structure of attentional control: Contingent attentional capture by apparent motion, abrupt onset, and color. *Journal of Experimental Psychology: Human Perception and Performance* 20, 317–329.

Friston, K. J. (1997). Another neural code? *NeuroImage* 5, 213–220.

Friston, K. J. (1998). Imaging neuroscience: Principles or maps? *Proceedings of the National Academy of Sciences USA* 95, 796–802.

Gomez Gonzalez, C. M., Clark, V. P., Fan, S., Luck, S. J., & Hillyard, S. A. (1994). Sources of attention-sensitive visual event-related potentials. *Brain Topography* 7, 41–51.

Green, V., Handy, T. C., Klein, R., & Mangun, G. R. (1998). The neural locus of attentional spotlight masking. *Abstracts of the Cognitive Neuroscience Society*, 1998 Program, 135.

Handy, T. C. (in press). Capacity theory as a model of cortical behavior. *Journal of Cognitive Neuroscience*.

Handy, T. C., Kingstone, A., & Mangun, G. R. (1996). Spatial distribution of visual attention: Perceptual sensitivity and response latency. *Perception & Psychophysics* 58, 613–627.

Handy, T. C., & Mangun, G. R. (2000). Attention and spatial selection: Electrophysiological evidence for modulation by perceptual load. *Perception & Psychophysics* 62, 175–186.

Hawkins, H. L., Hillyard, S. A., Luck, S. J., Mouloua, M., Downing, C. J., & Woodward, D. P. (1990). Visual attention modulates signal detectability. *Journal of Experimental Psychology: Human Perception and Performance* 16, 802–811.

Haxby, J. V., Horwitz, B., Ungerleider, L. G., Maisog, J. M., Pietrini, P., & Grady, C. L. (1994). The functional organization of human extrastriate cortex: A PET-rCBF study of selective attention to faces and locations. *Journal of Neuroscience* 14, 6336–6353.

Heinze, H. J., Mangun, G. R., Burchert, W., Hinrichs, H., Scholz, M., Münte, T. F., Gös, A., Scherg, M., Johannes, S., Hundeshagen, H., Gazzaniga, M. S., & Hillyard, S. A. (1994). Combined spatial and temporal imaging of brain activity during visual selective attention in humans. *Nature* 372, 543–546.

Hillyard, S. A., Hinrichs, H., Templemann, C., Morgan, S. T., Hansen, J. C., Scheich, H., & Heinze, H. J. (1997). Combining steady-state visual evoked potentials and fMRI to localize brain activity during selective attention. *Human Brain Mapping* 5, 287–292.

Hillyard, S. A., & Münte, T. F. (1984). Selective attention to color and location: An analysis with event-related potentials. *Perception & Psychophysics* 36, 185–198.

Hillyard, S. A., & Picton, T. W. (1987). Electrophysiology of cognition. In *Handbook of Physiology: The Nervous System*, F. Plum, cd., vol. 5, 519–584. Baltimore: Waverly Press.

Hillyard, S. A., Vogel, E. K., & Luck, S. J. (1998). Sensory gain control (amplification) as a mechanism of selective attention: Electrophysiological and neuroimaging evidence. *Philosophical Transactions of the Royal Society of London* B353, 1–14.

James, W. (1950). *The Principles of Psychology.* New York: Dover.

Jha, A. P., Buonocore, M., Girelli, M., & Mangun, G. R. (1997). fMRI and ERP studies of the organization of spatial selective attention in human extrastriate visual cortex. *Abstracts of the Society for Neuroscience* 23, 301.

Johnston, J. C., McCann, R. S., & Remington, R. W. (1995). Chronometric evidence for two types of attention. *Psychological Science* 6, 365–369.

Johnston, J. C., McCann, R. S., & Remington, R. W. (1996). Selective attention operates at two processing loci. In *Converging Operations in the Study of Visual Selective Attention*, A. F. Kramer, M. G. H. Coles, & G. D. Logan, eds. Washington, DC: American Psychological Association.

Jonides, J., Schumacher, E. H., Smith, E. E., Lauber, E. J., Awh, E., Minoshima, S., & Koeppe, R. A. (1997). Verbal working memory load affects regional brain activation as measured by PET. *Journal of Cognitive Neuroscience* 9, 462–475.

Just, M. A., & Carpenter, P. A. (1992). A capacity theory of comprehension: Individual differences in working memory. *Psychological Review* 99, 122–149.

Kastner, S., De Weerd, P., Desimone, R., & Ungerleider, L. G. (1998). Mechansims of directed attention in the human extrastriate cortex as revealed by functional MRI. *Science* 282, 108–111.

Kim, S. G., Richter, W., & Ugurbil, K. (1997). Limitations of temporal resolution in functional MRI. *Magnetic Resonance in Medicine* 37, 631–636.

Klein, R., Kingstone, A., & Pontefract, A. (1992). Orienting of visual attention. In *Eye Movements and Visual Cognition: Scene Perception and Reading*, K. Rayner, ed., 46–65. New York: Springer-Verlag.

Knight, R. T. (1997). Distributed cortical network for visual stimulus detection. *Journal of Cognitive Neuroscience* 9, 75–91.

Knight, R. T., Staines, W. R., Swick, D., & Chao, L. L. (in press). *Acta Psychologica.*

Kramer, A. F., & Hahn, S. (1995). Splitting the beam: Distribution of attention over noncontiguous regions of the visual field. *Psychological Science* 6, 381–386.

Kramer, A. F., & Spinks, J. (1991). Capacity views of human information processing. In *Handbook of Cognitive Psychophysiology: Central and Autonomic Nervous System Approaches*, J. R. Jennings & M. G. H. Coles, eds. New York: Wiley.

LaBerge, D. (1995). Computational and anatomical models of selective attention in object identification. In *The Cognitive Neurosciences*, M. S. Gazzaniga, ed., 649–663. Cambridge, MA: MIT Press.

Lavie, N., & Tsal, Y. (1994). Perceptual load as a major determinant of the locus of selection in visual attention. *Perception & Psychophysics* 56, 183–197.

Luck, S. J. (1995). Multiple mechanisms of visual-spatial attention: Recent evidence from human electrophysiology. *Behavioural Brain Research* 71, 113–123.

Mangun, G. R. (1995). Neural mechanisms of visual selective attention. *Psychophysiology* 32, 4–18.

Mangun, G. R., Buonocore, M. H., Girelli, M., & Jha, A. P. (1998). ERP and fMRI measures of visual spatial selective attention. *Human Brain Mapping* 6, 383–389.

Mangun, G. R., Hansen, J. C., & Hillyard, S. A. (1987). The spatial orienting of attention: Sensory facilitation or response bias? In *Current Trends in Event-Related Potential Research* (*EEG* suppl. 40), R. Johnson, Jr., J. W. Rohrbaugh, and R. Parasuraman, eds. Amsterdam: Elsevier.

Mangun, G. R., & Hillyard, S. A. (1991). Modulation of sensory-evoked brain potentials provides evidence for changes in perceptual processing during visual-spatial priming. *Journal of Experimental Psychology: Human Perception and Performance* 17, 1057–1074.

Mangun, G. R., & Hillyard, S. A. (1995). Mechanisms and models of selective attention. In *Electrophysiology of Mind: Event-Related Brain Potentials and Cognition*, M. D. Rugg & M. G. H. Coles, eds., 40–85. New York: Oxford University Press.

Mangun, G. R., Hillyard, S. A., & Luck, S. J. (1993). Electrocortical substrates of visual selective attention. In *Attention and Performance XIV*, D. E. Meyer and S. Kornblum, eds., 219–243. Cambridge, MA: MIT Press.

Mangun, G. R., Hopfinger, J. B., & Heinze, H. J. (1998). Integrating electrophysiology and neuroimaging in the study of human cognition. *Behavior Research Methods, Instruments, & Computers* 30, 118–130.

Mangun, G. R., Hopfinger, J. B., Kussmaul, C. L., Fletcher, E., & Heinze, H. J. (1997). Covariations in ERP and PET measures of spatial selective attention in human extrastriate visual cortex. *Human Brain Mapping* 5, 273–279.

Manoach, D. S., Schlaug, G., Siewert, B., Darby, D. G., Bly, B. M., Benfield, A., Edelman, R. R., & Warach, S. (1997). Prefrontal cortex fMRI signal changes are correlated with working memory load. *NeuroReport* 8, 545–549.

Martinez, A., Anllo-Vento, L., Sereno, M. I., Frank, L. R., Buxton, R. B., Dubowitz, D. J., Wong, E. C., Hinrichs, H., Heinze, H. J., & Hillyard, S. A. (1999). Involvement of striate and extrastriate visual cortical areas in spatial attention. *Nature Neuroscience* 2, 364–369.

Mesulam, M. M. (1981). A cortical network for directed attention and unilateral neglect. *Annals of Neurology* 10, 309–325.

Morgan, S. T., Hansen, J. C., & Hillyard, S. A. (1996). Selective attention to stimulus location modulates the steady-state visual evoked potential. *Proceedings of the National Academy of Sciences USA* 93, 4770–4774.

Morrow, L. A., & Ratcliff, G. (1988). The disengagement of covert attention and the neglect syndrome. *Psychobiology* 16, 261–269.

Motter, B. C. (1993). Focal attention produces spatially selective processing in visual cortical areas V1, V2, and V4 in the presence of competing stimuli. *Journal of Neurophysiology* 70, 909–919.

Müller, H. J., & Humphreys, G. W. (1991). Luminance-increment detection: Capacity-limited or not? *Journal of Experimental Psychology: Human Perception and Performance* 17, 107–124.

Näätänen, R. (1992). *Attention and Brain Function.* Hillsdale, NJ: Erlbaum.

Navon, D., & Gopher, D. (1980). Task difficulty, resources, and dual-task performance. In *Attention and Performance VIII*, R. S. Nickerson, ed. Hillsdale, NJ: Erlbaum.

Nobre, A. C., Sebestyen, G. N., Gitelman, D. R., Mesulam, M. M., Frackowiak, R. S. J., & Frith, C. D. (1997). Functional localization of the system for visuospatial attention using positron emission tomography. *Brain* 120, 515–533.

O'Craven, K. M., Rosen, B. R., Kwong, K. K., Treisman, A., & Savoy, R. L. (1997). Voluntary attention modulates fMRI activity in human MT-MST. *Neuron* 18, 591–598.

Pashler, H. (1993). Dual-task interference and elementary mental mechanisms. In *Attention and Performance XIV*, D. Meyer and S. Kornblum, eds., 245–264. Cambridge, MA: MIT Press.

Pashler, H. E. (1998). *The Psychology of Attention.* Cambridge, MA: MIT Press.

Pashler, H., & Johnston, J. C. (1998). Attentional limitations in dual-task performance. In *Attention*, H. Pashler, ed. Hove, UK: Psychology Press.

Petersen, S. E., van Mier, H., Fiez, J. A., & Raichle, M. E. (1998). The effects of practice on the functional anatomy of task performance. *Proceedings of the National Academy of Sciences USA* 95, 853–860.

Polson, M. C., & Friedman, A. (1988). Task-sharing within and between hemispheres: A multiple-resources approach. *Human Factors* 30, 633–643.

Posner, M. I. (1980). Orienting of attention. *Quarterly Journal of Experimental Psychology* 32, 3–25.

Posner, M. I. (1988). Structures and functions of selective attention. In *Master Lectures in Clinical Neuropsychology and Brain Function: Research, Measurement, and Practice*, T. Boll and B. Bryant, eds., 171–202. Washington, DC: American Psychological Association.

Posner, M. I. (1995). Attention in cognitive neuroscience. An overview. In *The Cognitive Neurosciences*, M. S. Gazzaniga, ed., 615–624. Cambridge, MA: MIT Press.

Posner, M. I., & Cohen, Y. (1984). Components of visual orienting. In *Attention and Performance X*, H. Bouma & D. G. Bouwhuis, eds., 531–556. Hillsdale, NJ: Erlbaum.

Posner, M. I., Cohen, Y., & Rafal, R. D. (1982). Neural systems control of spatial orienting. *Transactions of the Philosophical Society of London* B298, 187–198.

Posner, M. I., & Dehaene, S. (1994). Attentional networks. *Trends in Neuroscience* 2, 75–79.

Posner, M. I., & Driver, J. (1992). The neurobiology of selective attention. *Current Opinion in Neurobiology* 2, 165–169.

Posner, M. I., & Petersen, S. E. (1990). The attention system of the human brain. *Annual Review of Neuroscience* 13, 25–42.

Posner, M. I., Rafal, R. D., Choate, L., & Vaughn, J. (1985). Inhibition of return: Neural basis and function. *Cognitive Neuropsychology* 2, 211–228.

Posner, M. I., & Raichle, M. E. (1994). *Images of Mind*. New York: Scientific American Books.

Posner, M. I., Walker, J. A., Friedrich, F. J., & Rafal, R. D. (1984). Effects of parietal injury on covert orienting of attention. *Journal of Neuroscience* 4, 1863–1874.

Posner, M. I., Walker, J. A., Friedrich, F. J., & Rafal, R. D. (1987). How do the parietal lobes direct covert attention? *Neuropsychologia* 25, 135–145.

Prinzmetal, W. (1995). Visual feature integration in a world of objects. *Current Directions in Psychological Science* 4, 90–94.

Rafal, R. D. (1996). Visual attention: Converging operations from neurology and psychology. In *Converging Operations in the Study of Visual Selective Attention*, A. F. Kramer, M. G. H. Coles, & G. D. Logan, eds., 139–192. Washington, DC: American Psychological Association.

Rafal, R. D., & Henik, A. (1994). The neurology of inhibition: Integrating controlled and automatic processes. In *Inhibitory Processes in Attention, Memory, and Language*, D. Dagenbach & T. H. Carr, eds., 1–52. San Diego: Academic Press.

Raichle, M. E. (2000). The neural correlates of consciousness: An analysis of cognitive skill learning. In *The Cognitive Neurosciences*, M. S. Gazzaniga, ed. 2nd ed., 1305–1318. Cambridge, MA: MIT Press.

Rees, G., Frackowiak, R., & Frith, C. (1997). Two modulatory effects of attention that mediate object categorization in human cortex. *Science* 275, 835–838.

Rees, G., Frith, C., & Lavie, N. (1997). Modulating irrelevant motion perception by varying attentional load in an unrelated task. *Science* 278, 1616–1619.

Schneider, W., Worden, M., Shedden, J., & Noll, D. (1995). Assessing the distribution of exogenous and endogenous attentional modulation in human visual cortex with fMRI. Paper presented at the meeting of the Cognitive Neuroscience Society, San Francisco.

Sereno, M. I., Dale, A. M., Reppas, J. B., Kwong, K. K., Belliveau, J. W., Brady, T. J., Rosen, B. R., & Tootell, R. B. (1995). Borders of multiple visual areas in humans revealed by functional magnetic resonance imaging. *Science* 268, 889–893.

Shah, P., & Miyake, A. (1996). The separability of working memory resources for spatial thinking and language processing: An individual differences approach. *Journal of Experimental Psychology: General* 125, 4–27.

Shiu, L., & Pashler, H. (1994). Negligible effects of spatial precuing on identification of single digits. *Journal of Experimental Psychology: Human Perception and Performance* 20, 1037–1054.

Shulman, G. L., Corbetta, M., Buckner, R. L., Raichle, M. E., Fiez, J. A., Miezin, F. M., & Petersen, S. E. (1997). Top-down modulation of early sensory cortex. *Cerebral Cortex* 7, 193–206.

Sperling, G. (1984). A unified theory of attention and signal detection. In *Varieties of Attention*, R. Parasuraman & D. R. Davies, eds., 103–181. Orlando, FL: Academic Press.

Swick, D., & Knight, R. T. (1998). Cortical lesions and attention. In *The Attentive Brain*, R. Parasuraman, ed., 143–162. Cambridge, MA: MIT Press.

Tootell, R. B. H., Hadjikhani, N., Hall, E. K., Marrett, S., Vanduffel, W., Vaughan, J. T., & Dale, A. (1998). The retinotopy of visual spatial attention. *Neuron* 21, 1409–1422.

Treisman, A. M., & Gelade, G. (1980). A feature-integration theory of attention. *Cognitive Psychology* 12, 97–136.

Tsal, Y. (1983). Movements of attention across the visual field. *Journal of Experimental Psychology: Human Perception and Performance* 9, 523–530.

Van Voorhis, S., & Hillyard, S. A. (1977). Visual evoked potentials and selective attention to points in space. *Perception & Psychophysics* 22, 54–62.

Watanabe, T., Sasake, Y., Miyauchi, S., Putz, B., Fujimaki, N., Nielsen, M., Takino, R., & Miyakawa, S. (1998). Attention-regulated activity in human primary visual cortex. *Journal of Neurophysiology* 79, 2218–2221.

Wickens, C. D. (1992). *Engineering Psychology and Human Performance*, 2nd ed. New York: HarperCollins.

Wojciulik, E., Kanwisher, N., & Driver, J. (1998). Covert visual attention modulates face-specific activity in the human fusiform gyrus: fMRI study. *Journal of Neurophysiology* 79, 1574–1578.

Woldorff, M. G., Fox, P. T., Matzke, M., Lancaster, J. L., Veeraswamy, S., Zamarripa, F., Seabolt, M., Glass, T., Gao, J. H., Martin, C. C., & Jerabek, P. (1997). Retinotopic organization of early visual spatial attention effects as revealed by PET and ERPs. *Human Brain Mapping* 5, 280–286.

Yantis, S. (1998). Control of visual attention. In *Attention*, H. Pashler, ed., 223–256. Hove, UK: Psychology Press.

5 Functional Neuroimaging of Visual Recognition

Nancy Kanwisher, Paul Downing, Russell Epstein, and Zoe Kourtzi

INTRODUCTION: THE MODULARITY OF VISUAL RECOGNITION

The Problem of Visual Recognition

Visual recognition is one of the mind's most impressive accomplishments. The computational complexity of this task is illustrated by the fact that even after several decades of research in computer vision, no algorithms exist that can recognize objects in anything but the most restricted domains. Yet the human visual system is not only highly accurate but also extremely fast (Thorpe et al., 1996), recognizing objects and scenes at rates of up to about eight items per second (Potter, 1976). How is this accomplished?

Although multiple cues to visual recognition are available—including color, characteristic motion, and kind of stuff or material (Adelson & Bergen, 1991)—shape is widely considered to be the most important. The fundamental challenge for cognitive and computational theories of shape-based object recognition is to explain how we are able to recognize objects despite the substantial variation across the different images of each object caused by changes in viewpoint, lighting, occlusion, and other factors (Ullman, 1996).

A complete cognitive theory of human shape-based visual recognition would specify the precise sequence of computations that intervene between the retinal image and the matching of the input to a stored visual description in long-term memory, along with a characterization of the intervening representations that are computed along the way. While we are still far from attaining this goal, behavioral research has made significant progress. Several findings support the idea that object recognition is accomplished by the construction of viewpoint-invariant structural descriptions of visually presented objects, which are then matched to similar representations stored in long-term memory (Marr, 1982; Biederman & Gerhardstein, 1993; Ellis et al., 1989). On the other hand, numerous experiments have implicated the storage of multiple views for each object (e.g., Tarr & Bülthoff, 1995; Ullman & Basri, 1991) to which incoming perceptual information can be matched. Most researchers agree that variants of each of these types of representations are probably used in at least some conditions and/or for some levels of visual expertise (Diamond & Carey, 1986).

An important question for any theory of object recognition is whether different kinds of visual stimuli are recognized in the same basic way, or whether qualitatively different algorithms are involved in the recognition of different classes of stimuli, such as faces, objects, and words. Given the very different natures of the computational problems posed by the recognition of each of these stimulus types, it would be unsurprising if somewhat different mechanisms were involved in each. Indeed, behavioral findings have shown that face recognition differs from object recognition in that it is more dependent on stimulus orientation (Yin, 1969), more "holistic" as opposed to part-based (Tanaka & Farah, 1993), and more dependent on information about surface pigmentation and shading (Bruce, 1988). These and other findings suggest that a general-purpose algorithm which recognizes visual stimuli of all types may not constitute the best theory of human visual recognition.

Thus, one way to gain traction on the problem of understanding how visual recognition works is to attempt to discover the fundamental components of the process. One very rich source of information on the functional components of visual recognition comes from the lucky fact that the functional architecture of visual information processing is mirrored at least in part by the modular organization of visual cortex. As Marr (1982, p. 102) put it: "The idea that a large computation can be split up and implemented as a collection of parts that are as nearly independent of one another as the overall task allows, is so important that I was moved to elevate it to a principle, the principle of modular design.... The existence of a modular organization of the human visual processor proves that different types of information can be analyzed in relative isolation." A long tradition of cognitive neuropsychologists has exploited the modular structure of visual cortex in efforts to discover the functional components of vision. In this chapter we first review the evidence from neuropsychology for modularity of visual recognition. We then turn to the evidence from functional brain imaging before going on to consider the broader implications of these findings as well as the potential of brain imaging to elucidate visual cognition.

Modular Structure of Visual Recognition: Neuropsychological Evidence

Evidence for Dissociable Stages in Visual Recognition   The entire process of visual object recognition can be logically decomposed into (at last) four main components (see figure 5.1): (1) early image processing, including the extraction of features, edges, and contours; (2) extraction of higher-level information about object shape; (3) matching of that shape information to a particular stored visual representation in long-term memory; and (4) accessing of stored semantic/conceptual information about the object. Evidence that each of these processes may constitute a distinct component of human visual recognition comes from cases of people who (as a result of focal brain damage) are unable to carry out one or more of them (see Farah 1990; Humphreys & Bruce, 1989).

Cases of "apperceptive agnosia" have long been taken to suggest a distinction between the first and second components, that is, between the extraction of simple, low-level properties of the image, such as features and contours (preserved in this

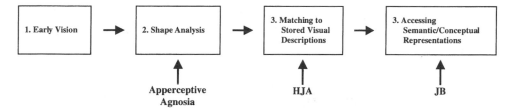

Figure 5.1
Four main candidate component processes of visual recognition, and the syndrome or patient suggesting
that each is dissociable from the others.

syndrome), and the appreciation of the shape or structure of an object (impaired).
Typical apperceptive agnosics can carry out simple visual tasks, such as discriminating curved lines from straight lines, but are impaired at discriminating different
shapes (whether novel or familiar). The precise definition of apperceptive agnosia
is a matter of ongoing debate (De Renzi & Lucchelli, 1993; Warrington, 1985). Researchers disagree on whether the inability to proficiently copy line drawings is a necessary criterion for diagnosis with this syndrome, or whether copying may sometimes
remain intact with the deficit affecting only higher-level tasks hinging on the perception of the three-dimensional structure of an object. Nonetheless, there is a consensus
that some agnosic patients fail to recognize objects not because of a deficit in either
low-level vision or in matching perceptual information to stored information in long-
term memory, but because of a failure to construct an adequate perceptual representation of the shape of the object from the retinal image. As such, these cases provide
evidence for a distinction between the first and second processes in figure 5.1.

Visual shape analysis (component 2 in figure 5.1) may itself have several distinct components. A particularly interesting dissociation was seen in patient DF
(Humphrey et al., 1996), who could discriminate the three-dimensional structure of
shapes defined by shading gradients, but was unable to discriminate similar shapes in
which the edges were depicted as luminance discontinuities or lines. This result suggests that extracting shape from shading may be a process distinct from extracting
shape from contours. Evidence that the extraction of viewpoint-invariant shape information entails distinct processes comes from patients with right posterior damage, who are often selectively impaired in recognizing objects from unusual views
(Warrington & Taylor, 1978). Further, a double dissociation between scene segmentation and shape extraction reported by Davidoff and Warrington (1993) suggests
that these processes may also be functionally distinct.

Evidence also exists for a dissociation between components 2 and 3 in figure 5.1.
For example, patient HJA, studied by Humphreys and Riddoch (1987), is able to

copy a line drawing of an object quite accurately, and can match two different views of an object, indicating a preserved ability to extract object-centered shape representations. HJA is also very good at drawing objects from memory, indicating intact memories for the appearances of objects. Yet HJA is grossly impaired at matching his perceptually derived shape representation to a stored representation in memory, and hence performs very poorly on object recognition tasks. Importantly, HJA is not simply impaired at *naming* the objects or understanding them at a semantic level. He is unable to perform an "object decision task" (introduced by Kroll & Potter, 1984), in which drawings depicting real familiar objects must be discriminated from similar drawings of possible but nonexistent objects. Because this task requires matching to stored visual descriptions, but not conceptual or verbal processes, it shows that HJA's impairment is due to an inability to recognize objects in the sense of matching visual information to a stored visual description (not subsequent stages). Thus this case demonstrates a dissociation between the construction of high-level representations of object shape (component 2) and the matching of shape information to a particular representation in long-term memory (component 3).

Finally, evidence that the process of matching perceptual representations to specific stored visual representations (component 3) is dissociable from accessing semantic representations of the recognized object (component 4) comes from cases of "optic aphasia." One such example is patient JB (Riddoch & Humphreys, 1987; see also Hillis & Caramazza, 1995), who performs the object decision task in the normal range, indicating the ability to match to stored descriptions. Yet JB frequently cannot provide any information about the objects he has correctly classified as real. This case demonstrates that matching to stored visual descriptions can be carried out independently of accessing semantic information about those objects (since he can do the former but not the latter). Note that this is not simply a problem of accessing the name of the object, but a more general problem of accessing any meaningful information about the object. Similarly, in the case of "word-meaning blindness," patient JO performs normally on a written lexical decision task, indicating preserved ability to recognize visually presented words. Yet she is severely impaired at accessing the meanings of the words so recognized (Lambon Ralph et al., 1996). Further, even normal subjects occasionally visually recognize a face (in the sense of being certain that it is familiar) without remembering anything about the person, indicating that for face recognition, too, matching to stored visual descriptions can proceed independently of access to semantic information about the recognized person. These examples demonstrate that the storage and accessing mechanisms for the *visual* form of familiar objects (component 3) is at least partly functionally distinct from the *knowledge* we have about those particular items (component 4). In this chapter we will use the word "recognition" to refer to the process of matching to the stored visual representation of an object, without assuming that this further entails accessing of semantic/conceptual information about the objects so recognized.

In sum, neuropsychological evidence supports the functional dissociation between the four main stages or components of object recognition depicted in figure 5.1. Next we consider the orthogonal question of whether different mechanisms are involved in recognizing different kinds of visual stimuli.

Evidence for Category-Specific Mechanisms for Visual Recognition   As mentioned above, the behavioral literature suggests that the visual recognition of distinct stimulus classes (e.g., faces versus objects) may involve qualitatively different mechanisms. This hypothesis is further strengthened by evidence from the syndrome of prosopagnosia (Bodamer, 1947), in which patients become unable to recognize previously familiar faces, sometimes in the absence of discernible impairments in the recognition of objects or words. One account of prosopagnosia argues that it is not a specific impairment in face recognition per se, but rather an impairment in the ability to make any fine-grained visual discriminations between different exemplars of the same class (Damasio et al., 1982), especially for highly overlearned "expert" discriminations (Diamond & Carey, 1986; Gauthier et al., 1997). Evidence against this hypothesis comes from several studies showing that at least some prosopagnosics retain a preserved ability to discriminate between different exemplars of a nonface class (De Renzi, 1986). For example, Sergent and Signoret (1992) reported a patient who was profoundly prosopagnosic despite showing an excellent ability to discriminate between different models of the same make of car, a category in which he had gained substantial premorbid visual expertise. Cases such as these suggest that prosopagnosia is not simply a general loss of expert subordinate-level discrimination.

Perhaps the strongest evidence for a dissociation between face and object recognition comes from the opposite case of agnosia for objects in the absence of an impairment in face recognition. Patient CK's general visual abilities are drastically disrupted, and he has great difficulty recognizing objects and words, yet he is completely normal at face recognition (Moscovitch et al., 1997). Moscovitch et al. argue that while most of the neural machinery necessary for object recognition is damaged in CK, face-specific recognition mechanisms are preserved. Strikingly, the face inversion effect (i.e., the decrement in face recognition performance when faces are presented upside down) is six times greater in patient CK than in normal subjects, consistent with the idea that the face-specific mechanisms preserved in this patient cannot process inverted faces.

These neuropsychological findings of localized face-specific mechanisms dovetail with results from intracranial recordings of face-specific responses from focal regions in the ventral occipitotemporal pathway in monkeys (Gross et al., 1972; Perrett et al., 1982) and humans (Fried et al., 1997; McCarthy et al., 1997; Allison et al., 1999), and with face-selective ERP (Bentin et al., 1996; Jeffreys, 1996) and MEG (Sams et al., 1997; Liu et al., 2000) responses recorded from the scalps of normal human subjects.

Further findings of alexia, or selective deficits in letter or word recognition, suggest that there may also be functional specialization for the recognition of letters or words (but see Shallice, 1988). This syndrome is of particular importance in the present context because reading has arisen so recently in evolution that any specialized mechanisms for this ability are very unlikely to be innately specified. However, Farah (1992) has argued that the pattern of co-occurrence of agnosia, alexia, and prosopagnosia suggests that there are only two, not three, processing components underlying these deficits (but see Rumiati et al., 1994; Farah, 1997).

Evidence for other fine-grained category-specific impairments in visual recognition has been reported. In the syndrome of "topographic agnosia" (Aguirre & D'Esposito, 1999), patients become unable to recognize previously familiar places. Reminiscent of prosopagnosic patients who know they are looking at a face but cannot tell who it is without a clue from a distinguishing feature, such as hairstyle or clothing, patients with topographic agnosia report that even their own house does not look familiar and can be recognized only by a distinguishing feature, such as the number on the door or the shape of the mailbox in front. Although topographic agnosia and prosopagnosia sometimes co-occur, the fact that each can occur without the other suggests that two distinct syndromes are involved, and that special-purpose mechanisms may exist for the visual recognition of familiar places (Aguirre & D'Esposito, 1999).

Further neuropsychological dissociations have been reported—for example, between the recognition of living things, such as animals, and nonliving things, such as tools and other artifacts (e.g., Hillis & Caramazza, 1991; Warrington & Shallice, 1984; Tranel et al., 1997; Caramazza & Shelton, 1998). How do these selective deficits fractionate along boundaries between visual recognition, lexical knowledge, and semantic knowledge? There is some evidence on this issue. For example, Sheridan and Humphreys (1993) describe a patient with relatively intact visual-structural representations, as assessed by an object decision task, who nonetheless has significant difficulty accessing semantic and lexical information about animals and foods, given pictures or verbal descriptions. In contrast, studies of other patients have suggested a category-specific deficit for living things with a locus in the visual-structural representation. For example, Sartori and Job (1988) tested a patient who showed difficulty on an object decision task on living things. Similarly, Silveri and Gainotti (1988) tested a patient's ability to name animals, given definitions; performance was worse when the definitions favored visual descriptions of the animals compared to abstract or functional descriptions.

Do these deficits necessarily imply category specificity in the neural organization of knowledge? In one of the earliest reports of a dissociation between living and non-living things, Warrington and Shallice (1984) suggested that the dissociation might be best explained not by a categorical division in semantic systems but rather by differences in the kinds of information involved in the representations of these categories. Specifically, it has been proposed that knowledge of animals is composed disproportionately of visual information, while knowledge of artifacts is dominated by functional (and perhaps motor) information. These differences are thought to arise from the kinds of experience we typically have with the objects in these categories—animals are generally observed from a distance, whereas tools and artifacts, manufactured for a specific purpose, typically are directly manipulated. However, a consensus has yet to emerge on this issue (see, e.g., Farah & McClelland, 1991; Farah, 1994, 1997; Farah et al., 1996; Caramazza & Shelton, 1998).

To sum up this section, the evidence from neuropsychology indicates that the mechanisms underlying visual recognition are characterized by a considerable degree of modularity. Patient studies implicate distinct mechanisms for different stages of visual recognition (i.e., the components illustrated in figure 5.1), and further suggest that distinct mechanisms may be involved in the visual recognition of stimulus classes such as faces, objects, words, animals, and tools. But although neuropsychological data are clearly important in evaluating theories of visual recognition, notorious difficulties arise when using data from brain-damaged patients to make inferences about cognition in the normal brain (Shallice, 1988). First, brain damage rarely affects a single focal area, so many functions are likely to be disrupted in any single case. Second, brain damage may result in the reorganization of cognition rather than in the deletion of a component from it. For these and other reasons, functional brain imaging in normal subjects provides an important complement to studies of patients with specific deficits resulting from focal brain damage. Next we outline the progress that functional brain imaging studies have made in discovering the fundamental components of the human visual recognition system.

FUNCTIONAL NEUROIMAGING OF VISUAL RECOGNITION

Early imaging work provided evidence that human visual cortex follows the same macroscopic organization reported earlier in the macaque, with a ventral/occipito-temporal pathway more engaged in visual recognition tasks and a dorsal/parietal pathway more engaged in tasks involving location and action. For example, Haxby et al. (1991, 1994) used PET to find occipitotemporal activations for a face-matching task but occipitoparietal activations for a location-matching task. A study by Köhler et al. (1995) used a similar technique with line drawings of objects, again finding greater activation in ventral regions for a task requiring encoding of the identities of objects, but greater activation in dorsal regions when location tasks had to be carried out on the same stimuli. These studies indicate that ventral occipitotemporal cortex is the general region where any modular components of visual recognition are most likely to be found. In this section we review the evidence that particular regions within this ventral pathway may be specialized for the perception of object shape, as well as the perception of faces, places, words, and other categories of visual stimuli.

Visual Shape Analysis

Evidence from a variety of sources indicates that a large region of lateral and inferior occipital cortex just anterior to retinotopic cortex (LO) responds more strongly to stimuli depicting shapes than to stimuli with similar low-level features which do not depict shapes (Malach et al., 1995; Kanwisher et al., 1996). Importantly, the three-dimensional shapes depicted in these studies were novel, so the activations in these conditions cannot be straightforwardly accounted for in terms of matching to stored visual representations, or semantic or verbal coding of the stimuli. Common areas within this lateral occipital region are activated by shapes defined by motion, texture, and luminance contours (Grill-Spector, Kushnir, Edelman, et al., 1998; Grill-Spector, Kushnir, Hendler, et al., 1998). Kourtzi and Kanwisher (2000a) have shown that 3D shapes defined primarily by shading information (grayscale photos) and those defined by contours (line drawings) activate largely overlapping regions in lateral occipital cortex. Further, Mendola et al. (1999) have shown that whereas simple forms defined by differences in luminance, color, or direction of motion largely activate regions in retinotopic cortex, stereoscopic and illusory-contour displays primarily activate the lateral occipital region, suggesting that this area may be particularly involved in extracting information about depth.

Several studies have shown a reduction in the response of a particular region of LO (and other regions of cortex) when stimuli are repeated (Malach et al., 1998). Grill-Spector et al. (1999) have further shown that in LO this effect can be observed even when the repeated shapes vary in size and position, thus demonstrating that the representations in this area are invariant with respect to changes in size and position. Importantly, this adaptation effect is not found across changes in object viewpoint, showing that the representations in this area are not viewpoint-invariant. As this work illustrates, fMRI adaptation is a potentially very powerful technique for characterizing the representations in particular regions of cortex.

Thus work on the lateral occipital complex is promising and suggests that regions of cortex may indeed exist which are specialized for some aspect/s of shape processing. However, several crucial questions have yet to be tackled. First, what specific aspect/s of shape analysis is/are computed in this region? Second, will the areas activated by different shape cues in different studies overlap if run on an individual subject, or will different but adjacent regions within lateral occipital cortex be activated by different shape cues? Third, a critical methodological point is that most of the prior work in this area has used passive viewing tasks (but see Grill-Spector et al., 1999). Will the greater activations to intact than to scrambled stimuli still be obtained when this attention confound is removed and similar attentional engagement in the two conditions is required? Research in this area has the potential to provide important insights about the nature of the intermediate representations of shape involved in object recognition (Kourtzi & Kanwisher, 2000a).

Faces

Faces may provide the strongest case for cortical specialization for a particular stimulus category. This is perhaps not too surprising, given that faces are enormously rich and biologically relevant stimuli, providing information not only about the identity of a person, but also about mood, age, sex, and direction of gaze. In this section we consider the evidence from functional brain imaging that a region of cortex is selectively involved in some aspect of face perception, and more specifically we ask what precise aspect of face perception might go on in this region.

Several early PET studies demonstrated that regions of the ventral pathway become active during face recognition tasks (Haxby et al., 1991, 1994; Sergent et al., 1992). Puce et al. (1995) and Clark et al. (1996) obtained similar results using fMRI, enabling them to more precisely localize the activations in the fusiform gyrus in individual subjects. Puce et al. (1996) used fMRI to demonstrate that a region in the fusiform gyrus was more active during face viewing than during letter-string viewing. They also found another region in the superior temporal sulcus that was more active for viewing of faces than of letter strings. While these findings are broadly consistent with the neuropsychological syndrome of prosopagnosia in suggesting that specialized neural mechanisms may exist for the perception of faces, they do not unequivocally demonstrate that the activated regions are selectively involved in face perception. To make such a case, it is necessary to quantify the response of the area to a large number of different conditions in order to show that it generalizes across widely different instances of faces, yet fails to generalize to nonfaces. Next we review the studies in our lab that have attempted to do exactly that.

A Distinct Face-Selective Region in the Mid Fusiform Gyrus   We began by scanning participants while they viewed a videotape composed of alternating 30-second periods, each containing a sequence of black-and-white photographs of either faces or objects (Kanwisher et al., 1997). To find parts of the brain that respond more

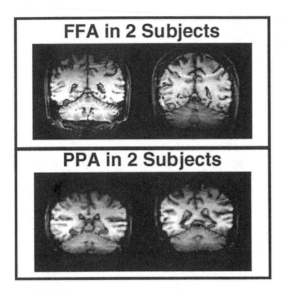

Figure 5.2
Coronal views of the brain showing the fusiform face area (FFA) in two subjects, and the parahippo-campal place area (PPA) in two subjects. Right hemisphere is shown on the left and vice versa. (See color plate 3.)

strongly to faces than to objects, we ran a statistical test on each voxel, asking whether its MR signal was significantly higher during face viewing than during object viewing. Although the exact location of the activation varied somewhat across subjects, in most participants a small region in the right fusiform gyrus (see color plates 3 and 4, figures 5.2 and 5.3a) responded significantly more strongly during face viewing than during object viewing.

Several aspects of this activation are striking. First, in most subjects the effect is strong enough that the pattern of large peaks for face epochs and much lower peaks for object epochs is clearly visible in the raw time course of MR signal intensity in this region in individual subjects (see figure 5.3c), and often even in individual voxels (figure 5.3d). Confirming this informal intuitive measure of significance, statistical tests comparing the response to faces against the response to objects reach p-levels (uncorrected for multiple spatial hypotheses) of $p < 10^{-4}$ or better on a Kolmogorov-Smirnov test (figure 5.3a), and t-tests on the same data tend to be even stronger (figure 5.3b). The signal increase (from a fixation baseline) is typically about 2% for faces and half that or less for nonfaces. In contrast, the ring of voxels immediately surrounding this region (figure 5.3e) typically exhibits little or no face selectivity, indicating that this region has sharp borders. Thus, the activation for faces versus objects is large,

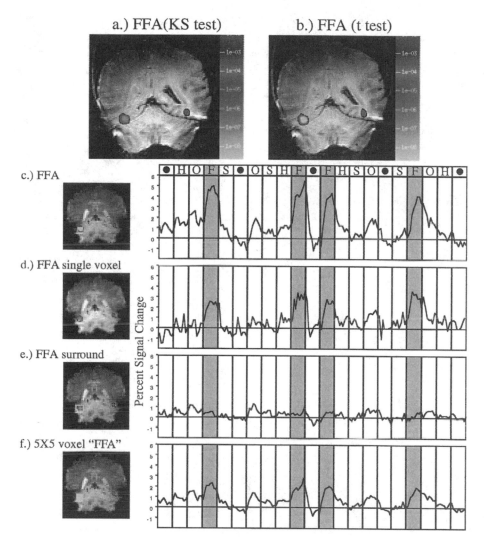

a.) FFA(KS test)   b.) FFA (t test)

c.) FFA

d.) FFA single voxel

Percent Signal Change

e.) FFA surround

f.) 5X5 voxel "FFA"

Figure 5.3
The fusiform face area in subject WB. (*a*, *b*) Regions responding significantly more strongly during face viewing than during object viewing on a Kolmogorov-Smirnov test (*a*), and the same data analyzed with a *t*-test (*b*). Although the Kolmogorov-Smirnov test is often criticized, we usually find that (as in this example) the results of the two tests are highly similar except that *t*-tests produce stronger *p* levels than KS tests on the same data. (*c*) The FFA as identified by our standard criterion ($p < 10^{-4}$ on a KS test, uncorrected) is shown in the yellow overlay on the slice at left. The time course of raw percent signal change (from the fixation baseline) in the FFA is shown at right. Note the obvious peaks in MR signal intensity corresponding to the face epochs (F); other epochs in this sequence contained houses (H), assorted objects (O), and scenes (S). (*d*) The time course of percent signal change from a single voxel within the FFA (shown as the yellow voxel in the slice at left), showing that face selectivity is often visible in the raw data from individual unsmoothed and unaveraged voxels. (*e*) The region immediately surrounding the FFA is not face-selective, as can be seen in the time course from this region at the right. (*f*) An illustration of the problem that can result when the FFA ROI is too large. In this case the face area is defined as a 5×5 voxel square centered on the voxel with maximal face versus object activation. Although some face selectivity is still visible in the raw data, the effect has clearly been diluted by averaging the nonface-selective surround with the FFA. (See color plate 4.)

highly significant, and spatially circumscribed. This region appears to reflect not simply a graded and continuous change from surrounding cortex, but a functionally distinct area.

Testing Alternatives to Face Selectivity   But what, exactly, does this area do? It was tempting to conclude that it is the face recognition mechanism that psychologists and neuropsychologists have long hypothesized to exist. But a greater response to faces than to objects is consistent with a number of alternative accounts. The activation for faces might simply reflect the possibility that faces are more interesting or attentionally engaging than objects. Or it could reflect the fact that faces are exemplars of a single category (face), whereas the objects we used came from many categories. Or perhaps this same area would respond similarly to animals, or to human hands, in which case it might be selective for animate objects or body parts, not faces. Before claiming that this region of the brain was specialized for face perception, it was necessary to test these alternatives.

Our strategy was first to find the candidate face region in each participant with our test comparing the activation for faces versus objects. Then we looked at this same region in each participant's data during several new tests. To see if the candidate face area simply responds whenever participants look at many different exemplars of any category of object, we looked again at each subject during a new test in which alternating sequences of faces and houses were presented. In this test, the average percent increase in MR signal in the candidate face area (from a baseline in which participants simply fixed their eyes on a dot) was several times greater during viewing of faces than during viewing of houses, indicating a high degree of stimulus selectivity. Clearly, this region does not simply respond maximally whenever a set of different exemplars of any category is presented. Other labs have also found greater responses in face selective regions during viewing of multiple exemplars of faces than during viewing of flowers (McCarthy et al., 1997), houses (Haxby et al., 1999), or cars (Halgren et al., 1999).

One could still argue that participants automatically categorize faces at the subordinate level (i.e., which specific face is this?), but they don't bother to do this when they look at houses or other objects. Further, participants may simply pay more attention to faces than to any other stimuli. So in another test we presented a sequence of 3/4-view faces with hair concealed, compared to a sequence of different people's hands all held in roughly the same position. We required participants to discriminate among the different exemplars in each case by asking them to press a button whenever they saw two consecutive images that were identical (a "1-back" task). This task is particularly difficult for the hand stimuli, so participants are likely to have paid at least as much attention to the hands as to the faces. The data showed that the candidate face region in all five participants responded more strongly to faces than to hands even in this task. So activation in this area does not reflect either general visual attention or effort, or subordinate-level classification of any visual stimuli. Instead, this area apparently responds specifically to faces.

After testing and rejecting the most plausible alternative accounts we could think of, we proposed that this area, which we named the "fusiform face area" (FFA), is selectively involved in the perception of faces (Kanwisher et al., 1997). By face "selectivity" or "specificity," we do not mean exclusivity. The FFA responds more to nonface objects than to a minimal stimulus like a fixation point (see also Haxby et al., 1999). Instead, we follow the definition used by single-unit physiologists (Tovee et al., 1993), in which selectivity means that the response must be at least twice as great for the preferred stimulus category as for any other stimulus category. Haxby et al. (1999: 196) have argued that the partial response to nonfaces is "problematic for [Kanwisher et al.'s] hypothesis that face-selective regions ... constitute a 'module specialized for face perception.'" We disagree. First, because of limitations on the spatial resolution due to voxel size, blood flow regulation, and other factors, the MR signal intensity from a particular ROI should not be expected to reflect a pure measure of the activity in a single functional module, but will include contributions from functionally distinct adjacent (and even interleaved) neural tissue. Second, there is no reason to expect even a strongly face-selective neural module to shut itself off completely when a nonface is presented (Carey & Spelke, 1994). Indeed, it is hard to imagine how this could occur without a special gating mechanism that discriminates between faces and nonfaces and allows only the face information into the FFA. In the absence of such a gating mechanism, it would be most natural to expect a much lower but still positive response to nonfaces in a region of cortex specialized for face processing. This is exactly what we observe.

In another line of experiments (Tong et al., 2000), we demonstrated that the FFA response is (1) equally large for cat, cartoon, and human faces despite very different image properties; (2) equal for front and profile views of human heads, but declining in strength as faces rotate away from view; and (3) weakest for nonface objects and houses. Finally, we have demonstrated (Kanwisher et al., 1999) that the response of the FFA is not selective for anything animate, because the response of this area to stimuli depicting animals with their heads not visible is not significantly greater than the response to inanimate objects (but see Chao et al., 1998).

At this point we have quantified the MR response of the FFA to over 20 different stimulus categories (figure 5.4). Each of these conditions has been run in both a passive viewing and a 1-back task, and we have never seen a different pattern of response between tasks, so we are reasonably confident that the results we have observed are

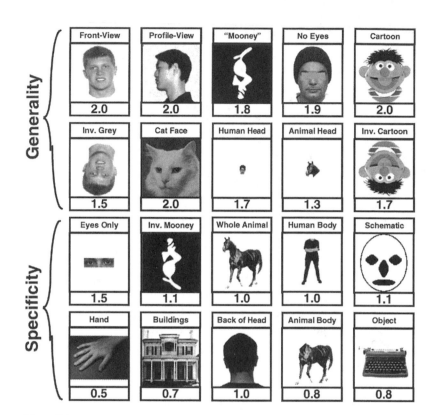

Figure 5.4
A summary of the main findings on the fusiform face area (FFA) from our lab. Each box contains an example of a stimulus from a different category; the number below it is the magnitude of the response of the FFA in that condition (in percent signal change from fixation). Each response magnitude is based on at least four subjects, and on the average over passive viewing and 1-back tasks. (In none of these experiments did we see a significant interaction of stimulus condition × task.) This summary is compiled from many different experiments. Because not all conditions were run within the same subjects and scans, the exact magnitudes of response across conditions should be considered illustrative only. In an effort to partially normalize for subject and scan differences, the magnitudes in each condition were normalized to the activation for front-view grayscale faces in the same scan.

not due to differences in attentional engagement between stimulus classes. Overall, our results indicate that the response of the FFA generalizes across very different face types, and so cannot be explained in terms of a specific response to a salient facial feature, such as the eyes, or a more general response to heads. Instead, the FFA appears to be optimally tuned to the broad category of faces.

A Role in Discrimination of Gaze, or Emotional Expression, or Semantic Processing? However, demonstrating the selectivity of this region to face stimuli is just the beginning. We still do not know what the FFA does with faces. Nonetheless, the data collected so far do provide some clues. We are very sensitive to subtle differences in the direction of another person's gaze, so one possibility is that the FFA is specifically involved in extracting this information. Evidence against this hypothesis comes from the fact that occluding the eyes does not produce a significant reduction in the FFA response to faces (Tong et al., 2000). One could imagine that subjects might occasionally infer the direction of gaze of a face even when the eyes are occluded, but it seems unlikely that this alternative can account for the nearly identical response to faces with eyes showing and faces with eyes occluded. Further, a study by Hoffman and Haxby (2000) found that regions in the STS responded more strongly during attention to direction of gaze, whereas regions in the fusiform gyrus were more active during attention to face identity (see also Wicker et al., 1998). The possibility that the FFA is specifically involved in extracting emotional expressions from faces also seems unlikely, given the consistently high response of the FFA during viewing of expressionless faces. Further, in studies directly manipulating the presence or absence of emotional expressions in face stimuli, the greatest activation is in the amygdala (Breiter et al., 1996; Morris et al., 1996) or anterior insula (Phillips et al., 1997), not the fusiform gyrus.

The further possibility that the FFA is involved in representing semantic information about particular individuals is also unlikely, given that in many of our experiments the faces are unfamiliar to the subjects, so little or no semantic information about the individuals should be available (and the rapid stimulus presentation rate of 1.5 faces per second would be likely to discourage imagination of the semantic details), yet the response magnitude and selectivity of the FFA does not appear to be any weaker for unfamiliar than for familiar faces (see below). Thus, while not definitive, the above considerations suggest that the FFA is unlikely to be involved in discriminating the direction of gaze or emotional expression in a face or in representing higher-level semantic information about individuals.

The FFA: Face Recognition Versus Face Detection? Is the FFA then involved in extracting the critical stimulus information necessary for the recognition of individuals, or is it simply engaged in detecting the presence of faces or finding them in complex images? At first glance it may seem implausible that a region of cortex would be dedicated to a computation as humble as face detection. However, Carey and Spelke (1994) have suggested that a face detection system might play a crucial role in cognition by selectively engaging the social cognition system when appropriate stimuli are present. From a very different perspective, research in computer vision suggests that finding faces in complex images may be one of the most computationally demanding components of the problem of face recognition (Hallinan et al., 1999). What makes the detection problem so challenging is the requirement to generalize across large within-class variations while maintaining fine between-class boundaries. This is a difficult balance to achieve, because increasing within-class generalization typically leads to blurring the distinction between classes (Yang and Huang 1994; Rowley et al., 1995).[1] These considerations lend plausibility to the idea that a region of cortex may be dedicated to face detection, and raise the question of whether that is the primary function of the FFA.

If, instead, the FFA is involved in face recognition, then we might expect to find a higher response when faces are successfully recognized than when they are not. However, several studies (Dubois et al., 1999; George et al., 1999; Gorno Tempini et al., 1998) have found no greater response in the FFA region to familiar than to unfamiliar faces (see also Haxby et al., 1996; Clark et al., 1998). Further evidence against a role in recognition comes from studies of face inversion. When grayscale faces are presented upside down, face detection remains easy (i.e., it is obvious that the stimulus is a face), but numerous behavioral studies have demonstrated that face recognition is impaired (e.g., Diamond & Carey, 1986). Thus, if the FFA is involved in face recognition (as opposed to face detection), we might expect the magnitude of the FFA response to be much lower for grayscale faces presented upside down, whereas if it is involved in face detection, the magnitude of the response may be similar for upright and inverted grayscale faces. In fact, although we did find significant reductions in the FFA response for inverted compared to upright faces, this effect was small in magnitude and was not consistent across subjects (Kanwisher et al., 1998). Further, two subsequent studies failed to find any significant reduction in the response of face-selective cortical regions to inverted compared to upright faces (Aguirre et al., 1999; Haxby et al., 1999). Given that the stimulus information extracted from inverted faces is not sufficient to support reliable face recognition, the failure to find a substantial reduction in the response magnitude for these stimuli provides some evidence against a role for the FFA in face recognition.

In a similar vein, preliminary results from our lab (Harris & Kanwisher, unpublished data; see also Halgren et al., 1999; Ishai et al., 1999) have found that the

FFA response to edge maps (i.e., line drawings) of faces is about as strong as the response to grayscale photos of faces, despite the fact that recognition of faces is much worse for edge maps than for grayscale photos (Bruce, 1988). Like the familiarity and face inversion results, these data provide another case in which a manipulation that prevents or severely disrupts recognition has little or no effect on the magnitude of the FFA response.

In contrast to the apparent lack of a correlation between the recognizability of a face stimulus and the FFA response, the detection of a face does seem to be correlated with the FFA response. First, inversion of two-tone ("Mooney") faces both drastically disrupts the ability to detect a face at all in the stimulus and produces a substantial reduction in the FFA response (Kanwisher et al., 1998). Second, Tong et al. (1998) demonstrated that a sharp rise in FFA activity occurs when subjects detect a face in an ambiguous rivalrous stimulus (with a face displayed to one eye and a house displayed to the other). In this study the same single face was used for the entire experiment, both within and across scans; it seems a bit strained to interpret this rise in activity as reflecting the recognition (as opposed to the detection) of the face. Given these clear fMRI responses during face detection, along with the apparent independence of the fMRI response from the recognizability of the face stimulus, the possibility that the FFA subserves face detection must be taken seriously.

Of course the FFA may be involved in both face detection and face recognition. This possibility is all the more plausible given that these two processes are often closely linked in current computational approaches to face recognition (Edwards et al., 1998; Hotta et al., 1998). In particular, detection can be thought of as the step that establishes correspondences between regions in an input image and parts of the internal representation—for instance, which image region corresponds to an eye and which to a mouth (Shakunaga et al., 1998). This step can serve to greatly simplify the subsequent recognition process.

The FFA: Origins and Role in Visual Expertise? In a landmark study, Diamond and Carey (1986) demonstrated that the behavioral cost of stimulus inversion, found originally for faces (Yin, 1969), is also found for dog stimuli in expert dog judges. Moreover, recent studies have shown that cells in monkey IT become selective for novel objects after extensive exposures to multiple views of these objects (Logothetis et al., 1994, 1995). These results suggest that visual expertise in any stimulus domain may lead to the creation or use of class-specific representations and subordinate-level discrimination mechanisms. Two important questions arise. First, is expertise alone (without a specific genetic blueprint) ever sufficient to create specialized mechanisms for the analysis of particular stimulus classes? If so, the face area may have originated through extensive experience with faces alone (in conjunction with cortical self-organization principles). We will discuss this question below. Second, can a single mechanism accomplish all expert within-class discrimination, or would one instead expect a functionally distinct mechanism for each stimulus category for which the subject gains substantial visual expertise? For example, in Diamond and Carey's subjects are the inversion-sensitive mechanisms for dog discrimination in dog experts merely qualitatively similar to, or actually identical to, those involved in face recognition? In two papers Gauthier and her colleagues (Gauthier et al., 1997; Gauthier et al., 2000a) have argued that they are identical. Specifically, these researchers have argued that the FFA is not in fact selective for faces per se, but is instead involved in subordinate-level (i.e., within-category) discrimination between members of any stimulus class for which the subject has gained visual expertise (see Kanwisher, 2000, and Tarr & Gauthier, 2000).

In one study testing the involvement of the fusiform gyrus in subordinate-level discrimination of nonface objects (Gauthier et al., 1997), the face area was not actually localized. Rather, the authors concluded that because subordinate-level discrimination of nonfaces activates regions of the fusiform gyrus, the FFA itself must be more generally involved in subordinate-level discrimination of nonface objects. However, the FFA is a small subset of the fusiform gyrus, which stretches for many centimeters from the occipital lobe well into the middle and anterior temporal lobe. Without localizing the FFA itself, one cannot determine to what extent the activations from subordinate-level categorization overlap with the FFA. In another study, Gauthier et al. (2000a) did functionally localize a face-selective region in the same subjects in whom they demonstrated activations for subordinate-level expertise. However, their criteria for defining the face area differed from those of Kanwisher et al. (1997), and were based on the assumption that the face area would constitute a square region of cortex. Thus, these studies cannot determine whether it is the FFA itself (as defined in this chapter), or nearby/overlapping cortex, that is activated by expert subordinate-level discrimination of nonface objects. However, the ambiguities in this work can be resolved by testing for expertise and subordinate-level categorization effects in individual subjects whose FFAs have been localized in the fashion we originally proposed (Kanwisher et al., 1997) and have used in all the subsequent studies in our lab (Wojciulik et al., 1998; Kanwisher et al., 1998; Tong et al., 1998; Kanwisher et al, 1999; Tong et al., 2000). Evidence from bird and car experts (Gauthier et al., 1999b) suggests that when the FFA is localized in this fashion, it does show effects of both level of categorization and visual expertise. However, the FFA response to cars in car experts (and birds in bird experts) was still only about half the magnitude of the response to faces in the same area. On the other hand, small differences in how the face area was defined led to substantial differences in the magnitude of the response to expert categories, so further study on this question is necessary.

Several findings from functional brain imaging also cast doubt on the idea that the FFA plays a general role in visual expertise and/or subordinate-level discrimination. First, the evidence in the section "The FFA: Face Recognition Versus Detection?," above, that the FFA may be more involved in face detection than in face recognition is also evidence against the role of this area in expert subordinate-level categorization of either faces or nonfaces. Further, letters and words may be the only stimulus class for which many people have an amount of visual experience comparable to what they have with faces. Yet letter strings do not strongly activate face-selective regions (Puce et al., 1996), so visual expertise with a particular visual category alone is not sufficient for strong activation of the FFA by that category. Further, within-class discrimination of structurally similar objects is not sufficient to produce a strong signal in the FFA, since Kanwisher et al. (1997) found a very low response in this area when subjects performed a difficult within-class discrimination task on human hands. Similarly, low responses in the FFA have also been found during discrimination tasks on houses, the backs of human heads, and human and animal bodies without heads visible (Tong et al., 2000; Kanwisher et al., 1999). Nonetheless, these studies do not rule out the possibility that the *combination* of expertise and within-class discrimination on structurally similar objects is sufficient to activate the FFA.

If indeed it does turn out that the FFA itself (as opposed to nearby neural populations) is activated to a similar extent by expert subordinate-level categorization of nonface objects, what will that mean? As noted in the section "Evidence for Category-Specific Mechanisms for Visual Recognition," above, the patient literature shows that prosopagnosia can occur in the apparent absence of deficits in expert subordinate-level categorization (but see Gauthier et al., 1999a). Thus one possibility is that the FFA is activated by, but is not necessary for, expert categorization. Alternatively, it could be that distinct but physically interleaved neural populations respond to faces and to nonface expert stimuli. Indeed, it would be surprising if neurons exist that respond strongly to both faces and cars (but not other complex objects) in car experts (for example). In Logothetis's work on monkeys (Logothetis et al., 1994, 1995), no cells have yet been found that are strongly responsive to both faces and exemplars from the "paperclip" stimulus set for which the monkey has gained expertise. Finally, even if it is eventually found that the identical neurons respond to both faces and non-face expert stimuli, it is worth noting that for most of us primates, faces remain the primary, if not the only, stimulus class on which we perform expert subordinate-level categorization. Thus the FFA would remain a face area in the sense that face perception has been its primary function in the lives of both our ancestors and ourselves (see also Kanwisher, 2000 and Tarr & Gauthier, 2000)

The FFA and Prosopagnosia   The apparent specificity of the FFA for face perception dovetails with the evidence from prosopagnosia that face perception is subserved by specialized cortical mechanisms. But is the FFA in fact the cortical region that is damaged in prosopagnosia? According to Damasio et al. (1990), prosopagnosia-producing lesions typically involve posterior and inferior regions especially of the right hemisphere. While consistent with the locus of the FFA, the large size of lesions in prosopagnosia underconstrains any effort to identify the FFA as the critical lesion site. However, we have taken another approach (De Gelder & Kanwisher, 1999) by scanning two prosopagnosic subjects with no brain damage visible on anatomical scans. Functional scans failed to reveal an FFA in either of these two subjects (though they both had clear PPAs; see below), consistent with our hypothesis that the lack of an FFA can produce prosopagnosia. Though promising, these results must be considered preliminary because we occasionally fail to find FFAs even in some apparently normal subjects.

In sum, a great deal of evidence suggests that the FFA constitutes a special-purpose mechanism subserving some aspect/s of face perception. Nonetheless, many questions remain about the precise functions carried out in this area. Luckily, many of these questions should be answerable with fMRI or related techniques.

The Parahippocampal Place Area

There were many prior reasons to expect that a face-selective region might exist in the human brain. Can functional brain imaging ever discover new functional components that were not predicted from prior work? In this section we describe a line of work in our lab that resulted in the discovery of a highly selective region of cortex that was a complete surprise to us.

While running the face experiments, we had noticed that in virtually every participant we ran on the standard faces-versus-objects comparison, a large region in bilateral parahippocampal cortex showed the reverse effect: it was more active during object viewing than face viewing. Epstein and Kanwisher (1998) tested the response of this region to complex scenes (such as landscapes, rooms, and outdoor campus scenes) in an experiment that also included epochs of faces, objects, and houses. Each of these four stimulus types was presented in both an intact version and a scrambled version in which the image was cut into small squares that were spatially rearranged. The results from this experiment were startling. The same region of parahippocampal cortex that had repeatedly shown a greater activation for objects than for faces showed a much stronger activation for scenes than for either faces or objects. This was true whether participants simply watched the stimuli without any specific task, or performed the 1-back task (forcing them to attend to all stimuli). All nine participants showed the identical bilateral brain region straddling the collateral sulcus to be much more active for scenes than for any of the other seven conditions (see figure 5.2, bottom).

Why should a region of cortex respond more to scenes than to other kinds of visual stimuli? The most obvious possibility was that the complexity, interest, or richness of the scenes was driving the response. The critical factor might also have been the presence of many different objects in the scenes. Another possibility was that this region of the brain was involved in extracting the layout of the local environment (Cheng, 1986; Hermer & Spelke, 1994). To test between these alternatives, we measured the response of this same area to photos of (1) furnished rooms, (2) the same rooms bare of all furniture and objects, and (3) edited photographs of the furnished room in which the furniture and objects were visible but the background (walls and floors) was blanked out. To our surprise, the response of the same region to fully furnished rooms was not reduced when the same rooms were shown empty of all furniture or other objects. In other words, the response of this region in parahippocampal cortex appeared to be entirely due to the presence of information about the layout of local space. Although all of our room stimuli were rectilinear, the data from another condition showed this was not critical for the response: photos of natural landscapes largely devoid of discrete objects also produced a strong response in the same area. In a third experiment, we showed that the response of this region to pictures of empty rooms was not diminished when the rooms were cut at their seams (leaving the shape of the room still clear), but dropped significantly when the resulting pieces were rearranged so that they no longer composed a coherent three-dimensional space.

We have named this region of cortex the "parahippocampal place area," or PPA (Epstein & Kanwisher, 1998; Epstein et al., 1999). In combination with preliminary results from several further experiments, we have now measured the response of this area to over 20 different stimulus types (figure 5.5). In these and other experiments we have continued to support our hypothesis that this region of the brain is selectively involved in processing visual information about places, particularly their spatial layout. We have also observed that the PPA generally responds more strongly to buildings than to other objects (including other large objects, such as ships and jumbo jets), though not as strongly as it does to full scenes.

The relationship between the PPA and other cortical regions that may also play a role in processing navigationally relevant information remains to be determined.

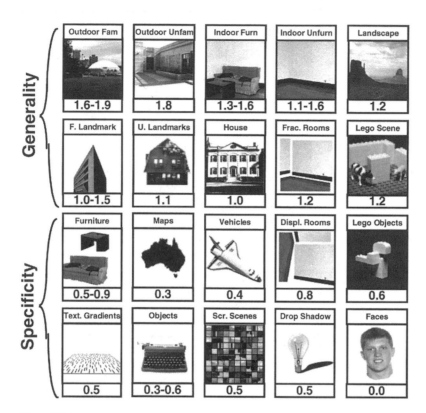

Figure 5.5
A summary of the main findings on the parahippocampal place area (PPA) from our lab. Each box contains an example of a stimulus from a different category; the number below it is the magnitude of the response of the PPA in that condition (in percent signal change from fixation). Each response magnitude is based on at least four subjects, and on the average over passive viewing and 1-back tasks. (In none of these experiments did we see a significant interaction of stimulus condition × task.) This summary is compiled from many different experiments. Because not all conditions were run within the same subjects and scans, the exact magnitudes of response across conditions should be considered illustrative only. In an effort to partially normalize for subject and scan differences, the magnitudes in each condition were normalized to the activation for front-view grayscale faces in the same scan.

Consistent with our results, other researchers have observed increased neural activity in parahippocampal cortex during virtual navigation through simple video-game environments (Aguirre et al., 1996; Maguire, Frith, et al., 1998). However, more anterior medial temporal regions appear to become active when subjects must plan routes through more complex environments (Maguire et al., 1997; Maguire, Burgess, et al., 1998). In addition, a number of researchers have observed voxels in ventral medial occipital-temporal cortex that respond more to buildings than to other stimuli, such as faces, chairs, and other objects (Ishai et al., 1999; Aguirre et al., 1998; Haxby et al., 1999). Some of these "house" activations appear to include the PPA as well as more posterior regions (Haxby et al., 1999), whereas others are circumscribed enough that they may be distinct from the PPA (Aguirre et al., 1998). It remains to be seen whether the PPA and these building-sensitive regions are distinct, and if so, how they interact in place perception and navigation.

Is the PPA a "place recognition" module? As noted above, patients with damage to parahippocampal cortex often suffer from topographical disorientation—difficulty finding their way around, particularly in novel environments (Habib & Sirigu, 1987; Landis et al., 1986; see Aguirre & D'Esposito, 1999, for review). For these patients, the core of the deficit seems to be an inability to use the overall appearance of places and buildings for purposes of orientation, which suggests that the PPA might be involved in place recognition. If this were the case, one might expect the PPA to respond more strongly to familiar places than to unfamiliar places. We tested this hypothesis (Epstein et al., 1999) and found that the PPA was just as active when subjects viewed photographs of places they knew as when they viewed photographs of places they had never visited. A follow-up experiment demonstrated that PPA response was very high even when viewing "scenes" made out of Legos, which seemed placelike but were clearly not real places in the world. The response to Lego scenes was much higher than the response to Lego objects, which were made out of the same materials. These experiments suggest that PPA activity does not covary with either successful or attempted recognition. Interestingly, the response to familiar buildings was higher than the response to unfamiliar buildings, perhaps because knowledge of the spatial context of a building makes it seem more "placelike" and less "objectlike."

An alternative to the place recognition hypothesis is that the PPA is primarily dedicated to perceptual or mnemonic encoding of place appearance, in which case deficits observed in parahippocampal patients would be the result of an encoding failure. This possibility would be generally consistent with evidence from other laboratories suggesting that parahippocampal cortex is involved in memory encoding (Stern et al., 1996; Wagner et al., 1998; Brewer et al., 1998). Specifically, Wagner et al. and Brewer et al. used an event-related technique to demonstrate greater activity in parahippocampal cortex for subsequently remembered, compared to subsequently forgotten, stimuli. To test whether the PPA is involved in encoding any visual stimuli, we examined the response of the PPA to scenes and faces under two conditions (Epstein et al., 1999). In the first ("all-novel") condition, subjects viewed a series of photographs that they had never seen before. In the second ("multiply repeated") condition, subjects viewed the same four photographs over and over again (though not necessarily in the same order). In both conditions, subjects performed a 1-back repetition task to ensure attention to each stimulus. We found that the PPA response was higher for scenes in the all-novel condition than in the multiply repeated condition. For faces, the PPA response was zero (i.e., the same as fixation) in both conditions. We conclude that the PPA is involved in encoding place information, but not face information.

But does this mean that the PPA plays a role in *memory* encoding? At present, the evidence is inconclusive. The greater response to novel compared to previously viewed scenes could be due either to greater perceptual *or* to greater memory encoding demands in the former condition. Similarly, the greater parahippocampal activation for encoding of subsequently remembered versus nonsubsequently remembered stimuli observed by other researchers (Brewer et al., 1998; Wagner et al., 1998) may simply indicate that stimuli which receive more perceptual processing are more likely to be remembered. It is quite possible that the PPA is involved in both kinds of encoding. Our evidence suggests that this encoding is specific to place information; however, it is interesting to note that Wagner et al. (1998) found memory effects for words in parahippocampal cortex (see also Kelley et al., 1998). This region of parahippocampal cortex may be distinct from the PPA. However, it may overlap, in which case Wagner et al.'s result may be evidence that the processing of place information performed in the PPA plays an indirect role in forming memories for other kinds of stimuli as well. Clearly, though, the absence of any response to faces in our experiments indicates that the PPA is involved in neither perceptual nor mnemonic encoding of face information.

Animals and Tools

A few neuroimaging studies have contrasted the perception of living things, including animals, with the perception of artifacts, such as tools. For example, Martin et al. (1996) directly compared naming of tools and animals in a PET study. They found a greater activation in the left medial occipital lobe for animals than for tools, and enhanced activations for tools in left premotor areas and the left middle temporal gyrus. A PET study by Damasio et al. (1996) tested naming of famous faces, animals, and tools (compared to a baseline consisting of a upright/inverted judgment on unfamiliar faces). They found an activation in the left inferotemporal region for animals, whereas tools produced a greater activation in posterior middle and inferior temporal gyri, regions that the same authors found to be implicated in specific deficits for these categories in a large population of patients with focal lesions. While some efforts were made to rule out accounts of these activations in terms of certain obvious confounds, such as visual complexity (e.g., Martin et al., 1996), more work will be needed before the evidence for the selectivity of these regions for animals or tools can be considered strong. The approach we favor involves the testing of the same cortical region on many different stimulus conditions to establish both the generality of the response (i.e., that many different instances of the category all produce a strong response) and its specificity (i.e., that a strong response is *not* found for noninstances of the category).

Biological Motion

Observers are particularly sensitive to human body movements. Numerous psychophysical studies suggest that observers can identify actions, discriminate the gender of the actor, and recognize friends from highly simplified point-light displays (Cutting, 1987; Cutting et al., 1978; Dittrich, 1993; Kozlowski & Cutting, 1977) generated by filming human actors with lights attached to their joints in a darkened environment (Marey, 1895/1972; Johansson, 1973). Interestingly, patients with damage to areas responsible for motion processing (i.e., MT) are impaired in detecting moving dots but can identify biological motions from point-light displays (McLeod et al., 1996; Vaina et al., 1990). Consistent with this observation, neurophysiological studies in monkeys provide evidence for cells in STPa that respond selectively to specific body movements (Oram & Perrett, 1994; Perrett et al., 1990). Imaging studies have shown activation in the superior temporal sulcus for biological motion stimuli, such as eye and mouth movements (Puce et al., 1998). Point-light displays of biological motions have also been shown to activate STS (Bonda et al., 1996; Howard et al., 1996). However STS seems to be activated more generally by structure from motion displays rather than selectively by biological motion displays (Howard et al., 1996). Thus cortical specializations for analyzing biological motion may exist in the region of the superior temporal sulcus, but the evidence is still inconclusive. Other regions of the brain may be involved in analyzing specific aspects of the information present in biological motion. For example, Decety et al. (1997) found activation in left frontal and temporal regions for observation of meaningful hand actions and activation of right occipitotemporal regions for meaningless actions. The same studies show that observing actions with the intent to recognize them later activates structures involved in memory encoding, while observing actions with the intent to imitate them activates regions involved in motor planning and execution of actions.

Regions of Cortex Specialized for the Perception of Letters and Words

What evidence is there for a cortical region specifically involved in the visual recognition of words and letters? Is there a localized "lexicon" in the brain, a place where visually presented words make contact with matching stored representations? In an early PET study by Petersen et al. (1990), subjects looked at a fixation cross while words and wordlike stimuli were presented just below. In different scans, subjects viewed sequences of either real English words, like HOUSE, pseudo words like TWEAL, consonant strings like NLPFZ, or "false fonts" (strings of unfamiliar letter-like stimuli). The activation that resulted from each of these four conditions was separately compared to that resulting from looking at a fixation point alone. Petersen et al. found a left medial extrastriate area that was significantly more active for words and pseudo words compared to fixation, but not for consonant strings and false fonts compared to fixation.

Petersen et al. argued that because this extrastriate area responded similarly to real words like HOUSE and pseudo words like TWEAL, it is unlikely to be involved in processing the meanings of words. Nor does the area seem to qualify as a visual "lexicon": HOUSE should have an entry in the mental dictionary but TWEAL should not. (Note, however, that Petersen et al. did not directly compare the word and pseudo word conditions, which would have been the strongest way to test for a distinct lexicon.) Petersen et al. suggested that this extrastriate region is a "visual word form area," meaning that it is involved in the visual recognition of words at some processing stage before final recognition of complete words.

Subsequent neuroimaging work on word recognition has not always supported the same role for the region of extrastriate cortex described by Petersen et al. Howard et al. (1992) and Price et al. (1994) have failed to find extrastriate activation for words when compared to false-font controls (as opposed to fixation-only controls as used by Petersen et al.). Indefrey et al. (1997) suggest string length (or total amount of visual stimulation) is the key to these conflicting results. In a single experiment, they found extrastriate activity for either pseudo words or false-font strings compared to a single false-font character; this activation disappeared for pseudo words compared to length-matched false-font strings. Other evidence suggests a more general visual role for the region in question. For example, Bookheimer et al. (1995) had subjects name pictures and read words either silently or aloud. They found activity (compared to scrambled-object controls) in an extrastriate region near that identified by Petersen et al., but importantly found this activity both for words and for pictures. These authors suggested that the region in question responds to familiar visual forms regardless of the format of the representation.

Some evidence exists for localization of other functions related to word reading. An fMRI study by Polk and Farah (1998) revealed a specific neural response to strings of letters as compared to strings of digits and geometric shapes. This activation was generally observed in left lateral occipitotemporal cortex, though the precise location varied substantially across subjects.

A number of studies have focused on higher-level aspects of reading, such as word pronunciation and semantics. Several studies have converged to suggest a role of the left inferior frontal gyrus in representing both meaning and phonology of words. Petersen et al. (1990) found activity in this region for real words but not pseudo words; activations in this same area from an earlier study (Petersen et al., 1988) during semantic processing tasks suggests it may be involved in retrieval of meaning. Fiez (1997) has reviewed more recent evidence suggesting a division of this region, with more anterior regions reflecting semantic processing and more posterior activations contributing phonological processing.

Other studies have implicated the fusiform gyrus in analysis of word meaning. For example, Nobre et al. (1994) recorded directly from the inferior temporal lobes of patients undergoing evaluation for brain surgery. Two areas with different functional properties were identified on the fusiform gyrus. Both regions responded differently to words than to pictures and texture patterns. A posterior region showed equivalent responses to words and nonwords, suggesting a role in initial segregation of lexical from nonlexical visual input. A more anterior region was sensitive to lexical status as well as semantic context. Responses to words in this region were modulated by whether the words fit the semantic context provided by a preceding sentence.

Thus, while several suggestive results have been published (e.g., Polk & Farah, 1998), the imaging literature has yet to converge on a consensus that specialized regions of cortex exist which are selectively involved in the visual recognition of letters and/or words. This will be a particularly important question to resolve in future research because of its implications for the origins of cortical specialization.

In summary, the evidence from functional brain imaging reviewed in this section strongly supports the existence of several modular components of visual recognition (see color plate 5, figure 5.6): area LO, which is involved in some aspect/s of the analysis of visual object shape; the fusiform face area, which is apparently specialized for face perception; and the parahippocampal place area, implicated in the perception and/or memory encoding of the appearance of places. Further, some evidence suggests that additional areas may exist which are selectively involved in the perception of words and/or letters, as well as areas for perceiving animals, tools, and biological motion. These findings from functional brain imaging dovetail with the results from

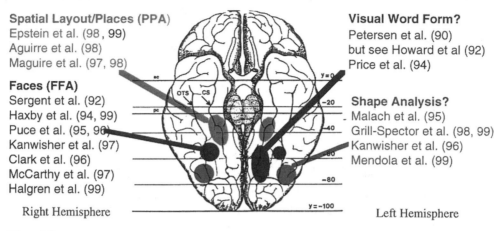

Figure 5.6
A schematic diagram showing the approximate cortical loci of some of the functionally localized components of visual recognition, including area LO, the FFA, the PPA, and the "visual word form area," with representative references to functional imaging studies supporting each (see text). Line drawing of ventral view of brain adapted from Allison et al. (1994). (See color plate 5.)

neuropsychology. Collectively, they suggest that visual recognition is accomplished not by way of a single general-purpose system, but instead through the operation of multiple mechanisms, each specialized for the analysis of a different kind of visual information. It will be an important mission of cognitive neuroscience over the next few years to advance this line of research by identifying and functionally characterizing the main modular components of visual recognition.

ISSUES

Implications for Visual Recognition

What are the implications of cortical modularity for theories of visual recognition? Does the selectivity of certain cortical areas for the recognition of different stimulus classes imply that qualitatively distinct processing mechanisms are involved in each? One might argue that special-purpose mechanisms for processing a particular stimulus class would be expected only if the recognition of stimuli from that class poses new computational problems that could not be handled by existing general-purpose mechanisms. Connectionist researchers have noted the computational efficiency gained by the decomposition of a complex function into natural parts (Jacobs et al., 1991; Jacobs, 1997, 1999), and cortical specializations for components of visual recognition are plausible candidates for such task decomposition. If visual cortex is organized in such a computationally principled fashion, then the modular components of the system we discover with functional imaging can be expected to provide important insights about visual recognition.

However, an alternative hypothesis is that visual cortex contains a large number of stimulus-selective regions (like the feature columns in inferotemporal cortex reported by Tanaka, 1997), but that the underlying computations which go on in each of these regions are very similar. On this view, cortical specialization might be found in future for virtually any stimulus class, and these specializations might not, after all, imply qualitative differences in the processing of different stimulus classes. Some support for this interpretation comes from a report (Ishai et al., 1999) that localized regions in human extrastriate cortex responding more strongly to apparently arbitrary categories such as chairs (compared to faces and houses). A critical goal for future research is to determine whether the functional organization of visual recognition is better characterized by such "shallow specialization" or suggests a deeper form of modularity in which each of a small number of functionally specific regions carries out a qualitatively distinct computation in the service of an evolutionarily or experientially fundamental visual process.

Origins of Cortical Specialization

Where do cortical specializations come from? Does the modular organization of visual recognition arise from experience-dependent, self-organizing properties of cortex (Jacobs, 1997, 1999), or are these cortical specializations innately specified? For faces and places, this question is hard to answer because both experiential and evolutionary arguments are plausible. However, preliminary evidence for cortical specializations for visually presented letters (Polk & Farah, 1998) suggests that at least in some cases, experience may be sufficient. Further evidence for experience-induced cortical specialization comes from Logothetis and Pauls (1995), who found that after training monkeys with a specific class of stimuli, small regions in AIT contained cells selectively responsive to these stimuli. An alternative view is that cortical specialization will arise only for perceptual tasks which have been of long-standing importance to our primate ancestors. In *How the Mind Works*, Pinker (1997, p. 315) argues, on the basis of evolutionary considerations, that "There are modules for objects and forces, for animate beings, for artifacts, for minds, and for natural kinds like animals, plants, and minerals ... [and] modes of thought and feeling for danger, contamination, status, dominance, fairness, love, friendship, sexuality, children, relatives, and the self." For the case of visual recognition, it is not yet clear whether it is the experience of the individual or the experience of the species (or both) that is critical for the construction of cortical modules. However, fMRI has opened up new ways to answer this question—for example, searching for cortical modules predicted by one hypothesis or the other (Downing & Kanwisher, 1999).

Beyond Mere Localization: (How) Can fMRI Inform Cognition?

Despite the considerable progress that has been made in functional brain imaging (e.g., the work summarized in the section "The Modular Structure of Visual Recognition," above), it is still true that most of the important insights we have about human visual cognition derive from behavioral work. Is there reason to hope that imaging studies will be able to contribute more significantly to our understanding of visual recognition in the future? In this final section we step back to take a broader look at the ways in which fMRI may be able to address not only visual recognition but also other areas of visual cognition, such as attention, imagery, and perceptual awareness.

In general, we agree with critics who argue that the brain locus of a particular mental process is not in itself of great importance for theories of cognition. However, functional localization need not be an end in itself, but can provide a means to tackle some of the long-standing and classic questions about cognition. Consider, for example, the finding that viewing static photos with implied motion (compared to photos without) produces activity in a particular region of lateral occipital cortex (Kourtzi & Kanwisher, 2000b). The location of this activation is not in itself of great interest. But when combined with a convincing argument that this same region is the human homologue of the well-studied visual area MT/MST (Tootell et al., 1995), the result takes on a whole new meaning. Now the great wealth of knowledge about visual area MT that has resulted from decades of neuroanatomical and physiological work on monkeys becomes directly relevant to the investigation of human perceptual inferences. Thus, when the locus of a particular activation is in a part of the brain about which we already know a great deal from other techniques (or from other imaging studies), the answer to the "where" question is not simply an arbitrary fact, but a powerful connection to a richly relevant literature.

Even when activations land in relatively uncharted cortical territories where the prior literature is less detailed and informative, imaging data have the potential to constrain cognitive theories in other ways that do not rely heavily on the significance of the particular locus of the activation. In this final section we outline the ways in which fMRI may be able to make important contributions to our understanding of visual cognition by (1) discovering the functional components of human visual cognition and characterizing them in detail, (2) identifying the precise stage of processing at which specific phenomena occur, and (3) testing particular cognitive theories by using the signals from brain regions with strong functional specificity as markers for the engagement of those specific functions. These points will be illustrated with recent examples from imaging research on visual attention, mental imagery, and perception without awareness.

Discovering Functional Components   One of the most fundamental questions one can ask about human cognition concerns the functional architecture of the mind: What are its basic components, and what does each of them do? Thus, many core questions about human cognition are of the following form: Is mental process A distinct from mental process B, or do the two processes share underlying mechanisms? Over the last few decades, experimental psychologists have developed a number of elegant techniques to address such questions. Brain imaging presents yet another tool, enabling us to tackle these questions by asking whether common or distinct brain areas are engaged in different tasks. For example, the evidence on the face area described previously suggests that different neural (and hence presumably cognitive) mechanisms are involved in the perception of faces and objects. While this result was anticipated on the basis of many other sources of evidence that predated functional brain imaging, the imaging data serve at the very least to strengthen the evidence for this dissociation. Further, the discovery of the parahippocampal place area demonstrates that fMRI can be used to discover new functional components of the mind/brain that few would have predicted. But beyond strengthening the evidence for long anticipated cognitive/cortical modules and discovering unanticipated new ones, we can also use fMRI to test for the existence of cognitive mechanisms about which current cognitive theories make contrasting predictions. This point is illustrated with the example of a recent study from our lab.

VISUAL ATTENTION: ONE THING OR MANY?   Hundreds of papers and decades of behavioral research have been devoted to an attempt to understand visual attention. In these experiments, participants typically carry out one of a wide variety of tasks designed to tax visual attention, from reporting the identities of letters to the side of fixation, to searching an array of colored shapes for the one green square, to watching a very rapid sequence of words presented at the center of gaze while monitoring for the occurrence of a particular word. The very heterogeneity of tasks used to study attention raises an important question: Is visual attention really one general-purpose mechanism, engaged in each of these different tasks, or is it just a term that has been used to stand for a disjunctive set of distinct mechanisms? In his book *The Psychology of Attention*, Hal Pashler (1998:1) argues that "no one knows what attention is, and ... there may even not be an 'it' there to be known about."

fMRI provides a way to test whether there is an "it" of visual attention. Wojciulik and Kanwisher (1999) reasoned that if there is a common visual attentional mechanism which is invoked by a wide variety of attention-requiring tasks, then there should be some place in the brain that should be activated by each of these tasks. Three very different attention-requiring tasks were designed, each of which was compared with a less demanding task that could be carried out on the same stimuli. Participants were then run in all six conditions in a single scanning session. In each voxel of the resulting fMRI data set for each individual, we tested whether a significant activation was found in that voxel for each of the three attentional tasks, each compared to its own identical-stimulus control condition. The key finding was that there was one region (in roughly the same location in the intraparietal sulcus in all seven participants tested) that showed a significant activation in the attention-demanding version of each of the three tasks. In a final comparison, a difficult language task (compared to an easier task carried out on the same stimuli) did not activate the same area. Thus, a part of the brain exists that is active across three very different attention-requiring tasks, but not during a difficult nonvisual task. These data suggest that visual attention may not simply be a collection of distinct special-purpose mechanisms, but instead that a unitary general-purpose attentional mechanism may exist.

This result bears importantly on a question that cognitive psychologists have long wondered about but have not been able to answer satisfactorily with behavioral measures. It suggests in a very concrete way that there is an "it" for visual attention. This work shows that fMRI can be used not only to show when two different processes are distinct (e.g., face recognition versus place recognition), but also to show when several very different tasks are carried out using a common underlying mechanism.

Pinpointing the Stage of Processing at Which a Particular Phenomenon Occurs   An enumeration and characterization of the basic components or modules of the mind is useful, but an understanding of cognition further requires knowledge of how each of these components works and how each becomes engaged during cognition. Our guess is that unless major advances are made in increasing the spatial and temporal resolution of the technique, fMRI will not be sufficient for understanding the internal workings of individual modules. However, it provides a powerful new way to answer a number of classic questions in visual cognition that concern the stage of processing at which a given mental process occurs. Indeed, the direct link to known neuro-anatomy (and physiology) afforded by fMRI enables us to define particular stages of visual processing with greater richness and precision than has been possible before.

We illustrate this point with examples from research on visual attention and mental imagery.

VISUAL ATTENTION   One of the classic questions about visual attention is whether information is selected "early" or "late." The distinction between early and late is notoriously vague, and depends on the perspective of the particular researcher. But with fMRI we can specify particular stages of processing by identifying the particular visual area where an attentional effect is observed. This localization of a particular attentional phenomenon to specific cortical areas further allows us to make the link to the known neuroanatomy and physiology of that area established from animal studies. In this vein, a number of neuroimaging studies have demonstrated clear modulatory effects of visual attention on a variety of extrastriate regions, including area MT/MST and the fusiform face area (O'Craven et al., 1997; Wojciulik et al., 1998; Clark et al., 1997; Beauchamp et al., 1997). Moreover, several groups have reported attentional modulation of processing in human area V1 (e.g., Somers et al., 1999; Gandhi et al., 1999). These effects certainly count as instances of early selection on anyone's definition, thereby providing a clear and crisp answer to one of the most long-standing questions about visual attention.

Of course this result leaves open many further questions. Does attention always select early, or does the stage of selection depend on other factors, as many theorists have suggested? Rees et al. (1997) showed that attentional modulation of activity in MT/MST depends on the processing load of a primary task, as predicted by Lavie's (1995) theory of attention. Another question about the stage of attentional selection may be more difficult to answer with fMRI, however. Early selection is often taken to refer to selection that occurs at short latencies after stimulus onset, rather than selection that happens in anatomical regions early in the processing pathway. The two definitions are not equivalent because feedback from later stages can produce effects in an anatomically early area at a temporally late stage. Currently fMRI does not have sufficient temporal resolution to distinguish these possibilities, but in combination with other techniques, such as ERPs and MEG, it may be possible to answer these questions.

MENTAL IMAGERY   Research on mental imagery (Kosslyn, 1980) has long focused on the question of whether visual mental images are really visual (like percepts) or whether they are more abstract (like propositions). Because behavioral data on this question proved ultimately ambiguous, more recent work has attempted to resolve the matter using the techniques of cognitive neuroscience (Kosslyn, 1994). In particular, Kosslyn has used PET to argue that V1 is activated during visual imagery and that, given the known topographic organization of this cortical area, this finding provides strong evidence for the visual/perceptual nature of the representations underlying mental imagery. In the absence of a clear neutral baseline condition known to involve neither visual processing nor its suppression, such demonstrations remain difficult to interpret. Nonetheless, if these issues could be resolved, activation of retinotopic regions during mental imagery would provide compelling evidence that mental images both share processing machinery with visual perception and, further, involve retinotopically organized representations. Evidence that these regions are not only activated during imagery but also are critical for it comes from demonstrations that disruption of these cortical regions (Farah et al., 1992; Kosslyn et al., 1999) interferes with mental imagery. Together, these findings provide fairly compelling evidence that mental imagery involves topographic cortex (and hence, presumably, imagelike representations). Thus these data constitute one of the strongest cases in which a cognitive question is answered by brain-based data.

Using fMRI Signals as Markers for Particular Processes   When the selectivity of a given area (e.g., for faces or places) is well characterized, then the signal coming from that area can serve as a marker for a particular visual process. This strategy can provide traction on a number of different questions in cognition. Just as single-unit physiologists have used the differential responses of single cells to preferred versus nonpreferred stimuli in various conditions as an indication of whether a particular stimulus is processed, we can use the differential response in a selective region of cortex to preferred versus nonpreferred stimuli (for that region of cortex) to the same end. This technique provides a powerful way to investigate visual attention, by enabling us to answer questions about the processing fate of unattended information.

The same technique can also provide a method for determining whether perception without awareness is possible, a topic of long-standing interest in cognitive psychology. fMRI is particularly useful in approaching this question for two main reasons. First, the dependent measure (fMRI signal intensity in particular regions of the brain) does not direct the subject's attention to the unseen item, a problem that has plagued some behavioral efforts to demonstrate perception without awareness. Second, the neural locus of any activations that occur outside of awareness provides some information about the nature of the information represented.

In one elegant study, for example, Whalen et al. (1998) showed that when masked presentations of emotionally expressive faces are presented to subjects in the scanner, the amygdala produces a stronger activation than when neutral faces are presented, despite the fact that most subjects reported never having seen any expressive faces in the course of the entire experiment. This study nicely demonstrates that some kind of perception without awareness is possible, and further specifies the anatomical locus where the relevant representations are likely to reside. Another impressive study used fMRI responses in motor cortex to demonstrate not only perception but also response selection and even motor planning for unseen stimuli (Dehaene et al., 1998).

In sum, cognitive neuroscientists using fMRI do not have to stop with the "where" question any more than cognitive psychologists measuring reaction times have to stop with the "when" question. fMRI research can transcend the narrow localizationist agenda by using the technique to discover and characterize the fundamental components of cognition, to link these components to known physiology and anatomy, and to watch these components in action as people carry out complex cognitive tasks. The literature reviewed above suggests that visual recognition is likely to be a particularly fertile area for this enterprise because the available evidence suggests a high degree of functional specialization in the neural mechanisms by which it is accomplished.

NOTE

1. We thank Pawan Sinha for this observation.

REFERENCES

Adelson, E. H., & Bergen, J. R. (1991). The plenoptic function and the elements of early vision. In *Computational Models of Visual Processing*, M. Landy and J. A. Movshon, eds., 3–20. Cambridge, MA: MIT Press.

Aguirre, G. K., & D'Esposito, M. (1999). Topographical disorientation: A synthesis and taxonomy. *Brain* 122, 1613–1628.

Aguirre, G. K., Detre, J. A., Alsop, D. C., & D'Esposito, M. (1996). The parahippocampus subserves topographical learning in man. *Cerebral Cortex* 6, 823–829.

Aguirre, G., Singh, R., & D'Esposito, M. (1999). Stimulus inversion and the responses of face and object-sensitive cortical areas. *NeurOreport* 10, 189–194.

Aguirre, G. K., Zarahn, E., & D'Esposito, M. (1998). An area within human ventral cortex sensitive to "building" stimuli: Evidence and implications. *Neuron* 21(2), 373–383.

Allison, T., Ginter, H., McCarthy, G., Nobre, A. C., Puce, A., Luby, M., & Spencer, D. D. (1994). Face recognition in human extrastriate cortex. *Journal of Neurophysiology* 71, 821–825.

Allison, T., Puce, A., Spencer, D. D., & McCarthy, G. (1999). Electrophysiological studies of human face perception. I. Potentials generated in occipitotemporal cortex by face and non-face stimuli. *Cerebral Cortex* 9, 415–430.

Beauchamp, M. S., Cox, R. W., & DeYoe, E. A. (1997). Graded effects of spatial and featural attention on human area MT and associated motion processing areas. *Journal of Neurophysiology* 78(1), 516–520.

Bentin, S., Allison, T., Puce, A., Perez, E., & McCarthy, G. (1996). Electrophysiological studies of face perceptions in humans. *Journal of Cognitive Neuroscience* 8, 551–565.

Biederman, I., & Gerhardstein, P. C. (1993). Recognizing depth-rotated objects: Evidence and conditions for three-dimensional viewpoint invariance. *Journal of Experimental Psychology: Human Perception and Performance* 19, 1162–1182.

Bodamer, J. (1947). Die Prosopagnosie. *Archiv für Psychiatrie und Nervenkrankheiten* 179, 6–53.

Bonda, E., Petrides, M., Ostry, D., & Evans, A. (1996). Specific involvement of human parietal systems and the amygdala in the perception of biological motion. *Journal of Neuroscience* 16, 3737–3744.

Bookheimer, S. Y., Zeffiro, T. A., Blaxton, T., Gaillard, W., & Theodore, W. (1995). Regional cerebral blood flow during object naming and word reading. *Human Brain Mapping* 3, 93–106.

Breiter, H. C., Etcoff, N. L., Whalen, P. J., Kennedy, W. A., Rauch, S. L., Buckner, R. L., Strauss, M. M., Hyman, S. E., & Rosen, B. R. (1996). Response and habituation of the human amygdala during visual processing of facial expression. *Neuron* 17, 875–887.

Brewer, J. B., Zhao, Z., Desmond, J. E., Glover, G. H., & Gabrieli, J. D. E. (1998). Making memories: Brain activity that predicts how well visual experience will be remembered. *Science* 281, 1185–1187.

Bruce, V. (1988). *Recognizing Faces*. London: Erlbaum.

Caramazza, A., & Shelton, J. R. (1998). Domain-specific knowledge systems in the brain: The animate/inanimate distinction. *Journal of Cognitive Neuroscience* 10, 1–34.

Carey, S., & Spelke, E. (1994). Domain-specific knowledge and conceptual change. In *Mapping the Mind*, L. A. Hirschfeld, & S. A. Gelman, eds., Cambridge: Cambridge University Press.

Chao L., Martin, A., & Haxby, J. (1999). Are face-responsive regions selective only for faces? *Neuroreport* 10, 2945–50.

Cheng, K. (1986). A purely geometric module in the rat's spatial representation. *Cognition* 23, 149–178.

Clark, V.P., Keil, K., Maisog, J. M., Courtney, S., Ungerleider, L. G., & Haxby, J. V. (1996). Functional magnetic resonance imaging of human visual cortex during face matching: A comparison with positron emission tomography. *NeuroImage* 4, 1–15.

Clark, V. P., Maisog, J. M., & Haxby, J. V. (1998). fMRI study of face perception and memory using random stimulus sequences. *Journal of Neurophysiology* 79, 3257–3265.

Clark, V. P., Parasuraman, R., Keil, K., Kulansky, R., Fannon, S., Maisog, J. M., Ungerleider, L. G., & Haxby, J. V. (1997). Selective attention to face identity and color studied with fMRI. *Human Brain Mapping* 5, 293–291.

Cutting, J. E. (1987). Perception and information. *Annual Review of Psychology* 38, 61–90.

Cutting, J. E., Proffitt, D. R., & Kozlowski, L. T. (1978). A biomechanical invariant of gait perception. *Journal of Experimental Psychology: Human Perception and Performance* 3, 357–372.

Damasio, A. R., Damasio, H., & VanHoesen, G. W. (1982). Prosopagnosia: Anatomic basis and behavioral mechanisms. *Neurology* 32, 331–341.

Damasio, A. R., Tranel, D., & Damasio, H. (1990). Face agnosia and the neural substrates of memory. *Annual Review of Neuroscience* 13, 89–109.

Damasio, H., Grabowski, T. J., Tranel, D., Hichwa, R. D., & Damasio, A. R. (1996). A neural basis for lexical retrieval. *Nature* 380, 499–505.

Davidoff, J., & Warrington, E. K. (1993). A dissociation of shape discrimination and figure-ground perception in a patient with normal acuity. *Neuropsychologia* 31, 83–93.

Decety, J., Grezes, J., Costes, N., Perani, D., Jeannerod, M., Procyk, E., Gassi, F., & Fazio, F. (1997). Brain activity during observation of actions: Influence of action content and subject's strategy. *Brain* 120, 1763–1776.

De Gelder, B., & Kanwisher, N. (1999). Absence of a fusiform face area in a prosopagnosic patient. Abstract for the Human Brain Mapping Conference.

Dehaene, S., Naccache, L., Le Clec, H. G., Koechlin, E., Mueller, M., Dehaene-Lambertz, G., van de Moortele, P. F., & Le Bihan, D. (1998). Imaging unconscious semantic priming. *Nature* 395, 597–600.

De Renzi, E. (1986). Current issues in prosopagnosia. In *Aspects of Face Processing*, H. D. Ellis, M. A. Jeeves, F. Newcombe, & A. W. Young, eds. Dordrecht, Netherlands: Martinus Nijhoff.

De Renzi, E., & Lucchelli, F. (1993). The fuzzy boundaries of apperceptive agnosia. *Cortex* 29, 187–215.

Diamond, R., & Carey, S. (1986). Why faces are and are not special: An effect of expertise. *Journal of Experimental Psychology: General* 115(2), 107–117.

Dittrich, W. H. (1993). Action categories and the perception of biological motion. *Perception* 22, 15–22.

Downing, P., & Kanwisher, N. (1999). Where do critical modules come from? Supplement of Journal of Cognitive Neuroscience, p. 89.

Dubois, S., Rossion, B., Schiltz, C., Bodart, J. M., Michel, C., Bruyer, R., & Crommelinck, M. (1999). Effect of familiarity on the processing of human faces. *NeuroImage* 9, 278–289.

Edwards, G. J., Taylor, C. J., & Cootes, T. F. (1998). Learning to identify and track faces in image sequences. In *Proceedings of the Third IEEE International Conference on Automatic Face and Gesture Recognition, Nara, Japan.*

Ellis, R., Allport, D. A., Humphreys, G. W., & Collis, J. (1989). Varieties of object constancy. *Quarterly Journal of Experimental Psychology* 41A, 775–796.

Epstein, R., Harris, A., Stanley, D., & Kanwisher, N. (1999). The parahippocampal place area: Recognition, navigation, or encoding? *Neuron* 23, 115–125.

Epstein, R., & Kanwisher, N. (1998). A cortical representation of the local visual environment. *Nature* 392, 598–601.

Farah, M. J. (1990). *Visual Agnosia: Disorders of Object Recognition and What They Tell Us About Normal Vision.* Cambridge, MA: MIT Press.

Farah, M. (1992). Is an object an object an object? *Current Directions in Psychological Science* 1, 164–169.

Farah, M. J. (1994). Neuropsychological inference with an interactive brain: A critique of the locality assumption. *Behavioral and Brain Sciences* 17(1), 43–61.

Farah, M. (1997). Distinguishing perceptual and semantic impairments affecting visual object recognition. *Visual Cognition* 2, 207–218.

Farah, M., & McClelland, J. L. (1991). A computational model of semantic memory impairment: Modality specificity and emergent category specificity. *Journal of Experimental Psychology: General* 120(4), 339–357.

Farah, M. J., Meyer, M. M., & McMullen, P. A. (1996). The living/nonliving dissociation is not an artifact: Giving a prior implausible hypothesis a strong test. *Cognitive Neuropsychology* 13, 137–154.

Farah, M. J., Soso, M. J., & Dasheiff, R. M. (1992). Visual angle of the mind's eye before and after unilateral occipital lobectomy. *Journal of Experimental Psychology: Human Perception and Performance* 18, 241–246.

Fiez, J. A. (1997). Phonology, semantics, and the role of the left inferior prefrontal cortex. *Human Brain Mapping* 5, 79–83.

Fried, I., MacDonald, K., & Wilson, C. (1997). Single neuron activity in human hippocampus and amygdala during recognition of faces and objects. *Neuron* 18, 753–765.

Gandhi, S. P., Heeger, D., & Boynton, G. M. (1999). Spatial attention affects brain activity in human primary visual cortex. *Proceedings of the National Academy of Sciences USA* 96, 3314–3319.

Gauthier, I., Anderson, A. W., Tarr, M. J., Skudlarski, P., & Gore, J. C. (1997). Levels of categorization in visual recognition studied using functional magnetic resonance imaging. *Current Biology* 7(9), 645–651.

Gauthier, I., Behrmann, M., & Tarr, M. (1999a). Can face recognition really be dissociated from object recognition? *Journal of Cognitive Neuroscience* 11, 349–371.

Gauthier, I., Tarr, M. J., Anderson, A., Skudlarski, P., & Gore, J. (1999b). Activation of the middle fusiform "face area" increases with expertise in recognizing novel objects. *Nature Neuroscience*, 2, 568–573.

Gauthier, I., Tarr, M. J., Anderson, A. W., Skudlarski, P., & Gore, J. (2000a). Does visual subordinate-level categorization engage the functionally-defined fusiform face area? *Cognitive Neuropsychology* 17, 143–164.

George, N., Dolan, R. J., Fink, G. R., Baylis, G. C., Russell, C., & Driver, J. (1999). Contrast polarity and face recognition in the human fusiform gyrus. *Nature Neuroscience* 2, 574–580.

Gorno Tempini, M. L., Price, C. J., Josephs, O., Vandenberghe, R., Cappa, S. F., Kapur, N., & Frackowiak, R. S. (1998). The neural systems sustaining face and proper-name processing. *Brain* 121, 2103–2118.

Grill-Spector, K., Kushnir, T., Edelman, S., Avidan-Carmel, G., Itzchak, Y., & Malach, R. (1999). Differential processing of objects under various viewing conditions in the human lateral occipital complex. *Neuron* 24, 187–203.

Grill-Spector, K., Kushnir, T., Edelman, S., Itzchak, Y., & Malach, R. (1998). Cue-invariant activation in object-related areas of the human occipital lobe. *Neuron* 21(1), 191–202.

Grill-Spector, K., Kushnir, T., Hendler, T., Edelman, S., Itzchak, Y., & Malach, R. (1998). A sequence of object-processing stages revealed by fMRI in the human occipital lobe. *Human Brain Mapping* 6(4), 316–328.

Gross, C. G., Roche-Miranda, G. E., & Bender, D. B. (1972). Visual properties of neurons in the infero-temporal cortex of the macaque. *Journal of Neurophysiology* 35, 96–111.

Habib, M., & Sirigu, A. (1987). Pure topographical disorientation: A definition and anatomical basis. *Cortex* 23, 73–85.

Halgren, E., Dale, A. M., Sereno, M. I., Tootell, R. B. H., Marinkovic, K., & Rosen, B. R. (1999). Location of human face-selective cortex with respect to retinotopic areas. *Human Brain Mapping* 7, 29–37.

Hallinan, P. L., Gordon, G. G., Yuille, A. L., Giblin, P. J., & Mumford, D. B. (1999). Two- and three-dimensional patterns of the face. Natwick, Mass.: A. K. Peters.

Haxby, J. V., Grady, C. L., Horwitz, B., Ungerleider, L. G., Mishkin, M., Carson, R. E., Herscovitch, P., Schapiro, M. B., & Rapoport, S. I. (1991). Dissociation of spatial and object visual processing pathways in human extrastriate cortex. *Proceedings of the National Academy of Sciences USA* 88, 1621–1625.

Haxby, J. V., Horwitz, B., Ungerleider, L. G., Maisog, J. M., Pietrini, P., & Grady, C. L. (1994). The functional organization of human extrastriate cortex: A PET-fCBF study of selective attention to faces and locations. *Journal of Neuroscience* 14, 6336–6353.

Haxby, J. V., Ungerleider, L. G., Clark, V. P., Schouten, J. L., Hoffman, E. A., & Martin, A. (1999). The effect of face inversion on activity in human neural systems for face and object perception. *Neuron* 22, 189–199.

Haxby, J. V., Ungerleider, L. G., Horwitz, B., Maisog, J. M., Rapoport, S. I., & Grady, C. L. (1996). Face encoding and recognition in the human brain. *Proceedings of the National Academy of Sciences USA* 93, 922–927.

Hermer, L., & Spelke, E. S. (1994). A geometric process for spatial reorientation in young children. *Nature* 370, 57–59.

Hillis, A. E., & Caramazza, A. (1991). Category-specific naming and comprehension impairment: A double dissociation. *Brain* 114, 2081–2094.

Hillis, A. E., & Caramazza, A. (1995). Cognitive and neural mechanisms underlying visual and semantic processing: Implications from "optic aphasia." *Journal of Cognitive Neuroscience* 7, 457–478.

Hoffman, E. A., & Haxby, J. V. (2000). Distinct representations of eye gaze and identity in the distributed human neural system for face perception. *Nature Neuroscience*, 3, 80–84.

Hotta, K., Kurita, T., & Mishima, T. (1998). Scale invariant face detection method using higher-order local autocorrelation features extracted from log-polar image. In *Proceedings of the Third IEEE International Conference on Automatic Face and Gesture Recognition, Nara, Japan.*

Howard, D., Patterson, K., Wise, R., Brown, W. D., Friston, K., Weiller, C., & Frackowiak, R. (1992). The cortical localization of the lexicons: Positron emission tomography evidence. *Brain* 115, 1769–1782.

Howard, R. J., Brammer, M., Wright, I., Woodruff, P. W., Bullmore, E. T., & Zeki, S. (1996). A direct demonstration of functional specialization within motion-related visual and auditory cortex of the human brain. *Current Biology* 6, 1015–1019.

Humphrey, K. G., Symons, L. A., Herbert, A. M., & Goodale, M. A. (1996). A neurological dissociation between shape from shading and shape from edges. *Behavioral Brain Research* 76, 117–125.

Humphreys, G. W., & Bruce, V. (1989). *Visual Cognition*. Hillsdale, NJ: Lawrence Erlbaum.

Humphreys, G. W., & Riddoch, J. (1987). *To See but Not to See: A Case Study of Visual Agnosia*. London: Lawrence Erlbaum.

Indefrey, P., Kleinschmidt, A., Merboldt, K.-D., Krüger, G., Brown, C., Hagoort, P., & Frahm, J. (1997). Equivalent responses to lexical and nonlexical visual stimuli in occipital cortex: A functional magnetic resonance imaging study. *NeuroImage* 5, 78–81.

Ishai, A., Ungerleider, L., Martin, A., Schouten, J. L., & Haxby, J. V. (1999). Distributed representation of objects in the human ventral visual pathway. *Proceedings of the National Academy of Sciences USA* 96, 9379–9384.

Jacobs, R. A. (1997). Nature, nurture, and the development of functional specializations: A computational approach. *Psychological Bulletin & Review* 4, 299–309.

Jacobs, R. A. (1999). Computational studies of the development of functionally specialized neural modules. *Trends in Cognitive Sciences* 3, 31–38.

Jacobs, R. A., Jordan, M. I., & Barto, A. G. (1991). Task decomposition through competition in a modular connectionist architecture: The what and where vision tasks. *Cognitive Science* 15, 219–250.

Jeffreys, D. A. (1996). Evoked potential studies of face and object processing. *Visual Cognition* 3, 1–38.

Johansson, G. (1973). Visual perception of biological motion and a model for its analysis. *Perception & Psychophysics* 14, 201–211.

Kanwisher, N. (2000). Domain specificity in face perception. *Nature Neuroscience*, 3, 759–763.

Kanwisher, N., McDermott, J., & Chun, M. M. (1997). The fusiform face area: A module in human extrastriate cortex specialized for face perception. *Journal of Neuroscience* 17, 4302–4311.

Kanwisher, N., Stanley, D., & Harris, A. (1999). The fusiform face area is selective for faces not animals. *NeuroReport* 10(1), 183–187.

Kanwisher, N., Tong, F., & Nakayama, K. (1998). The effect of face inversion on the human fusiform face area. *Cognition* 68, B1–B11.

Kanwisher, N., Woods, R., Iacoboni, M., & Mazziotta, J. (1996). A locus in human extrastriate cortex for visual shape analysis. *Journal of Cognitive Neuroscience* 91, 133–142.

Kelley, W. M., Miezin, F. M., McDermott, K. B., Buckner, R. L., Raichle, M. E., Cohen, N. J., Ollinger, J. M., Akbudak, E., Conturo, T. E., Snyder, A. Z., & Peterson, S. E. (1998). Hemispheric specialization in human dorsal frontal cortex and medial temporal lobe for verbal and nonverbal memory encoding. *Neuron* 20, 927–936.

Köhler, S., Kapur, S., Moscovitch, M., Winocur, G., & Houle, S. (1995). Dissociation of pathways for object and spatial vision: A PET study in humans. *NeuroReport* 6, 1865–1868.

Kosslyn, S. M. (1980). *Image and Mind*. Cambridge, MA: Harvard University Press.

Kosslyn, S. M. (1994). *Image and Brain*. Cambridge, MA: MIT Press.

Kosslyn, S. M., Pascual-Leone, A., Felician, O., Camposano, S., Keenan, J. P., Thompson, W. L., Ganis, G., Sukel, K. E., & Alpert, N. M. (1999). The role of area 17 in visual imagery: Convergent evidence from PET and rTMS [see comments] [published erratum appears in *Science* 1999, 284, 197]. *Science* 284, 167–170.

Kourtzi, Z., & Kanwisher, N. (2000a). Cortical regions involved in perceiving object shape. *Journal of Neuroscience*, 20, 3310–3318.

Kourtzi, Z., & Kanwisher, N. (2000b). Activation in human MT/MST for static images with implied motion. *Journal of Cognitive Neuroscience* 12, 48–55.

Kozlowski, L. T., & Cutting, J. E. (1977). Recognizing the sex of a walker from a dynamic point-light display. *Perception & Psychophysics* 21, 575–580.

Kroll, J. F., & Potter, M. C. (1984). Recognizing words, pictures, and concepts: A comparison of lexical, object, and reality decisions. *Journal of Verbal Learning and Verbal Behavior* 23, 39–66.

Lambon Ralph, M. A., Sage, K., & Ellis, A. W. (1996). Word meaning blindness: A new form of acquired dyslexia. *Cognitive Neuropsychology* 13, 617.

Landis, T., Cummings, J. L., Benson, D. F., & Palmer, E. P. (1986). Loss of topographic familiarity: An environmental agnosia. *Archives of Neurology* 43, 132–136.

Lavie, N. (1995). Perceptual load as a necessary condition for selective attention. *Journal of Experimental Psychology: Human Perception and Performance* 21, 51–68.

Liu, J., Higuchi, M., Marantz, A., & Kanwisher, N. (2000). The selectivity of the occipitotemporal M170 for faces. *Neuroreport*, 11, 337–341.

Logothetis, N. K., & Pauls, J. (1995). Psychophysical and physiological evidence for viewer-centered object representations in the primate. *Cerebral Cortex* 3, 270–288.

Logothetis N., Pauls, J., Bülthoff, H. H., & Poggio, T. (1994). Viewpoint-dependent object recognition by monkeys. *Current Biology* 4, 401–414.

Logothetis N., Pauls, J., & Poggio, T. (1995). Shape representation in the inferior temporal cortex of monkeys. *Current Biology* 5, 552–563.

Maguire, E. A., Burgess, N., Donnett, J. G., Frackowiak, R. S. J., Frith, C. D., & O'Keefe, J. (1998). Knowing where and getting there: A human navigational network. *Science* 280, 921–924.

Maguire, E. A., Frackowiak, R. S. J., & Frith, C. D. (1997). Recalling routes around London: Activation of the right hippocampus in taxi drivers. *Journal of Neuroscience* 17, 7103–7110.

Maguire, E. A., Frith, C. D., Burgess, N., Donnett, J. G., & O'Keefe, J. (1998). Knowing where things are: Parahippocampal involvement in encoding object locations in virtual large-scale space. *Journal of Cognitive Neuroscience* 10, 61–76.

Malach, R., Grill-Spector, K., Kushnir, T., Edelman, S., & Itzchak, Y. (1998). Rapid shape adaptation reveals position and size invariance. *NeuroImage* 7, S43.

Malach, R., Reppas, J. B., Benson, R. R., Kwong, K. K., Jiang, H., Kennedy, W. A., Ledden, P. J., Brady, T. J., Rosen, B. R., Tootell, R. B. H. (1995). Object-related activity revealed by functional magnetic resonance imaging in human occipital cortex. *Proceedings of the National Academy of Sciences USA* 92, 8135–8139.

Marey, E. J. (1895/1972). *Movement*. New York: Arno Press New York Times. (Originally published in 1895.)

Marr, D. (1982). *Vision*. San Francisco: W. H. Freeman.

Martin, A., Wiggs, C. L., Ungerleider, L. G., & Haxby, J. V. (1996). Neural correlates of category-specific knowledge. *Nature* 379, 649–652.

McCarthy, G., Puce, A., Gore J., & Allison, T. (1997). Face-specific processing in the human fusiform gyrus. *Journal of Cognitive Neuroscience* 9, 605–610.

McLeod, P., Dittrich, W., Driver, J., Perrett, D., & Zihl, J. (1996). Preserved and impaired detection of structure from motion by a "motion-blind" patient. *Visual Cognition* 3, 363–391.

Mendola, J. D., Dale, A. M., Fischl, B., Liu, A. K., & Tootell, R. B. H. (1999). The representation of real and illusory contours in human cortical visual areas revealed by fMRI. *Journal of Neuroscience* 19, 8540–8572.

Morris, J. S., Frith, C. D., Derrett, D. I., Rowland, D., Young, A. W., Calder, A. J., & Dolan, R. J. (1996). A different neural response in the human amygdala to fearful or happy facial expressions. *Nature* 383, 812–815.

Moscovitch, M., Winocur, G., & Behrmann, M. (1997). What is special about face recognition? Nineteen experiments on a person with visual object agnosia and dyslexia but normal face recognition. *Journal of Cognitive Neuroscience* 9, 555–604.

Nobre, A. C., Allison, T., & McCarthy, G. (1994). Word recognition in the human inferior temporal lobe. *Nature* 372, 260–263.

O'Craven, K. M., Rosen, B. R., Kwong, K. K., Treisman, A., & Savoy, R. L. (1997). Voluntary attention modulates fMRI activity in human MT-MST. *Neuron* 18, 591–598.

Oram, M. W., & Perrett, D. I. (1994). Responses of anterior superior temporal polysensory (STPa) neurons to "biological motion" stimuli. *Journal of Cognitive Neuroscience* 6, 99–116.

Pashler, H. E. (1998). *The Psychology of Attention*. Cambridge, MA: MIT Press.

Perrett, D. I., Harries, M., Mistlin, A. J., & Chitty, A. J. (1990). Three stages in the classification of body movements by visual neurons. In *Images and Understanding*, H. B. Barlow & M. Weston-Smith, eds., 94–107. Cambridge: Cambridge University Press.

Perrett, D. I., Rolls, E. T., & Caan, W. (1982). Visual neurones responsive to faces in the monkey temporal cortex. *Experimental Brain Research* 47, 329–342.

Petersen, S. E., Fox, P. T., Posner, M. I., Mintun, M. A., & Raichle, M. E. (1988). Positron emission tomographic studies of the cortical anatomy of single-word processing. *Nature* 331, 585–589.

Petersen, S. E., Fox, P. T., Snyder, A. Z., & Raichle, M. E. (1990). Activation of extrastriate and frontal cortical areas by visual words and word-like stimuli. *Science* 249, 1041–1044.

Phillips, M. L., Young, A. W., Senior, C., Brammer, M., Andrews, C., Calder, A. J., Bullmore, E. T., Perrett, D. I., Rowland, D., Williams, S. C. R., Gray, J. A., & David, A. S. (1997). A specific neural substrate for perceiving facial expressions of disgust. *Nature* 389, 495–498.

Pinker, S. (1997). *How the Mind Works*. New York: W. W. Norton.

Polk, T. A., & Farah, M. (1998). The neural development and organization of letter recognition: Evidence from functional neuroimaging, computational modeling, and behavioral studies. *Proceedings of the National Acadency of Sciences USA* 95(3), 847–852.

Potter, M. C. (1976). Short-term conceptual memory for pictures. *Journal of Experimental Psychology: Human Learning and Memory* 5, 509–522.

Price, C. J., Wise, R. J. S., Watson, J. D. G., Patterson, K., Howard, D., & Frackowiak, R. S. J. (1994). Brain activity during reading: The effects of exposure duration and task. *Brain* 117, 1255–1269.

Puce, A., Allison, T., Asgari, M., Gore, J. C., & McCarthy, G. (1996). Differential sensitivity of human visual cortex to faces, letter strings, and textures: A functional magnetic resonance imaging study. *Journal of Neuroscience* 16, 5205–5215.

Puce, A., Allison, T., Bentin, S., Gore, J. C., & McCarthy, G. (1998). Temporal cortex activation in human subjects viewing eye and mouth movements. *Journal of Neuroscience* 18, 2188–2199.

Puce, A., Allison, T., Gore, J. C., & McCarthy, G. (1995). Face-sensitive regions in human extrastriate cortex studied by functional MRI. *Journal of Neurophysiology* 74, 1192–1199.

Rees, G., Frith, C. D., & Lavie, N. (1997). Modulating irrelevant motion perception by varying attentional load in an unrelated task. *Science* 278, 1616–1619.

Riddoch, J., & Humphreys, G. W. (1987). Visual object processing in optic aphasia: A case of semantic access agnosia. *Cognitive Neuropsychology* 4, 131–185.

Rowley, H. A., Baluja, S., & Kanade, T. (1995) *Human Face Detection in Visual Scenes*. CMU-CS-95-158R. Pittsburgh: Carnegie-Mellon University.

Rumiati, R. I., Humphreys, G. W., Riddoch, M. J., & Bateman, A. (1994). Visual object agnosia without prosopagnosia or alexia: Evidence for hierarchical theories of visual recognition. *Visual Cognition* 1, 181–225.

Sams, M., Hietanen, J. K., Hari, R., Ilmoniemi, R. J., & Lounasmaa, O. V. (1997). Face-specific responses from the human inferior occipito-temporal cortex. *Neuroscience* 1, 49–55.

Sartori, G., & Job, R. (1988). The oyster with 4 legs: A neuropsychological study on the interaction of visual and semantic information. *Cognitive Neuropsychology* 5(1), 105–132.

Sergent, J., Ohta, S., & MacDonald, B. (1992). Functional neuroanatomy of face and object processing: A positron emission tomography study. *Brain* 115, 15–36.

Sergent, J., & Signoret, J. L. (1992). Varieties of functional deficits in prosopagnosia. *Cerebral Cortex* 2(5), 375–388.

Shakunaga, T., Ogawa, K., & Oki, S. (1998). Integration of eigentemplate and structure matching for automatic facial feature detection. In *Proceedings of the Third IEEE International Conference on Automatic Face and Gesture Recognition, Nara, Japan.*

Shallice, T. (1988). *From Neuropsychology to Mental Structure.* Cambridge: Cambridge University Press.

Sheridan, J., & Humphreys, G. W. (1993). A verbal-semantic category-specific recognition impairment. *Cognitive Neuropsychology* 10(2), 143–184.

Silveri, M. C., & Gainotti, G. (1988). Interaction between vision and language in category-specific semantic impairment. *Cognitive Neuropsychology* 5(6), 677–709.

Somers, D. C., Dale, A. M., Seiffert, A. E., & Tootell, R. B. H. (1999). Functional MRI reveals spatially specific attentional modulation in human primary visual cortex. *Proceedings of the National Academy of Sciences USA* 96, 1663–1668.

Stern, C. E., Corkin, S., Gonzalez, R. G., Guimaraes, A. R., Baker, J. R., Jennings, P. J., Carr, C. A., Sugiura, R. M., Vedantham, V., & Rosen, B. R. (1996). The hippocampal formation participates in novel picture encoding: Evidence from functional magnetic resonance imaging. *Proceedings of the National Academy USA* 93, 8660–8665.

Tanaka, J. W., & Farah, M. J. (1993). Parts and wholes in face recognition. *Quarterly Journal of Experimental Psychology* A46, 225–245.

Tanaka, K. (1997). Mechanisms of visual object recognition: Monkey and human studies. *Current Opinion in Neurobiology* 7, 523–529.

Tarr, M. J., & Bülthoff, H. H. (1995). Is human object recognition better described by geon structural descriptions or by multiple views? Comment on Biederman & Gerhardstein 1993. *Journal of Experimental Psychology: Human Perception and Performance* 21, 1494–1505.

Tarr, M. J., & Gauthier, I. (2000). FFA: A flexible fusiform area for subordinate-level visual processing automatized by expertise. *Nature Neuroscience,* 3, 764–769.

Thorpe, S., Fize, D., & Marlot, C. (1996). Speed of processing in the human visual system. *Nature* 381, 520–522.

Tong, F., Nakayama, K., Moscovitch, M., Weinrib, O., & Kanwisher, N. (2000). Response properties of the human fusiform face area. *Cognitive Neuropsychology* 17, 257–279.

Tong, F., Nakayama, K., Vaughan, J. T., & Kanwisher, N. (1998). Binocular rivalry and visual awareness in human extrastriate cortex. *Neuron* 21, 753–759.

Tootell, R. B. H., Reppas, J. B., Kwong, K. K., Malach, R., Brady, T., Rosen, B., & Belliveau, J. (1995). Functional analysis of human MT/V5 and related visual cortical areas using magnetic resonance imaging. *Journal of Neuroscience* 15(4), 3215–3230.

Tovee, M. J., Rolls, E. T., Treves, A., & Bellis, R. P. (1993). Information encoding and the responses of single neurons in the primate temporal visual cortex. *Journal of Neurophysiology* 70(2), 640–654.

Tranel, D., Damasio, H., & Damasio, A. R. (1997). A neural basis for the retrieval of conceptual knowledge. *Neuropsychologia* 35, 1319–1327.

Ullman, S. (1996). *High-level Vision.* Cambridge, MA: MIT Press.

Ullman S., & Basri, R. (1991). Recognition by linear combinations of models. *IEEE Trans Patt Anal and Mach Intel* 13, 992–1006.

Vaina, L. M., Lemay, M., Bienfang, D. C., Choi, A. Y., & Nakayama, K. (1990). Intact "biological motion" and "structure from motion" perception in a patient with impaired motion mechanisms: A case study. *Visual Neuroscience* 5, 353–369.

Wagner, A. D., Schacter, D. L., Rotte, M., Koutstaal, W., Maril, A., Dale, A. M., Rosen, B. R., & Buckner, R. L. (1998). Building memories: Remembering and forgetting of verbal experiences as predicted by brain activity. *Science* 281, 1188–1191.

Warrington, E. (1985). The impairment of object recognition. In *Handbook of Clinical Neurology: Clinical Neuropsychology*, J. A. M. Frederiks, ed. Amsterdam: Elsevier.

Warrington, E. K., & Shallice, T. (1984). Category-specific semantic impairments. *Brain* 107, 829–854.

Warrington, E. K., & Taylor, A. M. (1978). Two categorical stages of object recognition. *Perception* 7, 695–705.

Whalen, P. J., Rauch, S. L., Etcoff, N. L., McInerney, S. C., Lee, M. B., & Jenike, M. A. (1998). Masked presentations of emotional facial expressions modulate amygdala activity without explicit knowledge. *Journal of Neuroscience* 18, 411–418.

Wicker, B., Michel, F., Henaff, M. A., & Decety, J. (1998). Brain regions involved in the perception of gaze: A PET study. *NeuroImage* 8, 221–227.

Wojciulik, E., & Kanwisher, N. (1999). The generality of parietal involvement in visual attention. *Neuron* 4, 747–764.

Wojciulik, E., Kanwisher, N., & Driver, J. (1998). Modulation of activity in the fusiform face area by covert attention: An fMRI study. *Journal of Neurophysiology* 79, 1574–1579.

Yang, G. Z., & Huang, T. S. (1994). Human face detection in a complex background. *Pattern Recognition* 27, 53–63.

Yin, R. K. (1969). Looking at upside-down faces. *Journal of Experimental Psychology* 81, 141–145.

6 Functional Neuroimaging of Semantic Memory

Alex Martin

INTRODUCTION

It is now well recognized that memory is not a single, all-purpose, monolithic system, but rather is composed of multiple systems. Prominent among these systems is semantic memory (e.g., Tulving, 1983). "Semantic memory" refers to a broad domain of cognition composed of knowledge acquired about the world, including facts, concepts, and beliefs. In comparison to episodic or autobiographical memory, it consists of memories that are shared by members of a culture rather than those which are unique to an individual and are tied to a specific time and place. For example, whereas remembering what you had for breakfast yesterday is dependent on episodic memory, knowing the meaning of the word "breakfast" is dependent on semantic memory. Thus one component of semantic memory is the information stored in our brains about the meanings of objects and words.

Meaning, however, has proved to be a fairly intractable problem, especially regarding the meaning of words. One important reason why this is so is that words have multiple meanings. To cite one extreme example, the *Oxford English Dictionary* lists 96 entries for the word "run." The specific meaning of a word is determined by context, and comprehension is possible because we have contextual representations (see Miller, 1999, for a discussion of lexical semantics and context). One way to begin to get traction on the problem of meaning in the brain is to limit inquiry to concrete objects as represented by pictures and by their names (in which case the names are presented in a context that makes the reference clear (e.g., that "dog" refers to a four-legged animal, not a contemptible person).

Consider, for example, the most common meaning of two concrete objects, a camel and a wrench. Camel is defined as "either of two species of large, domesticated ruminants (genus camelus) with a humped back, long neck, and large cushioned feet"; wrench is defined as "any number of tools used for holding and turning nuts, bolts, pipes, etc." (*Webster's New World Dictionary*, 1988). Two things are noteworthy about these definitions. First, they are largely about features: camels are large and have a humped back, and wrenches hold and turn things. Second, different types of features are emphasized for different types of objects. The definition of the camel consists of information about its visual appearance, whereas the definition of the wrench emphasizes how it is used. I will return to this difference later in this chapter. For now, it should be noted that differences in the types of features that define different objects have played, and continue to play, a central role in thinking about disorders of semantic memory and in models of how semantic memory is organized in the human brain.

Another point about these brief definitions is that they include only part, perhaps only a small part, of the information we may possess about these objects. For example, we may know that camels are found primarily in Asia and Africa, that they are known as the "ships of the desert," and that the word "camel" can refer to a color as well as to a brand of cigarettes. Similarly, we also know that camels are larger than a bread box and weigh less than a 747 jumbo jet. Clearly, this information is also part of semantic memory. Unfortunately, little, if anything, is known about the brain bases of these associative and inferential processes. We are, however, beginning to gain insights into the functional neuroanatomy associated with our ability to identify objects and to retrieve information about specific object features and attributes. These topics will be the central focus of this review.

The chapter is divided into four main sections. In the first, I define semantic representations and review data from patients with selective but global (i.e., nonspecific) impairments of semantic memory. In the second, I review studies which show that many semantic tasks activate a broad network of cortical regions, most of which are lateralized to the left hemisphere. Prominent components of this network are the ventral and lateral surfaces of the temporal lobes. The third section concentrates on studies on retrieving information about specific features and attributes of objects. The results of these studies suggest that different regions of temporal cortex are active depending on the nature of the information retrieved. The final section concentrates on object category specificity, especially studies contrasting activity associated with animals and tools as represented by pictures and words. These studies suggest that object semantic representations consist of networks of discrete cortical regions ranging from occipital to left premotor cortices. The organization of these sites seems to parallel the organization of sensory and motor systems in the human brain. These networks may provide neurobiologically plausible mechanisms that function in the service of referential meaning.

Background

A semantic representation of an object is defined as the information stored in our brains which defines that object as a distinct entity (i.e., as a specific animal, food, item of furniture, tool, etc.). This information will include information shared by other category members, as well as information that makes it distinct from other exemplars of the same category. Thus the semantic representation of a particular object would include information about the object's typical shape. In addition, depending on the object, the semantic representation could include information about other visual attributes, such as color and motion, as well as features derived through other sensory modalities, and through visuomotor experience with the object. Finally, activation of these representations is dependent on an item's meaning, not on the physical format of the stimulus denoting that object. For example, the semantic representation of "dog" would be activated by a picture of a dog, the written word "dog," the heard name "dog," the sound of a dog's bark, or simply thinking about dogs. It is this claim that defines the representation as semantic. Thus, central to this model are the claims that there is a single semantic system which is accessed through multiple sensory channels, and that activation of at least part of the semantic representation of an object is automatic and obligatory.

A central question for investigators interested in the functional neuroanatomy of semantic memory is to determine where this information is represented in the brain. One particularly influential idea, and one that has guided much of my own work on this topic, is that the features and attributes which define an object are stored in the perceptual and motor systems active when we first learned about that object. Thus, for example, information about the visual form of an object, its typical color, its unique pattern of motion, would be stored in or near regions of the visual system that mediate perception of form, color, and motion. Similarly, knowledge about the sequences of motor movements associated with the use of an object would be stored in or near the motor systems active when that object was used. This idea, which I have referred to elsewhere as the sensory-motor model of semantic representations (Martin, 1998; Martin et al., 2000), has a long history in behavioral neurology. Indeed, many neurologists in the late nineteenth century assumed that the concept of an object was composed of the information about that object learned through direct sensory experience and stored in or near sensory and motor cortices (e.g., Broadbent, 1878; Freud, 1891; Lissauer, 1890/1988).

The modern era of the study of the organization of semantic memory in the human brain began with Elizabeth Warrington's seminal paper "The Selective Impairment of Semantic Memory" (Warrington, 1975). Warrington reported three patients with progressive dementing disorders that appeared to provide neurological evidence for Tulving's concept of a semantic memory system. (Pick's disease was later verified by autopsy for two of these patients.) There were three main components of the disorder. First, it was selective. The disorder could not be accounted for by general intellectual impairment, sensory or perceptual problems, or an expressive language disorder. Second, it was global rather than material-specific. Object knowledge was impaired regardless of whether objects were represented by pictures or by their written or spoken names. Third, the disorder was graded. Knowledge of specific object attributes (e.g., does a camel have two, four, or six legs?) was much more impaired than knowledge of superordinate category information (i.e., is a camel a mammal, bird, or insect?).

Following Warrington's report, similar patterns of semantic memory dysfunction have been reported. These have included patients with progressive dementias such as Alzheimer's disease (e.g., Martin & Fedio, 1983) and semantic dementia (e.g., Hodges et al., 1992), with herpes encephalitis (e.g., Pietrini et al., 1988), and with stroke (e.g., Hart & Gordon, 1990). In addition to the properties established by Warrington, these reports showed that these patients typically have a marked deficit in producing object names under a variety of circumstances, including difficulty naming pictures of objects, naming from the written descriptions of objects, and generating the names of objects that belong to a specific category (e.g., animals, fruits and vegetables, furniture, etc.). In addition, the deficits were primarily associated with damage to the left temporal lobe (see Martin et al., 1986, for evidence in patients with Alzheimer's disease; Hodges & Patterson, 1996, for semantic dementia; and Hart & Gordon, 1990, for focal brain injury cases).

FUNCTIONAL NEUROIMAGING OF SEMANTIC MEMORY

Object Naming and Word Reading

Difficulties in naming objects is a cardinal symptom of a semantic impairment. This is as expected. There is abundant evidence from the cognitive literature that semantic representations are automatically activated when objects are named, and even when they are simply viewed. When we see an object we cannot help but identify it. And in order to identify it, we must access previously stored information about that class of objects (e.g., Glaser, 1992; Humphreys et al., 1988).

Consistent with the clinical literature, functional neuroimaging studies of object naming suggest that semantic processing may be critically dependent on the left temporal lobe. Several studies have investigated silent object naming (Bookheimer et al., 1995; Martin et al., 1996) and object viewing (which also likely elicited silent naming; Zelkowicz et al., 1998) relative to viewing nonsense objects. The rationale behind this comparison is that both real and nonsense objects will activate regions which mediate perception of object shape, whereas only real objects will engage semantic, lexical, and phonological processes. Direct comparison of real object and nonsense object conditions revealed activity in a network of regions that included left inferior frontal cortex (Broca's area). Activation of left inferior frontal cortex was consistent with the clinical literature and with what is now a relatively large body of functional brain imaging studies, documenting the prominent role of this region in word selection and retrieval (see Caplan, 1992, for review of clinical literature; and Poldrack et al., 1999, for a review of brain-imaging studies). The other prominent site of activity was the

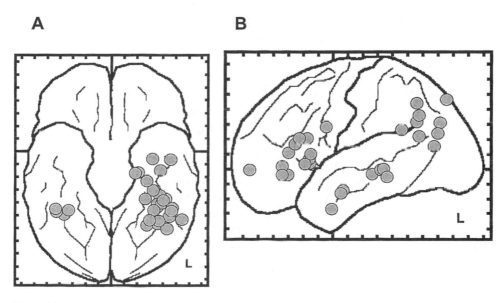

Figure 6.1
Schematic representation of the location of the main activations in temporal, left temporoparietal, and left prefrontal cortices, reported in object-naming, word-reading, semantic category fluency, semantic decision, and association tasks. Note the large number of activations in left ventral temporal cortex, clustered along fusiform and inferior temporal gyri (*A*), and left middle temporal gyrus (*B*).

posterior temporal lobes. These activations were centered on the fusiform gyrus, located on the ventral surface of the temporal lobes. The activity was bilateral in the Bookheimer et al. (1995) and Martin et al. (1996) studies, and on the left in Zelkowicz et al. (1998). Kiyosawa and colleagues (1996) also reported bilateral activation of this region when overt object naming was contrasted to rest, and to a counting condition to control for speech output (figure 6.1A).

Importantly, both real objects and nonsense objects produced equivalent activation of more posterior regions in ventrolateral occipital cortex, bilaterally (e.g., Malach et al., 1995; Martin et al., 1996). In contrast, the fusiform activations that were significantly greater for real, than for nonsense, objects were located further downstream in the ventral object-processing pathway. Because posterior temporal lobe lesions, especially to the left hemisphere, cause semantic deficits (including impaired object naming), the most likely explanation is that these temporal lobe activations reflect lexical and/or semantic processing.

If that is so, then this region should be active when single words are read in comparison to a baseline that presents physically similar stimuli devoid of semantic meaning. A number of studies have investigated this issue by comparing single-word reading to consonant strings. This baseline may be more appropriate than using non-sense words because the latter are often phonologically similar to real words, or contain legal words, and thus may produce unintended semantic processing. Price and colleagues (Price, Wise, et al., 1996) showed that reading words, relative to viewing consonant strings (and also relative to false font stimuli), activated the left fusiform gyrus of the temporal lobe slightly anterior to the regions active in the object-naming studies. A similar finding was reported by Herbster et al. (1997). In addition, and of particular relevance for the present discussion, Büchel and colleagues (1998) reported that this region of the left fusiform gyrus was active not only when normal individuals read words but also when congenitally blind subjects, and individuals blinded later in life, read Braille (Büchel et al., 1998). Based on these studies, it is apparent that both naming objects and reading words activate the ventral region of the posterior temporal lobes centered on the fusiform gyrus; this effect is greater on the left than on the right, especially during word reading. The data also suggest that activation of this region is independent of the physical form of the stimulus presented to the subjects.

Semantic Fluency

The findings from object naming and word reading are consistent with the view that the ventral region of the temporal lobes, in particular the fusiform gyrus, is engaged by lexical and/or semantic processing. One way to test whether these activations are purely lexical is to contrast word retrieval under conditions that emphasize semantic constraints (for example, asking subjects to generate a list of words denoting objects that belong to a specific semantic category) with conditions that emphasize lexical and phonological constraints (e.g., asking subjects to generate a list of words that begin with the same letter). If ventral temporal lobe activity reflects only lexical/phonological processes, then both of these tasks should activate this region to an equivalent degree. However, if activity in this region reflects semantic processes, then this region should be more active when word retrieval is driven by semantic, than by lexical, constraints.

Evidence in support of the semantic interpretation has been reported by Shaywitz et al. (1995) and Mummery et al. (1996). These studies were motivated by the findings that whereas lesions of the frontal lobes, especially of left lateral frontal cortex, disrupt word retrieval on both semantic and letter fluency tasks (e.g., Baldo & Shimamura, 1998), temporal lobe lesions produce greater impairment of semantic than of letter fluency (for a discussion of this issue, see Martin et al., 1994; Hodges et al., 1999). Mummery et al. (1996) compared semantic category fluency tasks to letter fluency tasks and reported that the semantically driven tasks produced greater activity of the left temporal lobe than lexically driven tasks, even though subjects produced a similar number of words under both retrieval conditions. The activations included both posterior and anterior regions of the inferior temporal gyrus and the anteromedial region of the left temporal lobe. Similarly, using fMRI, Shaywitz et al. (1995) reported that a semantic category fluency task produced greater activation of left posterior temporal cortex than a rhyme fluency task (generating words that rhymed with a target word). (Because fMRI is extremely sensitive to movement artifact, subjects generated words silently. As a result, output could not be monitored. Also, a "region of interest" analysis was employed that may have missed other activations.) Thus these findings suggest that activity in left ventral temporal cortex is modulated by semantic factors, and does not simply reflect lexical retrieval. As will be reviewed below, the importance of the temporal lobes, especially the posterior region of the left temporal lobe, has been confirmed by a number of studies directly aimed at evaluating the functional neuroanatomy of semantic processes.

Semantic Decision and Semantic Association Tasks

In one of the earliest functional brain-imaging studies of semantic processing, Sergent and colleagues (1992) asked subjects to make an overt semantic decision (living versus nonliving) about pictures of objects. Consistent with the reports reviewed above, this task produced activation of the left posterior fusiform gyrus, relative to a letter-sound decision task using visually presented letters. Using written words, Price and colleagues (1997) also reported activation of the left temporal lobe when a living/nonliving semantic judgment task was contrasted to a phonological decision task (two versus one or three syllables), using the same stimuli employed in the semantic decision condition. The activations included ventral temporal cortex, but were considerably anterior to those reported in the studies reviewed so far. The lack of activity in posterior regions of the ventral temporal lobe may have been due to the automatic engagement of semantic processing during the syllable decision baseline task (as had been demonstrated by these authors; Price, Wise, et al., 1996). Nevertheless, using a similar design, Chee et al. (1999) reported activation of the posterior left fusiform gyrus, as well as of the left middle temporal gyrus, when subjects made concrete/abstract decisions regarding aurally presented words, compared to a one- versus multiple-syllable decision task.

Activation of the left temporal lobe has also been found across a number of studies that have used more effortful and complex semantic decision tasks. Démonet and colleagues (1992) presented subjects with an adjective-noun word pair monitoring task. Subjects were instructed to monitor word pairs for a positive affect and a small animal (i.e., respond to "kind mouse" but not to "kind horse" or "horrible mouse.") The study was noteworthy because the stimuli were delivered aurally rather than visually (as in most of the previously reviewed studies), and the task required a rather detailed analysis of meaning. It also had some drawbacks, including the use of a highly unusual and complex task and limitation of words to two categories (animals and affective states). Nevertheless, relative to a task requiring subjects to monitor the order of phonemes in syllables (respond to /b/ when preceded by /d/), the semantic monitoring task activated the posterior region of the left ventral temporal cortex (fusiform and inferior temporal gyri). Other prominent regions of activity were in left posterior temporoparietal cortex (supramarginal and angular gyri), medial posterior parietal cortex (precuneus), posterior cingulate, and left prefrontal cortex.

This broad pattern of left hemisphere activation, including ventral and lateral regions of posterior temporal lobe, inferior parietal, and prefrontal cortices, has been replicated in nearly all studies using tasks that required effortful retrieval of semantic information. For example, Binder et al. (1997, 1999) used a semantic monitoring task similar to one employed by Démonet et al. (1992) (animals that are "native to the US and are used by people"). Relative to a tone detection task, the semantic decision task activated left ventral temporal cortex (including parahippocampal, fusiform, and inferior temporal gyri), left lateral temporal cortex (including middle and superior temporal gyri), left posterior parietal, and prefrontal regions. When these data were reanalyzed relative to a difficult phoneme monitoring task, the peak of the left ventral temporal lobe activation was located more medially in the parahippocampal gyrus (Binder et al. 1999; this study also demonstrated that the network active during the semantic monitoring task was also active when subjects were simply instructed to "rest" with eyes closed, i.e., when engaged in internally generated thought and daydreams).

Semantic association tasks requiring subjects to make subtle, within-category decisions have revealed a similar network of areas as well. Vandenberghe et al. (1996) tested subjects on a modified version of a semantic task, *The Pyramids and Palms Trees Test*, developed by Howard and Patterson (1992). In contrast to the semantic decision tasks reviewed above, this task was directly derived from the clinical literature. For example, patients with semantic dementia perform poorly on this test, whereas patients with nonfluent progressive aphasia do not (Hodges & Patterson, 1996). Subjects were shown triplets of pictures of objects with the target item on the top and two choice items below it to the left and right. Subjects indicated which of the two objects on the bottom was more similar to the object on top. For most trials, the objects were from the same semantic category, but one choice was more related to the target than the other choice. For example, the target may be a wrench and the choices pliers and a saw. Performance on this task activated a network of regions similar to those reported by Démonet et al. (1992), in comparison to a task that required subjects to make subtle visual distinctions (judging which object was more similar in size, as displayed on the screen, to the target object; Vandenberghe et al., 1996). Active regions included left posterior (fusiform gyrus) and anterior (inferior temporal gyrus) regions of ventral temporal cortex, left posterior lateral temporal cortex (middle temporal gyrus), left prefrontal, and left posterior parietal cortices. Importantly, these regions were also active when the objects were represented by their written names, thus providing evidence for a single semantic system engaged by pictures and words. Similar findings with *The Pyramids and Palms Trees Test* have been reported by Ricci et al. (1999; only pictures were used) and Mummery et al. (1999; for pictures and words).

The study by Mummery and colleagues (1999) is particularly noteworthy because it included patients with semantic dementia as well as normal individuals. The patients had prominent atrophy of the anterior temporal lobes, greater for the left than for the right hemisphere, as determined by volumetric analysis of the MRIs. Atrophy was not detected in more posterior temporal regions. Analysis of the PET data revealed activation of left anterior temporal lobe for the normal subjects during the semantic processing task (more strongly for words than for pictures). The dementia patients also showed activity in this region, but more variably than in normal individuals. This was not surprising, given that this was the area of greatest atrophy. However, whereas normal subjects also showed robust activation of posterior temporal cortex, the patients did not. One explanation for the patients' failure to activate left posterior temporal cortex was that this region was damaged, but the pathology was not detectable with present imaging technology. Alternatively, this region was intact, but inactive because of an absence of top-down influences from anterior temporal cortex. If that is the case, then this finding suggests that the effect of a lesion on task performance may be due not only to a disruption of processes normally performed by the damaged cortex but also to a disruption of processes performed at more distant sites within a processing network.

In summary, the studies reviewed to this point indicate a strong association between performance on a variety of semantic processing tasks and activation of a broad network of cortical regions, especially in the left hemisphere. This network includes prefrontal cortex, posterior temporoparietal cortex, and the ventral and lateral regions of the temporal lobes (fusiform, inferior, and middle temporal gyri; see figure 6.1A, B).

These temporal lobe sites accord well with the clinical literature reviewed previously that documented a strong association between semantic deficits and left temporal lobe pathology including, but certainly not limited to, posterior cortex. Studies of patients also have provided compelling evidence that semantic memory has a structure, and that this structure may, therefore, have anatomical boundaries. The goal of most of the studies reviewed above was to isolate "semantic processing regions" from brain areas that support perceptual and other language processes, not to reveal its structure. The studies considered next have direct bearing on the structure of semantic representations, from both a cognitive and a neuroanatomic perspective.

The Structure of Semantic Memory: Retrieving Information about Object Attributes

In 1988, Petersen and colleagues reported the first study of the functional neuroanatomy of semantic processing in the normal human brain. A word retrieval task was employed. However, unlike the previously discussed studies of semantic fluency that averaged brain activity across multiple retrieval cues (e.g., generating names of mammals and car parts; Shaywitz et al., 1995), the words generated in this study were all of the same type (action verbs). Subjects were presented with single words denoting concrete nouns (e.g., "cake") and asked to generate a single word denoting a use associated with the noun (e.g., "eat"). Comparison of activity recorded during this scan with activity recorded while the subjects simply read the words revealed activity in left lateral prefrontal cortex. Left prefrontal cortical activity was also found when the words were presented aurally, thus strengthening the authors' conclusion of an association between left prefrontal cortex and semantics.

There were two problems with this conclusion. First, many semantic models view meaning as compositional rather than unitary (e.g., Fodor & Lepore, 1996). As such, meaning in the brain has been viewed as a distributed system, involving many brain regions (e.g., Damasio, 1989). Second, even if semantic networks were confined to a single region, the neuropsychological evidence suggests that the critical area would be the left temporal, not the left frontal, lobe. As noted previously, damage to left prefrontal cortex often results in impaired word retrieval, thereby providing one explanation for the Petersen et al. finding (and see Thompson-Schill et al., 1997, 1998, for evidence of left prefrontal involvement in the selection of a specific word among competing alternatives). Alternatively, the left prefrontal site reported by Petersen and colleagues (1988) may have been associated with retrieval of verbs, relative to other word types (if that is the case, it would remain to be determined whether this was tied to the grammatical or to the semantic function of verbs). In support of this possibility, patients have been described with selective verb retrieval deficits (e.g., Caramazza & Hillis, 1991; Damasio & Tranel, 1993), and their lesions typically included left prefrontal cortex. (However, the damage often extended posteriorly to include much of the perisylvian region. See Gainotti et al., 1995, for review.)

We addressed some of these issues by comparing verb retrieval to retrieval of another object-associated feature, color (Martin et al., 1995). We decided on color and action because of evidence that the perception of these features, as well as knowledge about them, could be differentially impaired following focal damage to the human brain. Color blindness, or achromatopsia, is associated with lesions of the ventral surface of the occipital lobes (e.g., Damasio et al., 1980; Vaina, 1994). PET and fMRI studies of normal individuals had identified regions in ventral occipital cortex active during color perception (specifically, the fusiform gyrus and collateral sulcus in the occipital lobe) (e.g., Corbetta et al., 1990; McKeefry & Zeki, 1997; Sakai et al., 1995; Zeki et al., 1991). In contrast, impaired motion perception, or akinetopsia, is associated with a more dorsally located lesion at the border of occipital, temporal, and parietal lobes (e.g., Zihl et al., 1991; Vaina, 1994). This location has also been confirmed by imaging studies of normal subjects (e.g., Corbetta et al., 1990; A. Smith et al., 1998; Zeki et al., 1991; Watson et al., 1993) (see figure 6.2A, B).

In addition, focal lesions can result in selective deficits in retrieving information about object-associated color and object-associated motion. Patients have been de-

A   **B**

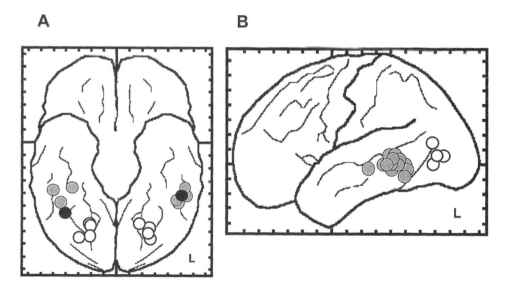

Figure 6.2
Schematic representation of the location of activations associated with perceiving and retrieving information about color and actions. (A) Ventral view of the left and right hemispheres showing occipital regions that responded to color (white circles), and temporal regions active when color information was retrieved (gray circles). Black circle on the left hemisphere shows location of the region active when color-word synethetes experienced color imagery. Black circle on the right hemisphere shows location of the region active in normal subjects during a color imagery task. (B) Lateral view of the left hemisphere showing sites at the junction of the occipital, temporal, and parietal lobes that responded to visual motion (white circles), and the region of the middle temporal gyrus active when verbs were retrieved (gray circles).

scribed with color agnosia who, for example, can neither retrieve the name of a color typically associated with an object nor choose from among a set of colors the one commonly associated with a specific object (e.g., De Vreese, 1991; Luzzati & Davidoff, 1994). And, as noted above, others have been described with selective verb comprehension and production impairments.

In our study, subjects were presented with black-and-white line drawings of objects. During one PET scan they named the object, during another scan they retrieved a single word denoting a color commonly associated with the object, and during a third scan they retrieved a single word denoting an action commonly associated with the object (Petersen et al's. verb generation condition). For example, subjects were shown a picture of a child's wagon and would respond "wagon," "red," and "pull" during the different scanning conditions (Martin et al., 1995).

In agreement with Petersen et al. (1988), retrieving object attribute information activated the left lateral prefrontal cortex, over and above that seen for object naming. However, this prefrontal activity did not vary with the type of information that subjects retrieved. Rather, the activation was similar for both the color and the action retrieval conditions, and thus consistent with the idea that left lateral prefrontal cortex is critically involved in retrieval from semantic memory (e.g., Gabrieli et al., 1998). In contrast, other brain regions were differentially active, depending on the type of information retrieved. Importantly, behavioral data collected during the scans (voice response times) confirmed that the color and action retrieval tasks were equally difficult to perform. As a result, differences in patterns of cortical activity associated with these tasks could be attributed to differences in the type of information retrieved rather than to differences in the ease of information retrieval.

Relative to action verbs, generating color words activated the ventral region of the temporal lobes bilaterally, including the fusiform and inferior temporal gyri, approximately 2 to 3 cm anterior to regions known to be active during color perception (figure 6.2A). In contrast, action word generation was associated with a broader pattern of activation that included left inferior frontal cortex (Broca's area), the posterior region of the left superior temporal gyrus (Wernicke's area), and the posterior region of the left middle temporal gyrus (figure 6.2B). Activation of the middle temporal gyrus was located approximately 1 to 2 cm anterior to the regions active during the motion perception, based on previous functional brain imaging findings. Thus, retrieving information about specific object attributes activated brain regions proximal to the areas that mediate perception of those attributes.

Given the claims of the sensory-motor model of semantic representations, it may be surprising that regions close to primary motor cortex were not active during action word generation. As we suggested in our initial report, this failure may have been related to our choice of objects. Few tools, or other small manipulable objects such as kitchen utensils, were presented because of their limited range of color associations (tools invariably elicit silver, black, and brown as color responses; Martin et al., 1995). However, as we will discuss later, left premotor cortex is indeed active when subjects generate action verbs exclusively to tools (Grafton et al., 1997).

Finally, a similar pattern of differential engagement of the fusiform gyrus (greater for color word generation than for action word generation) and left middle temporal gyrus (greater for action word generation than for color word generation) was seen when subjects responded to the written names of the objects rather than to pictures (Martin et al., 1995). Taken together, these results provided additional evidence that activity in these regions is related to meaning rather than to the physical characteristics of the stimuli.

It is also noteworthy that the activation in the ventral temporal cortex associated with retrieving color words, and the activation in the left middle temporal gyrus associated with retrieving action words, overlap with the regions active during performance of many of the semantic processing tasks reviewed previously (compare figures 6.1 and 6.2). Thus, the color/action word generation studies suggest that these posterior temporal regions may not serve a uniform function in the service of "semantics." Rather, temporal cortex may be segregated into distinct areas that serve different functions. Specifically, qualitatively different types of information are stored in ventral temporal and lateral temporal cortices.

We have now reported two additional studies of color word generation that provide supportive evidence for an association between retrieving information about object color and activity in posterior ventral temporal cortex. One experiment addressed whether activation of the ventral temporal lobe when color words are retrieved was specifically tied to retrieving information from semantic memory. Subjects generated the names of typical object colors in one condition (retrieval from semantic memory), and generated the names of recently taught object-color associations in another condition (retrieval from episodic memory). For example, subjects responded "red" to an achromatic picture of a child's wagon in one condition and "green" in another condition. (However, no subject saw the same objects in the semantic and episodic memory conditions. See Wiggs et al., 1999, for details.) In a second study, retrieving color information from semantic memory was evaluated in relation to color naming and color perception in order to more precisely map the functional neuroanatomy engaged by these processes (Chao & Martin, 1999). The results of these studies replicated our initial finding. Retrieving object-color information from semantic memory activated a region of ventral temporal cortex, bilaterally in Chao and Martin (1999) and lateralized to the left in Wiggs et al. (1999), that was located anterior to the occipital areas active during color perception (figure 6.2A). Thus, we interpreted these findings as identifying a region where object-associated color information is stored.

Additional evidence in support of this claim comes from functional brain-imaging studies of individuals with color-word synesthesia (Paulesu et al., 1995) and color imagery in normal individuals (Howard et al., 1998). Color-word synesthetes are individuals who claim that hearing words often triggers the experience of vivid color imagery. Using PET, Paulesu and colleagues reported that listening to words activated a site in the left ventral temporal lobe in color-word synesthetes, but not in the normal individuals. The region active in the synesthetes when they heard words and experienced colors was the same area active when normal subjects retrieved object-color information (figure 6.2A). Howard et al. (1998) also reported fusiform activity, but on the right rather than the left, when normal subjects answered questions designed to elicit color imagery (e.g., "Is a raspberry darker red than a strawberry?"). Thus, the vivid experience of color imagery automatically elicited in the synethestes —the effortful and conscious generation of color imagery, and effortful retrieval of verbal, object-color information—activated similar regions of the ventral temporal lobes (see figure 6.2A).

Interestingly, although the word-color synesthesia subjects experienced color when they heard words, they did not show activation of sites in ventral occipital cortex typically active during color perception. This finding is in accord with the Chao and Martin (1999) study of color word generation and color perception, and with the Howard et al. (1998) study of color imagery and color perception. In those reports, neither color word retrieval nor color imagery activated occipital regions that were active during color perception. These negative findings are consistent with clinical reports which suggest that color perception and color knowledge can be doubly dissociated. For example, Shuren et al. (1996) reported intact color imagery in an achromatopsic patient, while De Vreese (1991) reported impaired color imagery in a patient with intact color perception (case II). Taken together, the functional brain imaging and clinical literature provide converging evidence that information about object color is stored in the ventral temporal lobe, and that the critical site is close to, but does not include, more posterior occipital sites that respond to the presence of color.

In contrast to these reports on retrieving color information from semantic memory, there is now considerable evidence that retrieving a different type of object-associated information (as represented by action verbs) is associated with activity in a different region of the posterior temporal lobe; specifically, the left middle temporal gyrus. To date, there are at least 26 functional brain-imaging studies in the literature that have used the action word generation task. In addition to the studies discussed above (one in Petersen et al., 1988; and two in Martin et al., 1995), these include one study reported in Wise et al. (1991), one in Raichle et al. (1994), four reported in Warburton et al. (1996), 12 studies (from 12 different laboratories) in Poline et al. (1996), four studies (from different laboratories) in Tatsumi et al. (1999), and one in Klein et al. (1999). (All used PET. McCarthy et al., 1993, studied verb generation using fMRI, but only the frontal lobes were imaged.)

The stimuli used in these studies have included pictures of objects (Martin et al., 1995), words presented visually (Martin et al., 1995; Petersen et al., 1988; Raichle et al., 1994), and words presented aurally (the remaining studies). Stimulus presentation rates ranged from one per sec (Petersen et al., 1988) to one per 6 sec (Poline et al., 1996; Tatsumi et al., 1999). Subjects responded aloud in some studies (Klein et al., 1999; Martin et al., 1995; Petersen et al., 1988; Raichle et al., 1994) and silently in the others, and produced a single response to each item in some studies (Klein et al., 1999; Martin et al., 1995; Petersen et al., 1988; Raichle et al., 1994) and multiple responses to each item in the others. Finally, subjects have been tested in a variety of native languages, including English, German, French, Italian, Dutch, Danish, Swedish, Chinese, and Japanese. Given these and numerous other differences between studies (including baseline comparison tasks), the findings have been remarkably consistent. In particular, retrieving information about object-associated actions activated the left middle temporal gyrus in 19 of 25 studies that imaged this region. Two of the remaining studies reported peak activity at a slightly more superior location in the superior temporal gyrus (Wise et al., 1991, and one study in Warburton et al., 1996; superior temporal activity was also observed in several data sets analyzed in Poline et al., 1996). The locations of the left middle temporal gyrus activations relative to regions active during motion perception are illustrated in figure 6.2B.

Taken together, the findings provide clear and compelling evidence against the idea that information about object attributes and features is stored in a single region of the brain, and thus within an undifferentiated semantic system. Rather, the color/ action word retrieval data suggest that information is distributed throughout the cerebral cortex. In addition, the locations of the sites appear to follow a specific plan that parallels the organization of sensory systems and, as will be reviewed below, motor systems, as well. Thus, within this view, information about object features and attributes, such as form, color, and motion, would be stored within the processing streams active when that information was acquired, but downstream from (i.e., anterior to) regions in occipital cortex that are active when these features are physically present.

The Structure of Semantic Memory: Object Category-Specific Representations

Background Investigations of the functional neuroanatomy engaged by different categories of objects provide additional evidence for this view. As with many of the studies reviewed above, these investigations were motivated by the clinical literature.

Specifically, patients have been described with relatively selective deficits in recognizing, naming, and retrieving information about different object categories. The categories that have attracted the most attention are animals and tools. This is because of a large and growing number of reports of patients with greater difficulty naming and retrieving information about animals (and often other living things) than about tools (and often other man-made objects). Reports of the opposite pattern of dissociation (greater for tools than animals) are considerably less frequent. However, enough carefully studied cases have been reported to provide convincing evidence that these categories can be doubly dissociated as a result of brain damage. The impairment in these patients is not limited to visual recognition. Deficits occur when knowledge is probed visually and verbally, and therefore are assumed to reflect damage to the semantic system or systems (see Forde & Humphreys, 1999, for a review).

While it is now generally accepted that these disorders are genuine, their explanation, on both the cognitive and the neural level, remains controversial. Two general types of explanations have been proposed. The most common explanation focuses on the disruption of stored information about object features. Specifically, it has been proposed that knowledge about animals and tools can be selectively disrupted because these categories are dependent on information about different types of features stored in different regions of the brain. As exemplified by the definitions provided in the introduction to this chapter, animals are defined primarily by what they look like. Functional attributes play a much smaller role in their definition. In contrast, functional information—specifically, how an object is used—is critical for defining tools. As a result, damage to areas where object form information is stored leads to deficits for categories that are overly dependent on visual form information, whereas damage to regions where object use information is stored leads to deficits for categories overly dependent on functional information. The finding that patients with category-specific deficits for animals also have difficulties with other visual form-based categories, such as precious stones, provides additional support for this view (e.g., Warrington & Shallice, 1984; and see Bunn et al., 1998, for a reevaluation of this patient).

This general framework for explaining category-specific disorders was first proposed by Warrington and colleagues in the mid-to-late 1980s (e.g., Warrington & McCarthy, 1983, 1987; Warrington & Shallice, 1984). Influential extensions and re-formation of this general idea have been provided by a number of investigators, including Farah (e.g., Farah & McClelland, 1991), Damasio (1990), Caramazza (Caramazza et al., 1990), and Humphreys (Humphreys & Riddoch, 1987), among others (see Forde & Humphreys, 1999, for an excellent discussion of these models).

The second type of explanation focuses on much broader semantic distinctions (e.g., animate versus inanimate objects), rather than on features and attributes, as the

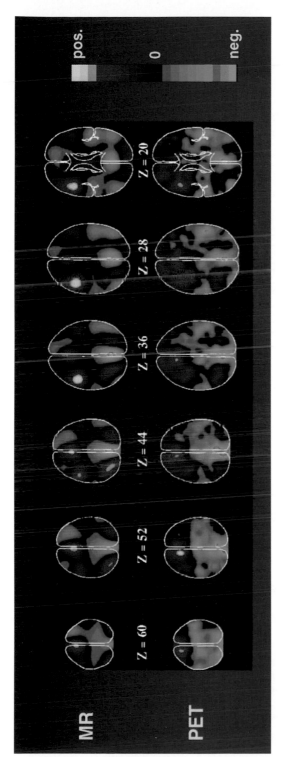

Plate 1 Functional magnetic resonance images (fMRI; top row) of the BOLD signal (Ogawa et al., 1990) and positron emission tomography (PET; bottom row) images of blood flow change. These images were obtained during the performance of a task in which subjects viewed three-letter word stems and were asked to speak aloud (PET) or think silently (fMRI) the first word to come to mind whose first three letters corresponded to the stems (e.g., *see you*, say or think *couple*; Buckner et al., 1995). The color scale employed in these images shows activity increases in reds and yellows and activity decreases in greens and blues. Note that both PET and fMRI show similar increases as well as decreases. The fMRI images were blurred to the resolution of the PET images (18-mm FWHM) to facilitate comparison. (See chapter 1.)

A. Attend Left   Attend Right

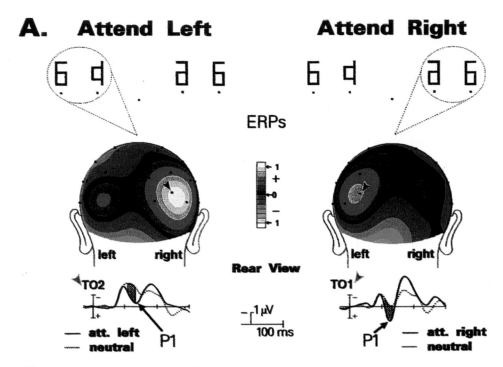

ERPs

Rear View

TO2 ─ att. left
─ neutral   P1

TO1 ─ att. right
─ neutral
P1

$-1\,\mu V$
$100\ ms$

B. Subtracted Attend Left Minus Right

PET   ERP

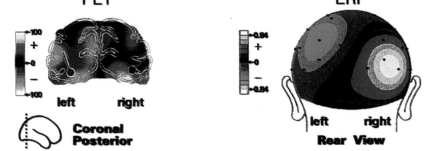

left   right

Coronal
Posterior

left   right
Rear View

C. Scalp Topographies of Dipole Models

Best Fit Inverse   Seeded Forward

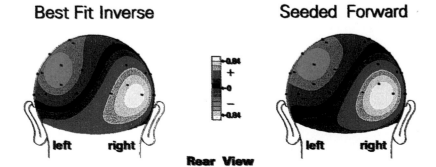

left   right   left   right

Rear View

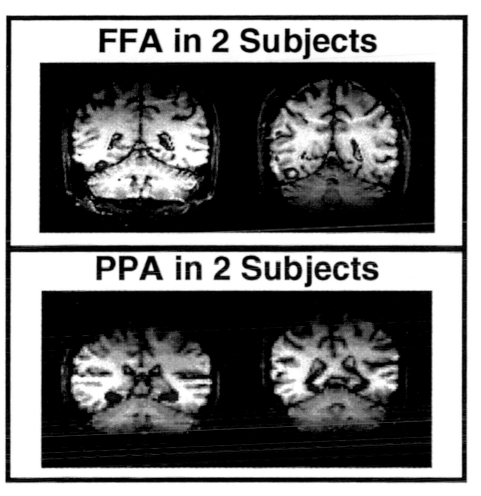

Plate 3 Coronal views of the brain showing the fusiform face area (FFA) in two subjects, and the parahippocampal place area (PPA) in two subjects. Right hemisphere is shown on the left and vice versa. (See chapter 5.)

◄ **Plate 2** Comparing PET and ERP attention effects from the combined study of Heinze et al. (1994). (*A*) Topographic isovoltage maps showing the lateral occipital focus of the P1 attention effect for both attend-left minus passive and attend-right minus passive conditions. The corresponding ERP waveforms, showing the associated attention effects, are below each map, along with the time-window of the shown scalp topography (shaded). (*B*) The attend-left minus attend-right ERP data are shown on the right, and a coronal section through the posterior occipital region in the PET data is shown on the left, for the same subtraction condition as the ERP data. The PET data reveal foci of activations in both the left and right fusiform gyrus (indicated by the dots), although the left activation appears as a decrease due to the subtraction condition. These data show that the attention effects in the PET and ERP data have similar spatial frames of reference. (*C*) Two different scalp topographies obtained using dipole modeling procedures. In the "seeded forward" solution (right) the dipole was held constant in the center of the fusiform PET activation, whereas in the "best fit" solution (left) the dipole was allowed to vary in position. The comparison demonstrates that the PET fusiform activation provides a good predictor of the actual dipole location. (Reprinted with permission from *Nature*, copyright 1994, Macmillan Magazines, Ltd.) (See chapter 4.)

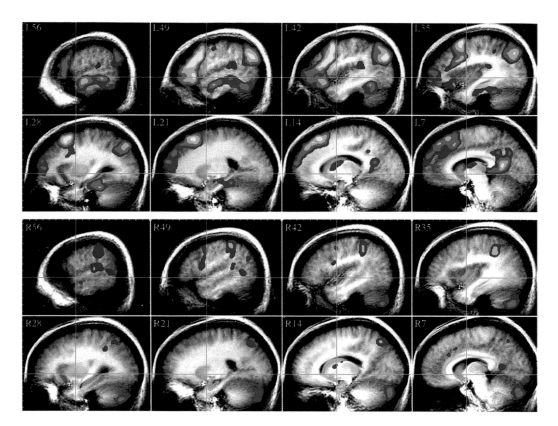

Plate 13 Serial sagittal sections showing significantly activated areas in the semantic processing study of Binder et al. Semantic processing areas, indicated in red–yellow, are strongly lateralized to the left cerebral hemisphere and right cerebellum. Blue shading indicates regions that were more active during the control (tone decision) task. Green lines indicate the standard stereotaxic y axis (AC–PC line) and z axis (vertical AC line). (Adapted with permission from Binder et al., 1997; copyright 1996 Society for Neuroscience.) (See chapter 7.)

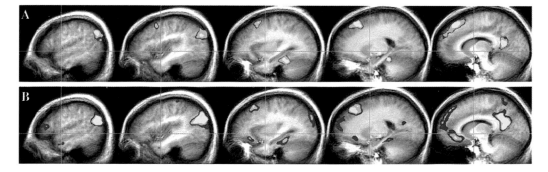

Plate 14 Left hemisphere areas associated with nonsensory semantic processing (Binder et al., 1999). Areas with higher signal during a semantic decision task compared to a phonemic decision task (*A*) are virtually identical to areas with higher signal during rest compared to a tone decision task (*B*). (Reproduced with permission from Binder, 1999.) (See chapter 7.)

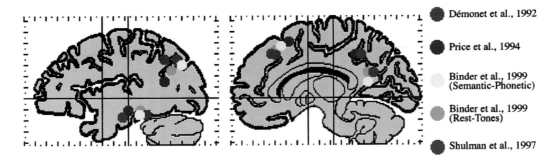

Plate 15 Convergence of results across four studies comparing either semantic to nonsemantic tasks (Binder et al., 1999; Démonet et al., 1992; Price et al., 1994) or resting to nonsemantic tasks (Binder et al., 1999; Shulman et al., 1997). (Reproduced with permission from Binder, 1999.) (See chapter 7.)

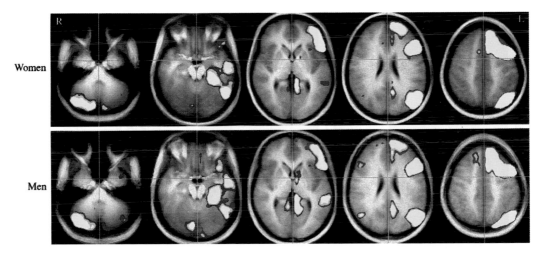

Plate 16 Serial axial sections showing average activation maps from 50 women and 50 men during a semantic word categorization task (Frost et al., 1999). Activation is strongly left-lateralized in both groups. There were no significant group differences at a voxel or regional level. (See chapter 7.)

Blocked Design

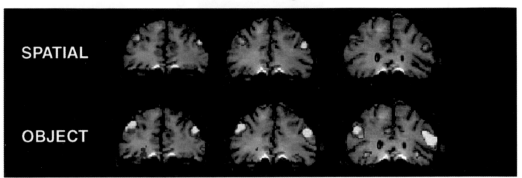

Event-related Design

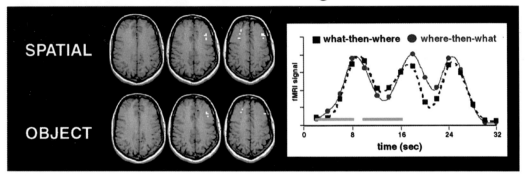

Plate 19 (*Top*) Data from a blocked design fMRI experiment by Postle et al. (1999) showing nearly identical bilateral PFC activation associated with spatial and object working memory in an individual subject. (*Bottom*) Data from an event-related fMRI experiment from Postle et al. (1999) study showing activation maps displaying suprathreshold activity in spatial and object delay periods in dorsolateral PFC in a single subject, illustrating the marked degree of overlap in PFC activity in the two conditions. The graph to the right shows the trial-averaged time series extracted from dorsolateral PFC voxels with object delay-period activity. Again, note the similarity of fMRI signal intensity changes in spatial and object delay periods. (See chapter 9.)

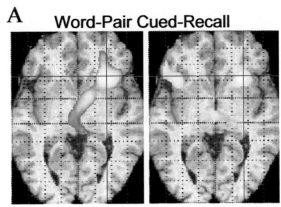

A Word-Pair Cued-Recall

Younger   Older

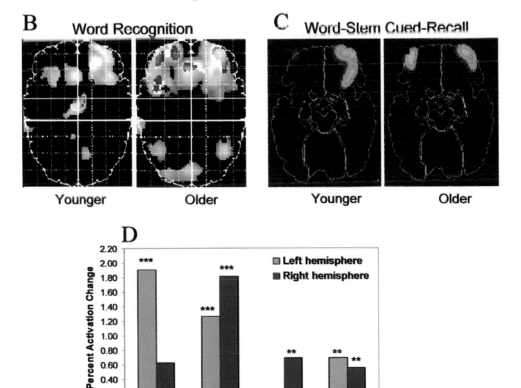

B Word Recognition

Younger   Older

C Word-Stem Cued-Recall

Younger   Older

D

Percent Activation Change

Legend:
- Left hemisphere
- Right hemisphere

Younger   Older   Younger   Older
Verbal Working Memory   **Spatial Working Memory**

Plate 20   Examples of an age-related attenuation in hemispheric asymmetry: unilateral activations in young adults coupled with bilateral activations in older adults. (*A*) Brain activity during recall (data from Cabeza et al., 1997a analyzed with SPM). (*B*) Brain activity during recognition (from Madden et al., 1999b, figure 5). (*C*) Brain activity during word-stem cued-recall (from Bäckman et al., 1997, figure 3). (*D*) Brain activity during verbal and spatial working memory (from Reuter-Lorenz, submitted, figure 3). (See chapter 10.)

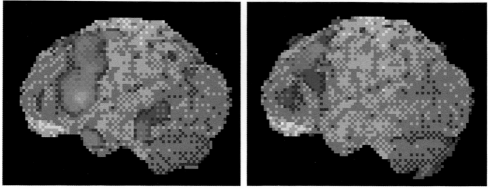

Younger   Older

Plate 21   Left PFC activation associated with inhibition in young and older adults (from Jonides et al., 2000). (See chapter 10.)

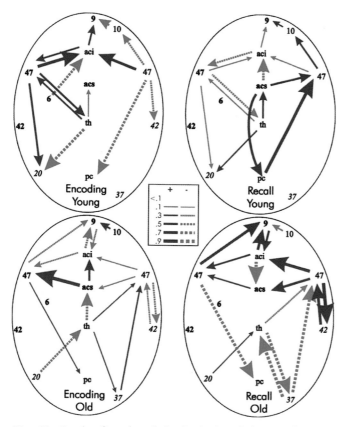

Plate 22   Results of a path analysis of activations during encoding and recall in young and older adults. Path coefficients that showed a difference of > 0.50 between encoding and recall conditions. Positive coefficients appear in solid red arrows and negative coefficients in segmented blue arrows, with the thickness of the arrow representing the strength of the coefficient (from Cabeza et al., 1997b). (See chapter 10.)

key to understanding category-specific deficits. A variant of this argument has been strongly presented by Caramazza and Shelton (1998) to counter a number of difficulties with feature-based formulations. Specifically, Caramazza and Shelton note that a central prediction of at least some feature-based models is that patients with a category-specific deficit for animals should have more difficulty answering questions that probe knowledge of visual information about animals (does an elephant have a long tail?) than about function information (is a elephant found in the jungle?). As Caramazza and Shelton show, at least some patients with an animal-specific knowledge disorder (and, according to their argument, all genuine cases) have equivalent difficulty with both visual and functional questions about animals. As a result of these and other findings, Caramazza and Shelton argue that category-specific disorders cannot be explained by feature-based models. Instead, they propose that such disorders reflect evolutionary adaptations for animate objects, foods, and, perhaps by default, tools and other man-made objects (the "domain-specific hypothesis").

We now turn to functional brain-imaging studies to see if they provide information that may help in sorting out these issues. Currently, there are 14 studies that have investigated object category specificity. Studies contrasting animals and tools (and other manipulable, man-made objects, such as kitchen utensils) have employed a variety of paradigms. Object naming has been investigated using detailed line drawings (Martin et al., 1996), silhouettes (Martin et al., 1996), and photographs (Chao, Haxby, et al., 1999; Damasio et al., 1996). Subjects responded silently, except in Damasio et al. Object comparison tasks have also been used in which subjects judged whether pairs of objects were different exemplars of the same object or different objects in the same category. Objects were represented by line drawings (Perani et al., 1995) and by written names (Perani et al., 1999). Other paradigms have included delayed match-to-sample using photographs (Chao, Haxby, et al., 1999), passive viewing of rapidly presented photographs (Chao, Haxby, et al., 1999), presentation of written yes/no questions probing knowledge of visual and associative features (objects represented by their written names; Cappa et al., 1998), and written yes/no questions about where objects are typically found (objects represented by their written names; Chao, Haxby, et al., 1999).

Other studies have investigated category specificity by averaging across multiple categories of living things and artifacts. These have employed verbal fluency tasks (land animals, sea animals, fruits, and vegetables, versus toys, tools, weapons, and clothes; Mummery et al., 1996); written yes/no questions about visual and nonvisual features (objects were represented by their written names; categories included, but were not limited to, animals, flowers, vegetables, versus clothing, furniture, kitchen utensils; Thompson-Schill et al., 1999); object comparisons based on similarity in color and similarity in location (place typically found), using visually presented word triads (living things versus artifacts, not further specified; Mummery et al., 1998); and naming and word-picture matching tasks using colored and black-and-white line drawings (animals, fruits, and vegetables versus vehicles, appliances, tools, and utensils; Moore and Price, 1999; only activations common to both the naming and the matching tasks were reported). All of the studies used PET except Chao, Haxby, et al. (1999) and Thompson-Schill et al. (1999), which used fMRI.

Category-Related Activations of Occipital Cortex The first studies to directly compare functional brain activity associated with animals versus tools were reported by Perani et al. (1995) and Martin et al. (1996). Both studies found greater activation of occipital cortex for animals relative to tools. These activations were lateralized to the left hemisphere and were located medially (Perani et al., 1995; Martin et al., 1996) and in ventrolateral cortex (fusiform gyrus and inferior occipital cortex; Perani et al., 1995). Using a naming task, Damasio et al. (1996) also reported greater medial occipital activity for animals, but lateralized to the right and superior to those in the above noted studies. Direct comparisons of animals and tools were not reported. Unlike the Martin and Perani studies, the tasks were not equated for difficulty, thus requiring the stimuli to be presented at different rates (see Grabowski et al., 1998, for details). Presentation rate, however, can influence the pattern of cortical activations (Price, Moore, et al., 1996). Moreover, the baseline comparison task consisted of judging whether photographs of faces were upright or inverted. As a result, the findings of Damasio et al. are difficult to interpret, especially in light of more recent data indicating substantial overlap in the network of regions activated by pictures of animals and human faces (Chao, Haxby, et al., 1999; Chao, Martin, et al., 1999).

Patients with category-specific deficits for living things most often have damage to the temporal lobes, usually as a result of herpes encephalitis (e.g., Pietrini et al., 1988). Thus, the finding that the occipital cortex was the main region activated for animals, relative to tools, was surprising and problematic. One possibility is that this heightened occipital activity simply reflected differences in the visual complexity of the stimuli. In this view, pictures of animals are visually more complex (e.g., Snodgrass & Vanderwart, 1980), and therefore require more visual processing than do pictures of tools (e.g., Gaffan & Heywood, 1993). This interpretation was weakened by the results of a study that used silhouettes of animals and tools, thereby eliminating stimulus differences with regard to internal visual detail. Naming animal silhouettes was associated with greater left medial occipital activity, relative to naming tool silhouettes, even though the stimuli were equated for naming speed and accuracy (Martin et al., 1996).

Recent reports have all but eliminated the visual complexity argument by showing greater occipital activity for animals, relative to tools, when the objects were represented by their written names rather than by pictures. Perani et al. (1999) reported greater left inferior occipital activity for animals than for tools using a same/different word-matching task, and Chao, Haxby, et al. (1999) reported greater bilateral inferior occipital activity for reading and answering questions about animals than about tools. Both of these studies also found greater animal-related than tool-related activity in inferior occipital cortex using object picture tasks (same/different judgments in Perani et al., 1999; viewing, delayed match-to-sample, and naming in Chao, Haxby, et al., 1999). However, Perani and colleagues also reported bilateral activation of the medial occipital region (lingual gyrus) for tools, relative to animals, in their reading task (but not in their object picture task). This exception notwithstanding, most of the evidence suggest that occipital cortex, especially around calcarine cortex and the inferior occipital gyrus, is more active when stimuli represent animals than when they represent tools (figure 6.3). Further support for this possibility is provided by a study of patients with focal cortical lesions. Tranel and colleagues identified 28 patients with impaired recognition and knowledge of animals, relative to tools, and famous people. All had posterior lesions that included medial occipital cortex, 14 on the right and 14 on the left (Tranel et al., 1997).

Given that occipital activity is unlikely to be due to differences in visual complexity, an alternative explanation is that it reflects top-down activation from more anterior sites (Martin et al., 1996, 2000). This may occur whenever retrieval of detailed information about visual features or form is needed to identify an object. However, if this were the case, then category-related differentiation should be found anteriorly in the ventral object-processing stream to drive this process. In addition, although, as noted above, there have been reports of patients with occipital lesions that had category-specific impairment for animals and other animate or living objects (Tranel et al., 1997), most cases have had lesions confined to the temporal lobes (see Gainotti et al., 1995, for review). Thus, one would expect to find animal-related activity farther downstream in the ventral object-processing pathway.

Ventral Temporal Cortex and the Representation of Visual Form   As reviewed previously, many studies of semantic processing have reported activity centered on the fusiform gyrus in posterior temporal cortex. For example, the naming studies reported by Martin et al. (1996) found bilateral fusiform activity for both animals and tools, relative to a lower-level baseline condition. However, these activations were not seen when the categories were directly contrasted, thus suggesting that category-related differences were not represented in this region of the brain. More recent studies, however, suggest that this failure may have been due to the limited spatial resolution of PET. Using fMRI, Chao, Haxby, et al. (1999) reported multiple, category-related sites in the ventral region of the posterior temporal lobes. These

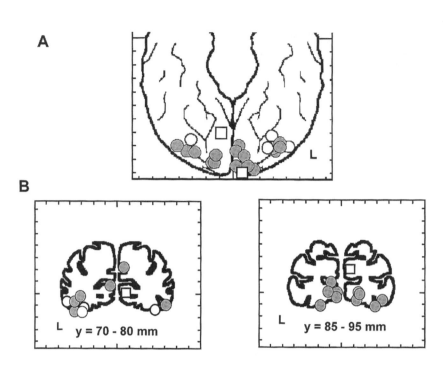

Figure 6.3
Schematic representation of category-related activations in occipital cortex reported by Perani et al. (1995), Martin et al. (1996), Damasio et al. (1996), Perani et al. (1999), and Chao, Haxby, et al. (1999). Circles represent sites more active for animals than for tools or other object categories; squares represent region more active for tools than for animals. Gray circles indicate tasks that employed pictures, and white circles indicate tasks that used words. Nearly all sites were activated more by animal than by tool stimuli. See text for description of paradigms. (*A*) Location of activations, represented as a see-through ventral view of the left and right hemispheres. (*B*) Coronal sections showing location of the same activations shown in A. Section on left depicts activations that were located approximately 70–80 mm posterior to the anterior commissure. Section on the right depicts activations located approximately 85–95 mm posterior to the anterior commissure.

ventral activations were located in the same region identified in many of the previously reviewed semantic tasks (fusiform gyrus, ~4.5–6.5 cm posterior to the anterior commissure) (figure 6.4 and color plate 6).

The location of these category-related activations was highly consistent across individual subjects, and different paradigms with pictures (passive viewing, delayed match-to-sample, and naming) and the written names of objects (Chao, Haxby, et al., 1999). In addition to animals and tools, the stimuli for the viewing and delayed match-to-sample tasks included pictures of human faces and houses. Faces and houses were included because previous studies had shown that these objects elicit highly consistent patterns of activation in ventral temporal cortex. Viewing faces has

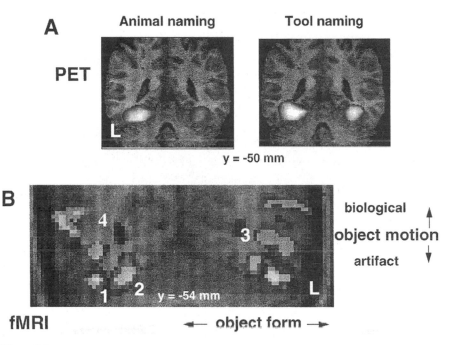

Figure 6.4
Coronal sections showing locations of animal- and tool-related activations in posterior temporal lobes. (*A*) Results from a study using PET (adapted from Martin et al., 1996). Both categories were associated with bilateral activity centered on the fusiform gyri. The only category-related activity seen with PET in this region was in the left middle temporal gyrus, greater for tools than for animals (not visible here because it was below the threshold used to make this picture, $p < .001$). (*B*) Category-related activity revealed by fMRI in the same region of the posterior temporal cortex shown in (*A*) (adapted from Chao, Haxby, et al., 1999). Regions depicted in the red-yellow color spectrum responded more to animals than to tools; regions in the blue-green spectrum responded more to tools than to animals. 1. lateral fusiform; 2. medial fusiform; 3. middle temporal gyrus; 4. superior temporal sulcus (see text and Chao, Haxby, et al., 1999, for details). The location of these activations in relation to the functions of more posterior regions leads to the suggestion that information about object form may be stored in ventral temporal cortex, and information about object-associated motion may be stored in lateral temporal cortex. (See color plate 6.)

been associated with activation of the more lateral portion of the fusiform gyrus (Haxby et al., 1999; Ishai et al., 1999; Kanwisher et al., 1997; McCarthy et al., 1997, Puce et al., 1996), whereas viewing houses and landmarks has activated regions medial to face-responsive cortex, including the medial aspect of the fusiform gyrus (Haxby et al., 1999; Ishai et al., 1999), lingual gyrus (Aguirre et al., 1998), and parahippocampal cortex (Epstein & Kanwisher, 1998).

In addition to the bilateral inferior occipital activation discussed above, Chao, Haxby, et al. (1999) found bilateral activation centered on the lateral half of the fusiform gyri for animals relative to tools (see figure 6.4B). This region could thus provide the purported top-down modulation of occipital cortex. In addition, consistent with reports cited above, this region also responded strongly to human faces. The peaks of the activation for animals and for human faces were essentially identical, even when the faces of the animals were completely obscured (Chao, Martin, et al., 1999). However, the animal- and face-related activations were not identical in all respects. Specifically, the neural response to faces was more focal than that to animals. This finding suggests that while recognition of animals and faces may be dependent, at least partially, on a common neural substrate, faces may be processed by a more discretely organized system. This finding, in turn, may explain why some patients may have selective deficit for faces (e.g., McNeil & Warrington, 1993), and also why impaired recognition of animals may be the most common co-occurring category-related deficit in prosopagnosic patients (Farah, 1990).

In contrast, the medial fusiform region responded more strongly to tools than to animals (see figure 6.4B). This region also responded strongly to houses, as previously reported. However, as was the case for the animals and faces, direct comparison of houses and tools revealed finer-grained distinctions between these object categories as well. The peak activity associated with processing tool stimuli was consistently lateral to the peak activation associated with houses (although still in the more medial section of the fusiform gyrus). These findings suggest that the pattern of response to different object categories varies continuously across the posterior ventral temporal cortex. For this reason, we suggested that the ventral temporal cortex may be organized according to object features that cluster together (Chao, Haxby, et al., 1999; Ishai et al., 1999; Martin et al., 2000). The nature of these features remains to be determined. However, because the fusiform gyrus is part of the ventral object vision pathway, this region may be tuned to the features of object form shared by members of a category.

Lateral Temporal Cortex and the Representation of Object-Related Visual Motion

Animal stimuli were also associated with activation of the lateral surface of the posterior temporal cortex centered on the superior temporal sulcus (STS). Again, the location of activity was consistent across individuals and tasks. However, in contrast to the fusiform activity, which was found in every subject, significant STS activity was found in only half the subjects for the picture-processing tasks, and only one quarter of the subjects (two of eight) for the word-reading task (Chao, Haxby, et al., 1999). Finally, as was the case for the lateral region of the fusiform gyrus, pictures of human faces also activated STS in approximately half the subjects, as previously reported by Kanwisher and colleagues (1997). Again, the peaks of the activations for animals and faces were essentially identical, but faces evoked a more focal pattern of activity in STS than did animals.

Single-cell recording studies in monkeys have shown activity in STS when viewing faces or face components, and when observing motion of people and other monkeys (see Desimone, 1991, for review). Consistent with these findings, human brain-imaging studies have revealed STS activity when viewing faces (Chao, Haxby, et al., 1999; Haxby et al., 1999; Ishai et al., 1999; Kanwisher et al., 1997), viewing mouth and eye movements (Puce et al., 1998), and observing human movements (Bonda et al., 1996; Rizzolatti, Fadiga, Matelli, et al., 1996). Thus, as we have suggested previously (Chao, Haxby, et al., 1999; Martin et al., 2000), STS may be involved not only in perception of biological motion but also in storing information about biological motion, perhaps in different parts of this region. If that is so, then the fact that viewing animals activates a portion of STS suggests that this information may be necessary, or at least available, to aid in identifying these stimuli.

In summary, the findings of the fMRI studies reported by Chao, Haxby, et al. (1999) revealed several category-related activations in the posterior region of the temporal lobes that were not seen in previous studies using PET. These included greater activation of the lateral portion of the fusiform gyrus and STS for animals (and human faces) than for tools (and houses), and greater activation of the medial fusiform region for tools (and houses) than for animals (and faces). In addition, these studies confirmed a finding that had been reported multiple times using PET: greater activity in the left posterior middle temporal gyrus for tools than for animals.

Activation of the left middle temporal gyrus in response to tools has been reported across a large number of paradigms using pictures of objects and their written names. These have included object naming of line drawings (Martin et al., 1996), silhouettes (Martin et al., 1996), and photographs (Chao, Haxby, et al., 1999); viewing rapidly presented pictures (Chao, Haxby, et al., 1999); delayed match-to-sample (Chao, Haxby, et al., 1999); answering written questions about object locations (Chao, Haxby, et al., 1999); verbal fluency (inanimate versus animate categories; Mummery et al., 1996); and answering written questions about visual and associative object features (Cappa et al., 1998). Other studies have employed a word triad task in which subjects judged the similarity of objects on different attributes (nonliving versus living categories; Mummery et al., 1998) and a same/different word-matching task (Perani et al., 1999). In addition, Perani and colleagues reported greater left middle temporal gyrus activity for a picture-matching task with tools, but not animals, relative to a low-level visual baseline task, and Moore and Price (1999) reported greater left middle temporal gyrus activity for tools versus a variety of other object categories using a picture-matching task (figure 6.5).

It is noteworthy that the location of these activations overlaps with the locations reported in verb generation studies reviewed previously (compare figures 6.2B and

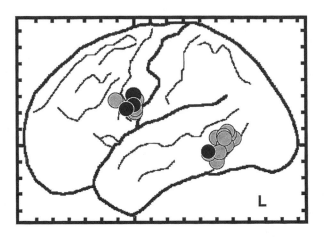

Figure 6.5
Schematic representation of the location of activations in the left middle temporal gyrus and left premotor cortex associated with tools, relative to animals or other object categories, across a variety of different paradigms (gray circles). Black circles indicate location of activations associated with imagined object grasping and imagined object manipulation (see text for details).

6.5). In addition, damage to this region has been linked to a selective loss of knowledge about tools (Tranel et al., 1997). These findings are consistent with the idea that information about object-associated motion is stored in the posterior region of the middle temporal gyrus.

As we suggested for the ventral region of the temporal lobe, the lateral region of the temporal lobes may also be tuned to different object features that members of a category share. The nature of these features remains to be determined. However, given the functional properties of posterior STS and middle temporal gyrus, one possibility may be that the lateral temporal cortex is tuned to the features of object motion. In the studies of Chao et al., biological objects (animals and faces) were associated with heightened activity in STS, whereas in Chao, Haxby, et al. (1999) and the studies listed above, tools were associated with heightened activity in the middle temporal gyrus. Objects, which by definition are stationary (houses), produced negligible activity in both regions. This pattern of activation suggests a superior-to-inferior gradient that may be tuned to the yet-to-be-determined features which distinguish biological motion from motion associated with the use of manipulable, man-made objects (see figure 6.4).

Left Premotor Cortex and the Representation of Object-Related Motor Sequences   In the view taken here, semantic representations of objects are assumed to include information about their defining attributes, and are automatically active when objects are identified. If that is so, one would expect to find selective activity near motor cortex for objects that we routinely manipulate manually (tools and utensils). Activation of one such area has been reported. Greater activation of the ventral region of left premotor cortex for tools than for animals has been reported for silent object naming of line drawings (Martin et al., 1996) and silhouettes (Martin et al., 1996). In addition, Grafton and colleagues (1997) reported left prefrontal activation for silently naming tools and tool-associated actions. Finally, Grabowski et al. (1998) reported that although left premotor and left prefrontal regions were active for naming animals and faces, as well as tools, an isolated region of left premotor cortex responded selectively to tools (this was a reanalysis of data from Damasio et al., 1996) (see figure 6.5).

These findings provide some support for an association between recognition of tools and activity in left premotor cortex. Tool-related activation of left premotor cortex, however, has not been nearly as consistent a finding as the association between tools and the left middle temporal gyrus. One possibility is that selective activity in left premotor cortex is difficult to identify with PET because many of the tasks employed have typically activated adjoining anterior sites in left lateral prefrontal cortex. In this regard, it may be noteworthy that the clearest findings have come from studies that used silent naming (Grafton et al., 1997; Martin et al., 1996) and silent verb generation (Grafton et al., 1997). Recent data from our laboratory using fMRI have replicated this finding. These studies have shown selective activation of left ventral premotor cortex for silent naming of tools relative to naming animal photographs and for viewing rapidly presented pictures of tools, but not of animals, faces, or houses (Chao & Martin, 2000). It is also noteworthy that activity in this region of premotor cortex has been found when subjects imagined grasping objects with their right hand (Decety et al., 1994; Grafton et al., 1997), and imagined performing a sequence of joystick movements with their right hand (Stephan et al., 1995) (figure 6.5).

Selective activation of left premotor cortex in response to manipulable objects is consistent with single-cell recording studies in monkeys. Rizzolatti and colleagues have identified neurons in the inferior region of monkey premotor cortex (area F5) that respond both during the execution of a movement and when observing the movement performed by others. Moreover, some cells that responded during movement execution also responded when the animals simply viewed objects they had previously manipulated (Murata et al., 1997). These and related findings have led to the suggestion that these neurons represent observed action, and form the basis for the understanding of motor events (see Jeannerod et al., 1995; Rizzollati, Fadiga, Gallese, et al., 1996). Thus, it may be that the left premotor region identified in the above noted functional brain-imaging studies carries out a similar function, specifically, storing information about the patterns of motor movements associated with the use of an object. If that is so, then the fact that naming tools, but not animals, activates this region further suggests that this information is automatically accessed when manipulable objects are identified.

Summary and Implications of Category-Specific Activations   Functional neuroimaging studies suggest that different types or classes of objects, such as animals and tools, are associated with different networks of discrete cortical regions. Tasks dependent on identifying and naming pictures of animals are associated with activity in the more lateral aspect of the fusiform gyrus, medial occipital cortex, and STS. These activations may be related to the automatic activation of stored information about object form, visual detail, and biological motion, respectively. In contrast, identifying and processing pictures of tools are associated with activation of the more medial aspect of the fusiform gyrus, left middle temporal gyrus, and left premotor cortex. These sites may be related to the automatic activation of stored information about object form, nonbiological motion, and object use-associated motor movements, respectively.

There is also evidence that reading the names of, and answering questions about, animals and tools produces category-related activity in some of the regions identified by the picture-processing tasks. This correspondence provides strong evidence that activity in temporal cortex reflects stored information about an object, not just the physical features of the material presented for processing. Moreover, in the Chao et al. study, the strongest activation was in the fusiform gyrus (a region assumed to represent object form) when answering questions about animals, and in the middle temporal gyrus (a region assumed to represent object motion) when answering questions about tools (see Chao, Haxby, et al., 1999, for details). Taken together with the studies of object picture-processing, these findings suggest that thinking about a particular object may require activation of the critical features that define that object. Thus, thinking about any characteristic of a particular animal would require activation of visual feature information. This finding could explain why some patients with a category-specific disorder for recognizing living things have difficulty answering questions that probe both visual and nonvisual information. In this view, these patients have damage to regions of the brain that store information about the visual form of animals, and activation of these representations may be necessary to gain access to other types of information about animals, assumed to be stored elsewhere. Consistent with this idea, Thompson-Schill and colleagues (1999) found increased activity in the left fusiform gyrus when subjects retrieved visual and nonvisual information about animals.

Viewed in this way, the evidence presented here appears to provide considerable support for feature-based models of semantic representation. However, some of the findings could be interpreted as evidence for Caramazza and Shelton's "domain-specific" hypothesis (1998) as well. For example, the clustering of activations associated with animals and faces, on the one hand, and tools and houses, on the other hand, reported by Chao, Haxby, et al. (1999) may be viewed as consistent with this interpretation. However, there is evidence to suggest that the representations of all nonbiological objects do not cluster together. For example, we have reported that the peak of activity associated with a category of objects of no evolutionary significance (chairs) was located laterally to the face-responsive region (in the inferior temporal gyrus) rather than medially (Ishai et al., 1999). Moreover, the domain-specific hypothesis does not make any predictions about where information about biological and nonbiological objects is represented in the brain. Clearly, different categories of objects activate different cortical networks. There does not seem to be a single region that maps onto whole categories. Nevertheless, it could be that there is a broader organization of these networks that reflects evolutionarily adapted, domain-specific knowledge systems for biological and nonbiological kinds. This possibility remains to be explored.

ISSUES

The evidence reviewed here suggests that we are beginning to make progress in understanding the neural substrate of some aspects of meaning. It is equally clear that we are only beginning to scratch the surface. Although I have tried to highlight agreements among studies, those familiar with this area of research may object that my focus has been overly narrow, and thus I have glossed over many puzzling discrepancies and contradictions in the literature. This is true. Time will tell whether the activations I chose to focus on, and the interpretations I have offered, are reasonable or not. Below I offer a brief list of some of the questions that may be worth pursuing in the future.

1. What is the role of the occipital lobes in object semantics? Specifically, does category-related activity in medial and ventral occipital cortex reflect top-down influences from more anterior regions in temporal cortex? If this activity is related to retrieving visual feature information, then why isn't occipital cortex active when information about color is retrieved? Integration of fMRI and MEG should help to sort out the temporal dynamics of activity within these networks.

2. How are category-related activations modified by experience? For example, what is the role played by expertise (e.g., Gauthier et al., 1999)? Will experience with motion and manipulation of novel objects result in the emergence of posterior middle temporal activity, and left premotor activity, respectively?

3. How is the lexicon organized? And how are lexical units linked to the networks of semantic primitives discussed in this chapter?

4. Similarly, where do we store associative information that comprises the bulk of semantic memory? How is this information linked to the networks of semantic primitives described here?

5. What neural structures mediate other aspects of meaning, such as the understanding of metaphor (e.g., Bottini et al., 1994)?

6. Do different structures within the medial temporal lobe declarative memory system (i.e., hippocampus, and entorhinal, perirhinal, and parahippocampal cortices) play different roles in the acquisition and/or retrieval of semantic and episodic memories (e.g., Maguire & Mummery, 1999)?

7. What brain structures are involved in categorizing objects? E. E. Smith and colleagues have shown that exemplar-based and rule-based categorizations activate different neural structures (E. E. Smith et al., 1999). Their study is an excellent example of how functional neuroimaging data can provide evidence germane to long-standing disputes in cognitive psychology.

ACKNOWLEDGMENTS

I thank my principal collaborators, Jim Haxby, Linda Chao, Cheri Wiggs, Alumit Ishai, and Leslie Ungerleider. This work was supported by the Intramural Research Program of the NIMH.

REFERENCES

Aguirre, G. K., Zarahn, E., & D'Esposito, M. (1998). An area within human ventral cortex sensitive to "building" stimuli: Evidence and implications. *Neuron* 21, 373–383.

Baldo, J. V., & Shimamura, A. P. (1998). Letter and category fluency in patients with frontal lobe lesions. *Neuropsychology* 12, 259–267.

Binder, J. R., Frost, J. A., Hammeke, T. A., Bellgowan, P. S. F., Rao, S. M., & Cox, R. W. (1999). Conceptual processing during the conscious resting state: A functional MRI study. *Journal of Cognitive Neuroscience* 11, 80–95.

Binder, J. R., Frost, J. A., Hammeke, T. A., Cox, R. W., Rao, S. M., & Prieto, T. (1997). Human brain language areas identified by functional magnetic resonance imaging. *Journal of Neuroscience* 17, 353–362.

Bonda, E., Petrides, M., Ostry, D., & Evans, A. (1996). Specific involvement of human parietal systems and the amygdala in the perception of biological motion. *Journal of Neuroscience* 16, 3737–3744.

Bookheimer, S. Y., Zeffiro, T. A., Blaxton, T., Gaillard, W., & Theodore, W. (1995). Regional cerebral blood flow during object naming and word reading. *Human Brain Mapping* 3, 93–106.

Bottini, G., Corcoran, R., Sterzi, R., Paulesu, E., Schenone, P., Scarpa, P., Frackowiak, R. S., & Frith, C. D. (1994). The role of the right hemisphere in the interpretation of figurative aspects of language: A positron emission tomography activation study. *Brain* 117, 1241–1253.

Broadbent, W. H. (1878). A case of peculiar affection of speech with commentary. *Brain* 1, 484–503.

Büchel, C., Price, C. J., & Friston, K. J. (1998). A multimodal language region in the ventral visual pathway. *Nature* 394, 274–277.

Bunn, E. M., Tyler, L. K., & Moss, H. E. (1998). Category-specific semantic deficits: The role of familiarity and property type reexamined. *Neuropsychology* 12, 367–379.

Caplan, D. (1992). *Language: Structure, Processing, and Disorders*. Cambridge MA: MIT Press.

Cappa, S. F., Perani, D., Schnur, T., Tettamanti, M., & Fazio, F. (1998). The effects of semantic category and knowledge type on lexical-semantic access: A PET study. *NeuroImage* 8, 350–359.

Caramazza, A., & Hillis, A. E. (1991). Lexical organization of nouns and verbs in the brain. *Nature* 349, 788–790.

Caramazza, A., Hillis, A. E., Rapp, B. C., & Romani, C. (1990). The multiple semantics hypothesis: Multiple confusions? *Cognitive Neuropsychology* 7, 161–189.

Caramazza, A., & Shelton, J. R. (1998). Domain-specific knowledge systems in the brain: The animate/inanimate distinction. *Journal of Cognitive Neuroscience* 10, 1–34.

Chao, L. L., & Martin, A. (1999). Cortical representation of perception, naming, and knowledge of color. *Journal of Cognitive Neuroscience* 11, 25–35.

Chao, L. L., & Martin, A. (2000). Representation of manipulable man-made objects in the dorsal stream. *NeuroImage*, in press.

Chao, L. L., Haxby, J. V., & Martin, A. (1999). Attribute-based neural substrates in temporal cortex for perceiving and knowing about objects. *Nature Neuroscience* 2, 913–919.

Chao, L. L., Martin, A., & Haxby, J. V. (1999). Are face-responsive regions selective only for faces? *NeuroReport* 2, 913–919.

Chee, M. W., O'Craven, K. M., Bergida, R., Rosen, B. R., & Savoy, R. L. (1999). Auditory and visual word processing studied with fMRI. *Human Brain Mapping* 7, 15–28.

Corbetta, M., Miezin, F. M., Dobmeyer, S., Shulman, G. L., & Petersen, S. E. (1990). Attentional modulation of neural processing of shape, color, and velocity in humans. *Science* 248, 1556–1559.

Damasio, A. R. (1989). Time-locked multiregional retroactivation: A systems-level proposal for the neural substrates of recall and recognition. *Cognition* 33, 25–62.

Damasio, A. R. (1990). Category-related recognition deficits as a clue to the neural substrates of knowledge. *Trends in Neurosciences* 13, 95–98.

Damasio, A. R., & Tranel, D. (1993). Nouns and verbs are retrieved with differently distributed neural systems. *Proceedings of the National Academy of Sciences of the United States of America* 90, 4957–4960.

Damasio, A., Yamada, T., Damasio, H., Corbett, J., & McKee, J. (1980). Central achromatopsia: Behavioral, anatomic, and physiologic aspects. *Neurology* 30, 1064–1071.

Damasio, H., Grabowski, T. J., Tranel, D., Hichwa, R. D., & Damasio, A. R. (1996). A neural basis for lexical retrieval. *Nature* 380, 499–505.

Decety, J., Perani, D., Jeannerod, M., Bettinardi, V., Tadary, B., Woods, R., Mazziotta, J. C., & Fazio, F. (1994). Mapping motor representations with positron emission tomography. *Nature* 371, 600–602.

Démonet, J. F., Chollet, F., Ramsay, S., Cardebat, D., Nespoulous, J. L., Wise, R., Rascol, A., & Frackowiak, R. (1992). The anatomy of phonological and semantic processing in normal subjects. *Brain* 115, 1753–1768.

Desimone, R. (1991). Face-selective cells in the temporal cortex of monkeys. *Journal of Cognitive Neuroscience* 3, 1–8.

De Vreese, L. P. (1991). Two systems for colour-naming defects: Verbal disconnection vs colour imagery disorder. *Neuropsychologia* 29, 1–18.

Epstein, R., & Kanwisher, N. (1998). A cortical representation of the local visual environment. *Nature* 392, 598–601.

Farah, M. (1990). *Visual Agnosia: Disorders of Object Recognition and What They Tell Us About Normal Vision*. Cambridge, MA: MIT Press.

Farah, M. J., & McClelland, J. L. (1991). A computational model of semantic memory impairment: Modality specificity and emergent category specificity. *Journal of Experimental Psychology: General* 120, 339–357.

Fodor, J., & Lepore, E. (1996). The red herring and the pet fish: Why concepts still can't be prototypes. *Cognition* 58, 253–270.

Forde, E. M. E., & Humphreys, G. W. (1999). Category-specific recognition impairments: A review of important case studies and influential theories. *Aphasiology* 13, 169–193.

Freud, S. (1891). *On Aphasia*, E. Stregel, trans. New York: International Universities Press.

Gabrieli, J. D. E., Poldrack, R. A., & Desmond, J. E. (1998). The role of left prefrontal cortex in language and memory. *Proceedings of the National Academy of Sciences USA* 95, 906–913.

Gaffan, D., & Heywood, C. A. (1993). A spurious category-specific visual agnosia for living things in normal human and nonhuman primates. *Journal of Cognitive Neuroscience* 5, 118–128.

Gainotti, G., Silveri, M. C., Daniele, A., & Giustolisi, L. (1995). Neuroanatomical correlates of category-specific semantic disorders: A critical survey. *Memory* 3, 247–264.

Gauthier, I., Tarr, M. J., Anderson, A. W., Skudlarski, P., & Gore, J. C. (1999). Activation of the middle fusiform "face area" increases with expertise in recognizing novel objects. *Nature Neuroscience* 2, 568–573.

Glaser, W. R. (1992). Picture naming. *Cognition* 42, 61–105.

Grabowski, T. J., Damasio, H., & Damasio, A. R. (1998). Premotor and prefrontal correlates of category-related lexical retrieval. *NeuroImage* 7, 232–243.

Grafton, S. T., Fadiga, L., Arbib, M. A., & Rizzolatti, G. (1997). Premotor cortex activation during observation and naming of familiar tools. *NeuroImage* 6, 231–236.

Hart, J., Jr., & Gordon, B. (1990). Delineation of single-word semantic comprehension deficits in aphasia, with anatomical correlation. *Annals of Neurology* 27, 226–231.

Haxby, J. V., Ungerleider, L. G., Clark, V. P., Schouten, J. L., Hoffman, E. A., & Martin, A. (1999). The effect of face inversion on activity in human neural systems for face and object perception. *Neuron* 22, 189–199.

Herbster, A. N., Mintun, M. A., Nebes, R. D., & Becker, J. T. (1997). Regional cerebral blood flow during word and nonword reading. *Human Brain Mapping* 5, 84–92.

Hodges, J. R., & Patterson, K. (1996). Nonfluent progressive aphasia and semantic dementia: A comparative neuropsychological study. *Journal of the International Neuropsychological Society* 2, 511–524.

Hodges, J. R., Patterson, K., Oxbury, S., & Funnell, E. (1992). Semantic dementia: Progressive fluent aphasia with temporal lobe atrophy. *Brain* 115, 1783–1806.

Hodges, J. R., Patterson, K., Ward, R., Garrard, P., Bak, T., Perry, R., & Gregory, C. (1999). The differentiation of semantic dementia and frontal lobe dementia (temporal and frontal variants of frontotemporal dementia) from early Alzheimer's disease: A comparative neuropsychological study. *Neuropsychology* 13, 31–40.

Howard, D., & Patterson, K. (1992). *Pyramids and Palm Trees: A Test of Semantic Access from Pictures and Words*. Bury St. Edmunds, UK: Thames Valley Test Company.

Howard, R. J., ffytche, D. H., Barnes, J., McKeefry, D., Ha, Y., Woodruff, P. W., Bullmore, E. T., Simmons, A., Williams, S. C. R., David, A. S., & Brammer, M. (1998). The functional anatomy of imagining and perceiving colour. *NeuroReport* 9, 1019–1023.

Humphreys, G. W., & Riddoch, M. J. (1987). On telling your fruit from your vegetables: A consideration of category-specific deficits after brain damage. *Trends in Neurosciences* 10, 145–148.

Humphreys, G. W., Riddoch, M. J., & Quinlan, P. T. (1988). Cascade processes in picture identification. *Cognitive Neuropsychology* 5, 67–103.

Ishai, A., Ungerleider, L. G., Martin, A., Schouten, J. L., & Haxby, J. V. (1999). Distributed representation of objects in the human ventral visual pathway. *Proceedings of the National Academy of Sciences USA* 96, 9379–9384

Jeannerod, M., Arbib, M. A., Rizzolatti, G., & Sakata, H. (1995). Grasping objects: The cortical mechanisms of visuomotor transformation. *Trends in Neurosciences* 18, 314–320.

Kanwisher, N., McDermott, J., & Chun, M. M. (1997). The fusiform face area: A module in human extrastriate cortex specialized for face perception. *Journal of Neuroscience* 17, 4302–4311.

Kiyosawa, M., Inoue, C., Kawasaki, T., Tokoro, T., Ishii, K., Ohyama, M., Senda, M., & Soma, Y. (1996). Functional neuroanatomy of visual object naming: A PET study. *Graefes Archives of Clinical and Experimental Ophthalmology* 234, 110–115.

Klein, D., Olivier, A., Milner, B., Zatorre, R. J., Zhao, V., & Nikelski, J. (1999). Cerebral organization in bilinguals: A PET study of Chinese-English verb generation. *NeuroReport* 10, 2841–2846.

Lissauer, H. (1890/1988). A case of visual agnosia with a contribution to theory. *Cognitive Neuropsychology* 5, 157–192. (First published in 1890.)

Luzzatti, C., & Davidoff, J. (1994). Impaired retrieval of object-colour knowledge with preserved colour naming. *Neuropsychologia* 32, 933–950.

Maguire, E. A., & Mummery, C. J. (1999). Differential modulation of a common memory retrieval network revealed by positron emission tomography. *Hippocampus* 9, 54–61.

Malach, R., Reppas, J. B., Benson, R. R., Kwong, K. K., Jiang, H., Kennedy, W. A., Ledden, P. J., Brady, T. J., Rosen, B. R., & Tootell, R. B. H. (1995). Object-related activity revealed by functional magnetic resonance imaging in human occipital cortex. *Proceedings of the National Academy of Sciences USA* 92, 8135–8139.

Martin, A. (1998). The organization of semantic knowledge and the origin of words in the brain. In *The Origins and Diversification of Language*, N. G. Jablonski & L. C. Aiello, Eds., 69–88. *Memoirs of the California Academy of Sciences*. no. 24. San Francisco: California Academy of Sciences.

Martin, A., Brouwers, P., Lalonde, F., Cox, C., Teleska, P., Fedio, P., Foster, N. L., & Chase, T. N. (1986). Towards a behavioral typology of Alzheimer's patients. *Journal of Clinical and Experimental Neuropsychology* 8, 594–610.

Martin, A., & Fedio, P. (1983). Word production and comprehension in Alzheimer's disease: The breakdown of semantic knowledge. *Brain and Language* 19, 124–141.

Martin, A., Haxby, J. V., Lalonde, F. M., Wiggs, C. L., & Ungerleider, L. G. (1995). Discrete cortical regions associated with knowledge of color and knowledge of action. *Science* 270, 102–105.

Martin, A., Ungerleider, L. G., & Haxby, J. V. (2000). Category-specificity and the brain: The sensory-motor model of semantic representations of objects. In *The Cognitive Neurosciences*, M. S. Gazzaniga, ed., 2nd ed. Cambridge, MA: MIT Press.

Martin, A., Wiggs, C. L., Lalonde, F. M., & Mack, C. (1994). Word retrieval to letter and semantic cues: A double dissociation in normal subjects using interference tasks. *Neuropsychologia* 32, 1487–1494.

Martin, A., Wiggs, C. L., Ungerleider, L. G., & Haxby, J. V. (1996). Neural correlates of category-specific knowledge. *Nature* 379, 649–652.

McCarthy, G., Blamire, A. M., Rothman, D., Gruetter, R., & Shulman, R. G. (1993). Echo-planar magnetic resonance imaging studies of frontal cortex activation during word generation in humans. *Proceedings of the National Academy of Sciences USA* 90, 4952–4956.

McCarthy, G., Puce, A., Gore, J., & Allison, T. (1997). Face-specific processing in the human fusiform gyrus. *Journal of Cognitive Neuroscience* 9, 605–610.

McKeefry, D. J., & Zeki, S. (1997). The position and topology of the human colour centre as revealed by functional magnetic resonance imaging. *Brain* 120, 2229–2242.

McNeil, J. E., & Warrington, E. K. (1993). Prosopagnosia: A face-specific disorder. *Quarterly Journal of Experimental Psychology* A46, 1–10.

Miller, G. A. (1999). On knowing a word. *Annual Review of Psychology* 50, 1–19.

Moore, C. J., & Price, C. J. (1999). A functional neuroimaging study of the variables that generate category-specific object processing differences. *Brain* 122, 943–962.

Mummery, C. J., Patterson, K., Hodges, J. R., & Price, C. J. (1998). Functional neuroanatomy of the semantic system: Divisible by what? *Journal of Cognitive Neuroscience* 10, 766–777.

Mummery, C. J., Patterson, K., Hodges, J. R., & Wise, R. J. S. (1996). Generating "tiger" as an animal name or word beginning with T: Differences in brain activation. *Proceedings of the Royal Society of London* B263, 989–995.

Mummery, C. J., Patterson, K., Wise, R. J. S., Vandenberghe, R., Price, C. J., & Hodges, J. R. (1999). Disrupted temporal lobe connections in semantic dementia. *Brain* 122, 61–73.

Murata, A., Fadiga, L., Fogassi, L., Gallese, V., Raos, V., & Rizzolatti, G. (1997). Object representation in the ventral premotor cortex (F5) of the monkey. *Journal of Neurophysiology* 78, 2226–2230.

Paulesu, E., Harrison, J., Baron-Cohen, S., Watson, J. D., Goldstein, L., Heather, J., Frackowiak, R. S., & Frith, C. D. (1995). The physiology of coloured hearing. A PET activation study of colour-word synaesthesia. *Brain* 118, 661–676.

Perani, D., Cappa, S. F., Bettinardi, V., Bressi, S., Gorno-Tempini, M., Matarrese, M., & Fazio, F. (1995). Different neural systems for the recognition of animals and man-made tools. *NeuroReport* 6, 1637–1641.

Perani, D., Schnur, T., Tettamanti, M., Gorno-Tempini, M., Cappa, S. F., & Fazio, F. (1999). Word and picture matching: A PET study of semantic category effects. *Neuropsychologia* 37, 293–306.

Petersen, S. E., Fox, P. T., Posner, M. I., Mintun, M. A., & Raichle, M. E. (1988). Positron emission tomographic studies of the cortical anatomy of single-word processing. *Nature* 331, 585–589.

Pietrini, V., Nertempi, P., Vaglia, A., Revello, M. G., Pinna, V., & Ferro-Milone, F. (1988). Recovery from herpes simplex encephalitis: Selective impairment of specific semantic categories with neuroradiological correlation. *Journal of Neurology, Neurosurgery and Psychiatry* 6, 251–272.

Poldrack, R. A., Wagner, A. D., Prull, M. W., Desmond, J. E., Glover, G. H., & Gabrieli, J. D. E. (1999). Functional specialization for semantic and phonological processing in the left inferior frontal cortex. *NeuroImage* 10, 15–35.

Poline, J. B., Vandenberghe, R., Holmes, A. P., Friston, K. J., & Frackowiak, R. S. J. (1996). Reproducibility of PET activation studies: Lessons from a multi-center European experiment. *NeuroImage* 4, 34–54.

Price, C. J., Moore, C. J., & Frackowiak, R. S. (1996). The effect of varying stimulus rate and duration on brain activity during reading. *NeuroImage* 3, 40–52.

Price, C. J., Moore, C. J., Humphreys, G. W., & Wise, R. J. S. (1997). Segregating semantic and phonological processes during reading. *Journal of Cognitive Neuroscience* 9, 727–733.

Price, C. J., Wise, R. J. S., & Frackowiak, R. S. J. (1996). Demonstrating the implicit processing of visually presented words and pseudowords. *Cerebral Cortex* 6, 62–70.

Puce, A., Allison, T., Asgari, M., Gore, J. C., & McCarthy, G. (1996). Differential sensitivity of human visual cortex to faces, letter strings, and textures: A functional magnetic resonance imaging study. *Journal of Neuroscience* 16, 5205–5215.

Puce, A., Allison, T., Bentin, S., Gore, J. C., & McCarthy, G. (1998). Temporal cortex activation in humans viewing eye and mouth movements. *Journal of Neuroscience* 18, 2188–2199.

Raichle, M. E., Fiez, J. A., Videen, T. O., MacLeod, A. M., Pardo, J. V., Fox, P. T., & Petersen, S. E. (1994). Practice-related changes in human brain functional anatomy during nonmotor learning. *Cerebral Cortex* 4, 8–26.

Ricci, P. T., Zelkowicz, B. J., Nebes, R. D., Meltzer, C. C., Mintun, M. A., & Becker, J. T. (1999). Functional neuroanatomy of semantic memory: Recognition of semantic associations. *NeuroImage* 9, 88–96.

Rizzolatti, G., Fadiga, L., Gallese, V., & Fogassi, L. (1996). Premotor cortex and the recognition of motor actions. *Cognitve Brain Research* 3, 131–141.

Rizzolatti, G., Fadiga, L., Matelli, M., Bettinardi, V., Paulesu, E., Perani, D., & Fazio, F. (1996). Localization of grasp representations in humans by PET: 1. Observation versus execution. *Experimental Brain Research* 111, 246–252.

Sakai, K., Watanabe, E., Onodera, Y., Uchida, I., Kato, H., Yamamoto, E., Koizumi, H., & Miyashita, Y. (1995). Functional mapping of the human colour centre with echo-planar magnetic resonance imaging. *Proceedings of the Royal Society of London* B261, 89–98.

Sergent, J., Zuck, E., Levesque, M., & MacDonald, B. (1992). Positron emission tomography study of letter and object processing: Empirical findings and methodological considerations. *Cerebral Cortex* 2, 68–80.

Shaywitz, B. A., Pugh, K. R., & Constable, R. T. (1995). Localization of semantic processing using functional magnetic resonance imaging. *Human Brain Mapping* 2, 149–158.

Shuren, J. E., Brott, T. G., Schefft, B. K., & Houston, W. (1996). Preserved color imagery in an achromatopsic. *Neuropsychologia* 34, 485–489.

Smith, A. T., Greenlee, M. W., Singh, K. D., Kraemer, F. M., & Hennig, J. (1998). The processing of first- and second-order motion in human visual cortex assessed by functional magnetic resonance imaging (fMRI). *Journal of Neuroscience* 18, 3816–3830.

Smith, E. E., Patalano, A. L., & Jonides, J. (1999). Alternative strategies of categorization. *Cognition* 65, 167–196.

Snodgrass, J. G., & Vanderwart, M. (1980). A standardized set of 260 pictures: Norms for naming agreement, familiarity, and visual complexity. *Journal of Experimental Psychology: Human Learning and Memory* 6, 174–215.

Stephan, K. M., Fink, G. R., Passingham, R. E., Silbersweig, D., Ceballos-Baumann, A. O., Frith, C. D., & Frackowiak, R. S. (1995). Functional anatomy of the mental representation of upper extremity movements in healthy subjects. *Journal of Neurophysiology* 73, 373–386.

Tatsumi, I. F., Fushimi, T., Sadato, N., Kawashima, R., Yokoyama E., Kanno, I., & Senda, M. (1999). Verb generation in Japanese: A multicenter PET activation study. *NeuroImage* 9, 154–164.

Thompson-Schill, S. L., Aguirre, G. K., D'Esposito, M., & Farah, M. (1999). A neural basis for category and modality specificity of semantic knowledge. *Neuropsychologia* 37, 671–676.

Thompson-Schill, S. L., D'Esposito, M., Aguirre, G. K., & Farah, M. J. (1997). Role of left inferior prefrontal cortex in retrieval of semantic knowledge: A reevaluation. *Proceedings of the National Academy of Sciences of the United States of America* 94, 14792–14797.

Thompson-Schill, S. L., Swick, D., Farah, M. J., D'Esposito, M., Kan, I. P., & Knight, R. T. (1998). Verb generation in patients with focal frontal lesions: A neuropsychological test of neuroimaging findings. *Proceedings of the National Academy of Sciences of the United States of America* 95, 15855–15860.

Tranel, D., Damasio, H., & Damasio, A. R. (1997). A neural basis for the retrieval of conceptual knowledge. *Neuropsychologia* 35, 1319–1327.

Tulving, E. (1983). *Elements of Episodic Memory*. New York: Oxford University Press.

Vaina, L. M. (1994). Functional segregation of color and motion processing in the human visual cortex: Clinical evidence. *Cerebral Cortex* 4(5), 555–572.

Vandenberghe, R., Price, C. J., Wise, R., Josephs, O., & Frackowiak, R. S. J. (1996). Functional anatomy of a common semantic system for words and pictures. *Nature* 383, 254–256.

Warburton, E., Wise, R. J., Price, C. J., Weiller, C., Hadar, U., Ramsay, S., & Frackowiak, R. S. (1996). Noun and verb retrieval by normal subjects: Studies with PET. *Brain* 119(1), 159–179.

Warrington, E. K. (1975). The selective impairment of semantic memory. *Quarterly Journal of Experimental Psychology* 27, 635–657.

Warrington, E. K., & McCarthy, R. (1983). Category specific access dysphasia. *Brain* 106, 859–878.

Warrington, E. K., & McCarthy, R. A. (1987). Categories of knowledge: Further fractionations and an attempted integration. *Brain* 110(5), 1273–1296.

Warrington, E. K., & Shallice, T. (1984). Category specific semantic impairments. *Brain* 107, 829–854.

Watson, J. D., Myers, R., Frackowiak, R. S., Hajnal, J. V., Woods, R. P., Mazziotta, J. C., Shipp, S., & Zeki, S. (1993). Area V5 of the human brain: Evidence from a combined study using positron emission tomography and magnetic resonance imaging. *Cerebral Cortex* 3, 79–94.

Webster's New World Dictionary, Third College Edition. (1988). New York: Simon & Schuster.

Wiggs, C. L., Weisberg, J., & Martin, A. (1999). Neural correlates of semantic and episodic memory retrieval. *Neuropsychologia* 37(1), 103–118.

Wise, R., Chollet, F., Hadar, U., Friston, K., Hoffner, E., & Frackowiak, R. (1991). Distribution of cortical neural networks involved in word comprehension and word retrieval. *Brain* 114, 1803–1817.

Zeki, S., Watson, J. D., Lueck, C. J., Friston, K. J., Kennard, C., & Frackowiak, R. S. (1991). A direct demonstration of functional specialization in human visual cortex. *Journal of Neuroscience* 11, 641–649.

Zelkowicz, B. J., Herbster, A. N., Nebes, R. D., Mintun, M. A., & Becker, J. T. (1998). An examination of regional cerebral blood flow during object naming tasks. *Journal of the International Neuropsychological Society* 4, 160–166.

Zihl, J., von Cramon, D., Mai, N., & Schmid, C. (1991). Disturbance of movement vision after bilateral posterior brain damage: Further evidence and follow up observations. *Brain* 114, 2235–2252.

7 Functional Neuroimaging of Language

Jeffrey Binder and Cathy J. Price

INTRODUCTION

Humans communicate using a variety of signals, including speech sounds, written symbols and other visual artifacts, axial and limb gestures, and facial expressions. "Language" refers to any system of communication involving arbitrary (symbolic or nonidentity) representation of information. While all of the communicative signals available to humans are thus used for languages of varying complexity, communication with spoken, written, and signed *words* is arguably the most extensive and uniquely human of these languages. Our capacity to maintain the arbitrary relationships linking a large number of words to underlying concepts is staggering, as is the capacity to combine these words in a virtually limitless number of different expressions. In this chapter we focus on the neuroanatomy of this verbal language system as it is revealed by functional brain imaging.

Defined in this way, the verbal language system in the brain is most concisely characterized as a complex system of knowledge (i.e., genetically inherited or learned information) about words. This knowledge base can be divided into conceptually distinct subsystems that may or may not have spatially distinct neural representations. The major traditional subsystems include (1) phonetics, information concerning articulatory and perceptual characteristics of speech sounds; (2) orthographics, information concerning written letter combinations; (3) phonology, the language-specific rules by which speech sounds are represented and manipulated; (4) lexicon, information about specific phoneme and grapheme combinations that form words in the language; (5) semantics, information regarding word meanings, names, and other declarative knowledge about the world; and (6) syntax, the rules by which words are combined to make well-formed sentences and sentences are analyzed to reveal underlying relationships between words.

Effective use of words also requires the interaction of these verbal knowledge stores with sensory input, motor output, attention, and short-term memory systems. Everyday conversation, for example, would not be possible without arousal systems to keep us awake, low-level auditory processors, short-term memory, and speech articulation mechanisms. Although language behavior is dependent on such systems, there is reason for a conceptual distinction between these systems and the verbal knowledge systems mentioned earlier. We can imagine engaging early sensory, motor, attention, and working memory processes during behaviors that are essentially nonverbal, such as in a task involving pressing a key every other time a sensory signal appears. To the extent that these systems are used in common to support both verbal and nonverbal behaviors, we regard them as nonlinguistic, general-purpose systems, while recognizing that they interact closely with verbal knowledge stores and may in some cases be partly specialized for language-related functions (for example, in the case of "verbal working memory").

Special Problems for Language Activation Imaging Studies

Functional imaging of language processes occurs in the context of more than a century of research on language localization using lesion-deficit correlation (Broca, 1861; H. Damasio, 1989; Geschwind, 1965; Goldstein, 1948; Henschen, 1920–1922; Luria, 1966; Nielsen, 1946; Penfield & Roberts, 1959; Shallice, 1988; Wernicke, 1874). Although much has been learned from lesion-deficit research, this approach also has important limitations. The overall extent and precise distribution of the lesions vary considerably across individuals, creating a large number of lesion variables that may or may not be related to the behavioral deficits. Meanwhile, commonly shared features of the vascular supply result in areas of lesion overlap across subjects independent of any shared deficits. Detection of deficits varies with the method and timing of testing, and with the a priori aims of the experimenter. Patients are not tested prior to occurrence of the lesion, so no baseline data are available. Finally, dysfunction of one processing subsystem may interfere with a wide range of observable behaviors, leading to overlocalization by false attribution of these behaviors to the lesioned area.

These and other problems have limited the ultimate spatial precision and interpretability of lesion-deficit correlation data. Despite these limitations, however, there are also broad points of consensus about the anatomical basis of certain aphasic symptoms, as well as a large number of carefully executed correlation studies from which reasonably firm conclusions can be drawn. These results thus provide important constraints for the interpretation of functional imaging data. Functional imaging techniques have the potential to provide localization information that is considerably more precise than what can be obtained by lesion analysis, and the potential to observe the full workings of the intact language system. On the other hand, several theoretical issues complicate the design and interpretation of language activation studies.

Interactive Coactivation of Linguistic Subsystems   Although conceptually distinct, the linguistic subsystems (phonological, semantic, syntactic, etc.) act together during everyday language behaviors. For example, "comprehension" of a spoken sentence engages speech sound perceptual mechanisms in concert with word recognition, semantic, and syntactic knowledge systems. Many lines of evidence suggest, for example, that lexical, semantic, and syntactic knowledges constrain phoneme and grapheme perception (Ganong, 1980; Miller, 1963; Reicher, 1969; Tulving & Gold, 1963; Warren & Obusek, 1971), and that word-level semantic processing interacts with knowledge of syntactic relationships during sentence interpretation (Marslen-Wilson & Tyler, 1981; McClelland & Kawamoto, 1986). The extent to which each component subsystem can be examined in isolation thus remains a major method-ological issue for functional activation imaging studies. By contrasting, for example, conditions in which attention is directed to either semantic or syntactic features of sentences, a large part of both processing subsystems might remain invisible because of interactive coactivation of both subsystems across both conditions. At issue here is the degree to which attentional shifts between contrasting knowledge subsystems can create activation contrasts in functional imaging tasks and, conversely, the degree to which activation in these subsystems is independent of selective attentional influences.

Preattentive (Automatic, Obligatory, or Implicit) Processing   A closely related issue concerns the degree to which linguistic attributes of stimuli are processed when there are no task demands related to these attributes. A familiar example is the Stroop effect, in which semantic processing of printed words occurs even when subjects are instructed to attend to the color of the print, and even when this semantic processing interferes with task performance (Macleod, 1991). Considerable converging evidence suggests that such preattentive processing is commonplace when the brain is pre-sented with stimuli that have phonological and semantic associations, and occurs out-side the control or conscious awareness of subjects (Carr et al., 1982; Macleod, 1991; Marcel, 1983; Price, Wise, & Frackowiak, 1996; Van Orden, 1987). Price, Wise, and Frackowiak (1996) demonstrated this general phenomenon in a PET study. Subjects were required to detect a target visual feature (vertical lines) in printed text stimuli. This task remained constant while the stimuli varied in terms of linguistic value. Compared to activation produced by nonsense characters and consonant strings, pronounceable (i.e., orthographically legal) nonwords and real words produced addi-tional activation in widespread, left-lateralized cortical areas, even though the explicit task was identical across all conditions (figure 7.1 and color plate 7).

If familiar stimuli such as words, pronounceable nonwords, and pictures evoke uncontrolled, automatic language processing, these effects need to be considered in the design and interpretation of language activation experiments. Use of such stimuli in a baseline condition could result in undesirable subtraction (or partial subtraction) of language-related activation. Such inadvertent subtraction may be particularly rel-evant in functional imaging studies of language processing, which frequently attempt to match, as closely as possible, the stimuli in the activation and control tasks. One notable example is the widely employed "word generation" task, which is frequently

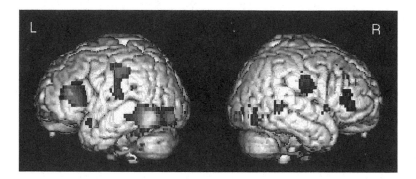

Figure 7.1
Regions demonstrating greater activation to words than to consonant letter strings during a nonlinguistic visual feature detection task. This activation represents preattentive (automatic) processing of linguistic information associated with the words. Very similar patterns resulted from contrasting words to false font, and pseudo words to letters (Price, Wise, & Frackowiak, 1996). (See color plate 7.)

paired with a control task involving repetition or reading of words (Buckner et al., 1995; Petersen et al., 1988; Raichle et al., 1994). In most of these studies, which were aimed at detecting activation related to semantic processing, there has been relatively little activation in temporal and temporoparietal structures that are known, on the basis of lesion studies, to be involved in semantic processing. In contrast, subtractions involving control tasks that use nonlinguistic stimuli generally reveal a much more extensive network of left hemisphere temporal, parietal, and frontal language-processing areas (Binder et al., 1997; Bookheimer et al., 1995; H. Damasio et al., 1996; Démonet et al., 1992; Price, Wise, & Frackowiak, 1996). Collectively, these results suggest that the word repetition control task used in the word generation studies elicits preattentive processing in many of the regions shown in figure 7.1, and that this control task activation obscures much of the activation in these areas that presumably occurs during word generation. These results also illustrate a more general point: that activation contrast maps are as dependent on properties of the *control* task and *control* stimuli as on the explicit requirements of the activation task.

Stimulus-Unrelated Language Processing   Verbal language, as we have defined it, is dependent on interactive systems of internally stored knowledge about words and word meanings. Although in examining these systems we typically use familiar stimuli or cues to engage processing, it seems quite likely that activity in these systems could occur independently of external stimulation and task demands. The idea that the conscious mind can be internally active independent of external events has a long history in psychology and neuroscience (Aurell, 1979; Hebb, 1954; James, 1890;

Miller et al., 1960; Picton & Stuss, 1994; Pope & Singer, 1976). When asked, subjects in experimental studies frequently report experiencing seemingly unprovoked thoughts that are unrelated to the task at hand (Antrobus et al., 1966; Pope & Singer, 1976; Teasdale et al., 1993). The precise extent to which such "thinking" engages linguistic knowledge remains unclear (Révész, 1954; Weiskrantz, 1988), but many researchers have demonstrated close parallels between behavior and language content, suggesting that at least some thought processes make use of verbally encoded semantic knowledge and other linguistic representations (Karmiloff-Smith, 1992; Révész, 1954; Vygotsky, 1962).

Stimulus-unrelated processing appears to require attentional resources. The frequency of reported "thoughts" and hallucinations increases as external stimulation decreases or becomes more static and predictable (Antrobus et al., 1966; Pope & Singer, 1976; Solomon et al., 1961). Conversely, the performance of effortful perceptual and short-term memory tasks suppresses these phenomena, indicating a direct competition between exogenous and endogenous signals for attentional and executive resources (Antrobus et al., 1966; Filler & Giambra, 1973; Pope & Singer, 1976; Segal & Fusella, 1970; Teasdale et al., 1993, 1995). These studies suggest that the "resting" state and states involving minimal attentional demands (such as passive stimulation and visual fixation tasks) may actually be very active states in which subjects frequently are engaged in processing linguistic representations (Binder et al., 1999). Use of such states as control conditions for language activation imaging studies may thus obscure similar processing that occurs during the language task of interest. This is a particularly difficult problem for language and conceptual processing studies because, for such studies, task-unrelated processing may be a profoundly important variable that cannot be directly measured or precisely controlled.

Some General Characteristics of PET and fMRI Language Activation Data

The functional imaging data to be considered in this chapter come primarily from O15 PET and fMRI studies of language processing. Although different in some respects, the two methods share a sufficient number of common features to warrant consideration of a combined review. Both methods measure signals associated with blood flow increases in metabolically active tissue rather than signals arising directly from neural activity. As typically practiced, both methods measure relative differences in signal (rather than absolute levels) across different activation conditions. Very similar or identical methods of statistical analysis within and among subjects have been applied in PET and fMRI research.

Essential differences between these methods also exist. For example, fMRI signals depend not only on changes in blood flow but also on changes in oxygen extraction fraction that alter intravascular oxygen concentration (known as blood oxygenation level dependency, or BOLD). fMRI appears to be more sensitive than PET to whole-head movement and soft tissue motion, which cause artifactual signals in fMRI data that may appear to be correlated with changes in task condition (Hajnal et al., 1994). PET methods typically sample larger volume elements (voxels) and produce fewer data points per subject compared to fMRI. At issue is whether or not these and other differences are large compared to the similarities, and therefore preclude direct comparisons between PET and fMRI language data. The most precise evidence on this issue includes direct comparisons of PET and fMRI data in the same subjects, using the same activation contrasts (Kraut et al., 1995; Ramsay et al., 1996), but no such studies have yet been published in the language activation literature. Many PET and fMRI studies show very similar patterns of activation in visual and auditory sensory areas during passive word presentation (e.g., compare superior temporal gyrus activation by speech sounds, in Wise et al., 1991, and Binder et al., 1996). Very similar PET and fMRI activation patterns have also been demonstrated using nearly identical language task contrasts (Binder et al., 1997, 1999; Buckner et al., 1995, 1996; Démonet et al., 1992; Howard et al., 1992; Small et al., 1996).

Figure 7.2 (and color plate 8) shows an example of such a replication across imaging modalities. In this example very similar activation foci associated with semantic processing are observed in the left angular gyrus, dorsal prefrontal cortex, and posterior cingulate cortex in both studies, despite use of different imaging modalities, different subjects, slightly different tasks and stimuli, and different statistical methods. The small differences between these and other matched PET/fMRI studies do not seem as large as some differences observed across supposedly similar experiments performed in the same imaging modality (Poeppel, 1996; Poline et al., 1996). While more such replication studies are needed, initial results like these suggest that under ideal circumstances it is reasonable to expect very similar results from PET and fMRI. Large differences are thus more likely to be due to lack of statistical power on the part of one or both studies, differences in task requirements or stimuli (either control or activation task), or some other unknown systematic bias.

Special Problems for PET Language Studies   The relatively lower spatial and temporal resolutions of PET compared to fMRI are well recognized and will not be discussed further here. These problems place limits on the level of observable detail and preclude use of PET to study short-term cognitive events, but do not impact on the valid use of this technique to address many other issues in the localization of language processes. Similarly, although the relatively smaller number of measurements obtainable from each subject using PET makes its application to studying individual vari-

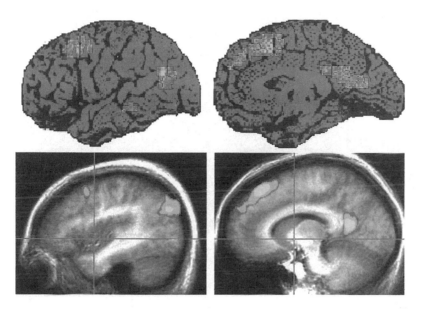

Figure 7.2
Similarity of activation patterns obtained by PET and fMRI in two studies contrasting semantic categorization of auditory words with phonetic categorization of nonwords. Top row shows surface projection PET images from Démonet et al. (1992). Bottom row shows sagittal fMRI slices from Binder et al. (1999). (See color plate 8.)

ability and changes that occur within individuals over time more difficult, PET is well suited to group studies, in which greater statistical certainty is obtained by studying more subjects rather than by studying each subject more.

PET data analysis typically includes considerable spatial smoothing of individual subject data prior to conducting group analyses in order to overcome misalignment of activation foci across subjects due to anatomical and functional variability, and to maximize within-subject signal-to-noise ratio by suppressing high-frequency spatial noise. Smoothing is typically performed with a Gaussian function applied over a kernel of 15–20 mm diameter. As a result of this process, the final activity level at a given voxel location is a sum of weighted activation values in the spatial neighborhood of the voxel. Depending on the proximity of different activation foci and the degree of smoothing used, activity from one focus may contribute significantly to the activation level of a neighboring focus.

This neighborhood influence can present a problem when investigators wish to make claims about interhemispheric asymmetry of activation, claims that are frequently of theoretical importance in language studies. In one report, for example, left-

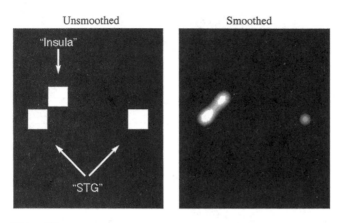

Figure 7.3
Illustration of neighborhood effects induced by spatial smoothing. Proximity of the left hemisphere "insula" and "STG" foci results in spurious STG asymmetry due to smoothing.

ward asymmetry of activation in the superior temporal gyrus (STG) was interpreted as evidence for linguistic-level processing in this region (Rumsey et al., 1997). However, this left STG activation was accompanied by activation in the neighboring left insula, whereas no such neighboring focus occurred near the right STG. Figure 7.3 illustrates a simulation of this situation, beginning with simulated cubical "activation foci" of equal size and magnitude, centered on the stereotaxic coordinates given for the STG and insular foci in the original study. These foci were then smoothed using a Gaussian filter with root mean square diameter of 20 mm. As shown on the right side of the figure, the simulated insular focus had a profound effect on the neighboring left STG focus, substantially increasing its peak magnitude and thresholded extent relative to the contralateral STG focus, and resulting in a degree of asymmetry very similar to that observed in the original study. Although they were actually identical, smoothing caused these two foci to appear quite asymmetric. The degree and significance of such effects depend on several factors, including the magnitude of any neighboring foci, the proximity of these foci to the focus in question, and the degree of smoothing employed. Unless all of these variables can be quantified and taken into consideration, it may be difficult to draw conclusions about magnitude differences between activation foci located in very different activity "environments."

Special Problems for fMRI Language Studies   fMRI enables imaging at greater spatial and temporal resolution than O15 PET, and there are no safety restrictions on the number of images than can be made of a given individual. These characteristics greatly increase the practicality of obtaining robust signals from individual subjects, of exploring a wider variety of activation conditions within each subject, and of detecting small areas or small differences between areas of activation. A disadvantage of fMRI for studies of speech perception is the unavoidable presence of noise generated by the scanner, caused by transduction of energy in the imaging coil during rapid magnetic field gradient switching. The characteristics of this noise depend on many variables, including the type of imaging pulse sequence, head coil and other hardware, rate of image acquisition, and image slice orientation used. Echoplanar imaging, probably the most common type of pulse sequence, is typically associated with a brief (e.g., <100 msec) broadband, harmonically complex noise pulse with peak intensity levels on the order of 110–130 dB SPL. Despite this noise, robust activation signals associated with intermittent presentation of experimental stimuli can be readily obtained from auditory cortex using fMRI (Binder et al., 1996; Binder, Rao, Hammeke, et al., 1994; Dhankhar et al., 1997; Jäncke et al., 1998). A study suggests that fMRI activation signals resulting from the scanner noise are confined primarily to Heschl's gyrus (Bandettini et al., 1997), although the extent to which this activation interferes with the detection of responses in other auditory regions has not yet been precisely determined.

A concern is that the scanner noise may raise baseline BOLD signal to varying degrees in auditory (and perhaps other) areas, thus decreasing the dynamic range available for stimulus-induced contrasts (Zatorre & Binder, 2000). A reasonable solution to this problem takes advantage of the fact that the BOLD signal response (which is dependent primarily on vascular events), resulting from a brief neural activation, typically reaches a peak within 5 or 6 sec and returns to baseline within 10–15 sec after the neural event (Buckner et al., 1996). To avoid imaging these BOLD responses arising from scanner noise stimulation thus requires separation of the image acquisitions in time by at least 10–15 sec. For multislice acquisitions, this means that all slice locations must be imaged quickly during the early portion of each repetition time (TR) interval, followed by a much longer interval (10–15 sec) until the next acquisition (Zatorre & Binder, 2000), in contrast to the conventional approach, in which image acquisitions at the selected slice locations are spaced evenly throughout the TR interval. Provided that these clustered image acquisitions are sufficiently separated in time, the resulting BOLD signals should reflect only the activation from experimental stimuli presented during the interval between acquisitions. A relative drawback of this method is that considerably fewer images are acquired in a given unit of time (because of the much longer TR), necessitating longer scanning sessions to obtain comparable statistical power.

A second issue regarding interpretation of fMRI language studies is the problem of artifactual signal loss in certain brain regions on T2*-weighted (particularly echo-

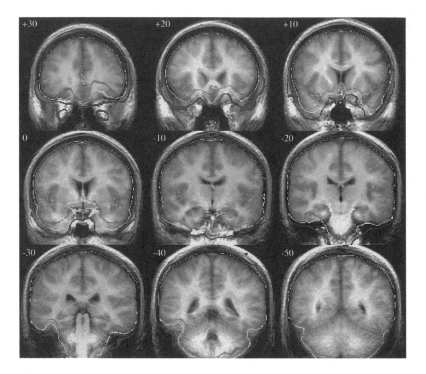

Figure 7.4
Coronal sections (stereotaxic y axis coordinates in upper left of section) illustrating areas of relative signal loss during echoplanar imaging (EPI). Single-shot EPI data (TE = 40 ms) were acquired at 1.5 T at 19 contiguous sagittal slice locations, with in-plane dimensions of 3.75 mm × 3.75 mm and slice thickness = 7 mm. Averaged, thresholded EPI data from 12 subjects are superimposed on averaged brain anatomy images. EPI signals are greatest in the ventricles and brain parenchyma (not shown). Colored lines represent iso-intensity contours at 30% (red), 20% (yellow), and 10% (blue) of maximum average signal. Regions of significant signal loss (<20% of maximum) occur particularly in posteromedial orbital frontal cortex and anteromedial temporal pole ($y = +30$ to 0), with a smaller region in mid-ventrolateral temporal cortex ($y = -30$ to -50). Contrary to common belief, the hippocampus is relatively unaffected. (See color plate 9.)

planar) images. As shown in figure 7.4 (and color plate 9) the problem is most evident in the posteromedial orbital frontal and medial anterior temporal regions (perhaps because of proximity to the nasal cavity and sphenoidal sinuses) and the midportion of the ventrolateral temporal lobe (perhaps because of proximity to the middle ear cavity and auditory canal). It is generally believed that natural air-tissue interfaces in these regions cause small, local distortions of the magnetic field. These distortions produce small, intravoxel field gradients that greatly reduce MR signal as a result of intravoxel spin dephasing (the macroscopic susceptibility or T2* effect). Because signal loss is proportional to the magnitude of this intravoxel gradient, the problem is worse at higher field strengths, when using larger voxels, and when the longest voxel diameter happens to be oriented along the gradient. Loss of baseline signal probably reduces sensitivity to activation-induced BOLD signal changes in these areas, although this putative reduction in sensitivity has not yet been demonstrated or quantified. Several research teams have developed techniques for recovering signal in these areas by applying information about the intravoxel gradients (Kadah & Hu, 1997; Yang et al., 1998). Thus, although a practical solution to the problem appears imminent, this may involve collection of additional data at each time point, with resulting trade-offs in temporal resolution.

Finally, as mentioned above, fMRI is very sensitive to whole-head and soft tissue motion. Even relatively small movements can significantly alter the composition of small voxels situated at tissue boundaries (e.g., gray matter/white matter junction or brain edge), thereby causing signal changes unrelated to blood flow, or may produce signal changes by altering the magnetic field itself (Birn et al., 1998). This problem can affect interpretation of fMRI data in three ways. First, as already mentioned, motion may be correlated for various reasons with changes in activation state, resulting in false positive "activation" at structural boundaries or in areas affected by magnetic field disturbances (Birn et al., 1999; Hajnal et al., 1994). Second, even very small head movements between successive scans may cause previously active voxels to appear inactive or less active, or previously inactive voxels to become active. This fact renders problematic any experimental design in which task conditions are not interleaved in time within subjects or order effects are not reduced by counterbalancing across subjects. Finally, random motion adds noise to the data, potentially causing false negative results and contributing to within-subject, intersubject, and between-center variability of activation patterns. This last problem is one of a number of phenomena that may variably affect signal-to-noise ratio in fMRI studies; other such variables include coil sensitivity, scanner stability, magnetic field homogeneity ("shim"), voxel size, field strength, and subject characteristics. Similar variability of hardware operating characteristics and data acquisition methods exists for PET studies, and probably explains some of the variability of results observed across different centers (Poline et al., 1996).

Several unique characteristics of fMRI suggest other potentially useful avenues of research. Temporal properties (latency, rise time, time to peak, etc.) of the hemodynamic BOLD response can be determined to a high degree of precision using high-resolution sampling in time and averaging over multiple trials (Buckner et al., 1996; De Yoe et al., 1992). Although the hemodynamic response is considerably slower (e.g., latency of 1–2 sec) than neural responses in primary and association sensory cortices, this technique may prove useful for discriminating different brain regions activated sequentially during complex, multicomponent cognitive tasks that evolve over several seconds (Cohen et al., 1997). fMRI is ideally suited to averaging of responses arising from relatively brief periods of neural activation, such as single sensory stimulations or single trials of a cognitive task (Buckner et al., 1996). This capability allows investigators to mix different kinds of trials during scanning and later analyze the brain responses according to a factor of interest (e.g., target vs. distractor stimuli, correct vs. incorrect responses, presence or absence of a stimulus feature). The significant methodological advantage of this technique is that trials of a given type need not be grouped in time (as is necessary in PET); hence otherwise identical task conditions and instructional sets can be held constant while the factor of interest is manipulated.

FUNCTIONAL NEUROIMAGING OF LANGUAGE

In the following sections we present a brief overview of some of the published PET and fMRI studies performed in speech and language processing. Although a complete survey is beyond the scope of this chapter, an attempt will be made to illustrate several notable areas of developing consensus and continued controversy. Because PET and fMRI data reflect *relative* changes in brain activity, it is of utmost importance to consider the characteristics of both activation and control states—that is, the nature of the task *contrast*—when attempting to make sense of this vast literature. For this reason, studies with similar task contrasts are presented together. Where possible, the data are interpreted in the context of functional localization models based on lesion-deficit correlation studies.

Spoken Speech Perception

Activation by Speech Sounds   Recognition that the superior temporal region plays a critical role in speech processing dates at least to the studies of Wernicke (1874), who observed patients with language comprehension deficits resulting from left temporo-parietal lesions that included the STG. Because his patients had deficits involving both spoken and written material, Wernicke hypothesized that the left STG contains not only neural representations of sounds but also the "sound images" of words, which he felt were critical for recognition of both spoken and written linguistic tokens. Although the functional and anatomical definitions of "Wernicke's area" have never been fully agreed upon, the association of word "comprehension" (variously envisioned as encompassing phonemic, lexical, and semantic representations) with the left STG has been a prevalent theme in neuroanatomical models of language organization (Bogen & Bogen, 1976; Geschwind, 1971; Lichtheim, 1885; Mesulam, 1990). Particular interest has focused in the last several decades on the posterior left STG and its posterior dorsal surface, or planum temporale (PT). This region shows interhemispheric morphological and cytoarchitectural asymmetries that roughly parallel language lateralization, suggesting that it plays a key role in language function (Foundas et al., 1994; Galaburda et al., 1978; Geschwind & Levitsky, 1968; Steinmetz et al., 1991).

Consistent with this model of STG function, PET and fMRI studies reliably demonstrate activation of the STG when subjects are presented with speech sounds in contrast to no sounds (Binder, Rao, Hammeke, et al., 1994; Dhankhar et al., 1997; Fiez, Raichle, et al., 1995, 1996; Hirano et al., 1997; Howard et al., 1992; Jäncke et al., 1998; Mazoyer et al., 1993; O'Leary et al., 1996; Price, Wise, Warburton, et al., 1996; Warburton et al., 1996; Wise et al., 1991). Stimuli used in these experiments included syllables, single words, pseudo words, foreign words, and sentences. Activated areas included Heschl's gyrus (HG), the PT, the dorsal STG anterior to HG (planum polare and dorsal temporal pole), the lateral STG, and the superior temporal sulcus (STS). The extent to which this activation spreads ventrally into the middle temporal gyrus (MTG) or dorsally into the inferior parietal lobe is not yet clear.

Other aspects of these data are less consistent with a specifically linguistic role for the STG. For example, although language functions are believed, on the basis of lesion studies, to be strongly lateralized to the left hemisphere in most people, STG activation by speech sounds occurs bilaterally. While some investigators have observed relatively small degrees of leftward asymmetry in such studies (Binder, Rao, Hammeke, et al., 1994; Mazoyer et al., 1993), most others have not (Fiez, Raichle, et al., 1996; Hirano et al., 1997; Howard et al., 1992; Jäncke et al., 1998; O'Leary et al., 1996; Warburton et al., 1996; Wise et al., 1991). Although most of the studies have involved only passive listening, performance of language tasks requiring semantic categorization or target detection does not alter this activation symmetry (Fiez et al., 1995; Grady et al., 1997; Wise et al., 1991). Also somewhat problematic is that STG activation by speech sounds is very sensitive to the number of sounds presented per unit of time (Binder, Rao, Hammeke, Frost, et al., 1994; Dhankhar et al., 1997; Price et al., 1992; Price, Wise, Warburton, et al., 1996; Wise et al., 1991), and generally does not occur during silent language tasks involving purely visual stimulation (Howard et al., 1992; Petersen et al., 1988; Price et al., 1994; Rumsey et al., 1997). These findings suggest that much of the activation observed in the STG during auditory presentation of words may arise from processing the complex auditory information present in speech stimuli rather than from activation of linguistic (phonemic, lexical, or semantic) representations.

Speech Sounds Contrasted with Nonspeech Sounds   While in the neurological literature the left STG has been associated with language processes, evidence from other sources points to a primarily auditory sensory function for this region. HG and PT are well established as the primary cortical projection areas for the ascending auditory pathway (Flechsig, 1908; Jones & Burton, 1976; Merzenich & Brugge, 1973; Mesulam & Pandya, 1973; von Economo & Horn, 1930). These primary sensory regions in turn provide the major input to surrounding cortical regions in lateral and anterior STG (Galaburda & Pandya, 1983; Hackett et al., 1998; Morel et al., 1993; Morel & Kaas, 1992). Electrophysiological recordings in monkeys (Baylis et al., 1987; Leinonen et al., 1980; Rauschecker et al., 1997) and in humans (Celesia, 1976; Creutzfeld et al., 1989) also corroborate the idea that most of the STG consists of unimodal auditory association cortex (Mesulam, 1985). Even the neurological literature provides little support for a higher language center in the STG. Lesions confined to this area (and not involving neighboring MTG or inferior parietal areas) do not appear to cause multimodal language comprehension disturbances, but rather an auditory speech perceptual deficit known as "pure word deafness," in which lexical, semantic, orthographic, phonologic, and syntactic knowledge is intact (Barrett, 1910; Henschen, 1918–1919; Tanaka et al., 1987). In almost all of these cases the lesions were bilateral (Buchman et al., 1986), suggesting that the speech perceptual processes damaged by the lesion can be carried out successfully by either STG alone.

In view of this evidence, an important issue is whether STG activation resulting from speech sounds reflects processing of the acoustic content (i.e., physical features such as frequency and amplitude information) or the linguistic content (phonemic, lexical, and semantic associations) of the stimuli. This problem was addressed in several functional imaging studies comparing activation with words or speech syllables to activation with simpler, nonspeech sounds like noise and pure tones. These studies included both passive listening and active target detection tasks. The consistent finding from these PET and fMRI studies is that speech and nonspeech sounds produce roughly equivalent activation of the dorsal STG, including the PT, in both hemispheres (Binder et al., 1996, 1997; Démonet et al., 1992; Zatorre et al., 1992). In contrast, more ventral areas of the STG within and surrounding the superior temporal sulcus (STS) are preferentially activated by speech sounds (figure 7.5 and color plate 10). Activation in this STS area, although bilateral, appears to be more left-lateralized than is the general STG activation observed in the speech-vs.-silence comparisons (Binder et al., 1997; Démonet et al., 1992; Zatorre et al., 1992).

There are, however, several possible interpretations of this differential STS activation. Because the stimuli used in the contrasting conditions differ in terms of both acoustic complexity and phoneme content, the resulting STS activation could represent early auditory, phoneme recognition, or word recognition processes. The fact that the STS response occurs with both word and nonword stimuli suggests a closer relationship to phonemic than to lexical-semantic processes. STS cortex receives

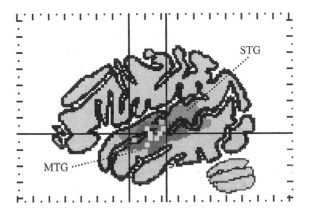

Figure 7.5
Left hemisphere superior temporal areas activated in three auditory studies. Blue indicates regions activated equally by tones and words (Binder et al., 1996). Areas activated more by speech than by nonspeech sounds are indicated by red shading (Binder et al., 1996), orange squares (Zatorre et al., 1992), and yellow squares (Démonet et al., 1992). All data are aligned in standard stereotaxic space at $x = -51$. (Reproduced with permission from Binder, 1999.) (See color plate 10.)

significant auditory input but is relatively distant from the primary auditory fields. These characteristics suggest that it may be involved in processing more specific and complex representations of auditory sensory information, as would be involved in phoneme recognition. Several other pieces of evidence, however, further complicate interpretation.

The STS in monkeys contains polymodal areas that receive visual and somatosensory as well as auditory projections (Baylis et al., 1987; Desimone & Gross, 1979; Hikosawa et al., 1988; Seltzer & Pandya, 1994), suggesting the possibility of a multimodal, integrative role for this region. Several studies using visual stimuli provide additional insights into this possibility. Calvert et al. (1997) studied brain areas involved in lip-reading. In the lip-reading condition, subjects watched a video of a face silently mouthing numbers and were asked to silently repeat the numbers to themselves. In the control condition a static face was presented, and subjects were asked to silently repeat the number "one" to themselves. The moving face condition produced activation in widespread extrastriate regions, but also in the vicinity of the STS bilaterally. The authors concluded that these areas, which were also activated by listening to speech, may be sites where polymodal integration of auditory and visual information occurs during speech perception, as demonstrated behaviorally by the McGurk effect (McGurk & MacDonald, 1976). Several investigators also found STS activation when subjects silently read printed words or pseudo words in comparison to reading meaningless letter strings or nonsense characters (Bavelier et al., 1997;

Howard et al., 1992; Indefrey et al., 1997; Price, Wise, & Frackowiak, 1996; Small et al., 1996). These activations were generally stronger in the left than the right STS and were more prominent in the posterior half of the sulcus. This STS activity might conceivably relate to activation of phoneme representations associated with the printed stimuli. Taken together, these data suggest that cortical areas in the STS receive inputs from both auditory and visual sensory cortices, and thus may be important sites for polymodal integrative functions such as those that underlie phoneme recognition and grapheme-to-phoneme translation.

Words Contrasted with Nonword Speech and Other Complex Sounds   One method of further examining these issues is to compare auditory stimuli that differ in linguistic content but are closely matched in terms of physical features. Several research groups, for example, compared activation with single words to activation with nonwords, nonword syllables, or reversed speech sounds that were acoustically matched to the single-word stimuli (Binder et al., 1999; Binder, Rao, Hammeke, et al., 1994; Dehaene et al., 1997; Démonet et al., 1992, 1994a; Hirano et al., 1997; Howard et al., 1992; Mazoyer et al., 1993; Müller et al., 1997; Perani et al., 1996; Price, Wise, Warburton, et al., 1996; Wise et al., 1991). By controlling for acoustic information processing, these comparisons should identify brain regions involved in processing nonphysical, linguistic representations associated with the word stimuli (i.e., lexical, semantic, and syntactic knowledge). In most of these comparisons, there was no difference in STG or STS activation between real words and these other sounds (Binder et al., 1999; Binder, Rao, Hammeke, et al., 1994; Démonet et al., 1992, 1994a; Hirano et al., 1997; Mazoyer et al., 1993; Perani et al., 1996; Wise et al., 1991). In contrast to these generally negative findings in the STG and STS, differences between words and nonwords have been observed in other neighboring regions, including the temporal poles (Brodmann area 38) (Mazoyer et al., 1993; Perani et al., 1996; Price, Wise, Warburton, et al., 1996), the MTG (Perani et al., 1996; Price, Wise, Warburton, et al., 1996), inferior temporal or fusiform gyrus (Démonet et al., 1992; Price, Wise, Warburton, et al., 1996), and angular gyrus (Binder et al., 1999; Démonet et al., 1992; Perani et al., 1996) (figure 7.6 and color plate 11). Howard et al. (1992) described an activation focus associated with word-level processing lying near the junction of superior and middle temporal gyri (i.e., in the STS), but a reanalysis of these data by Price, Wise, Warburton, et al. (1996) produced four foci, all of which were in the middle or inferior temporal gyri.

Interpretation of these word-specific activations is not yet entirely clear. Because the activation and control conditions in these studies differed in terms of the linguistic associations of the stimuli, the most straightforward interpretation is that the

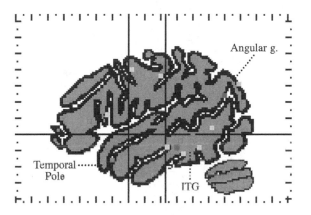

Figure 7.6
Left hemisphere foci of activation by auditory words greater than nonwords. Yellow = repeating words—
saying same word to reversed speech (Price, Wise, Warburton, et al., 1996); green = passive listening to
words—reversed speech (Price, Wise, Warburton, et al., 1996); cyan = passive listening to words—reversed
speech (Perani et al., 1996); red = semantic task on words—phonetic task on pseudo words (Démonet et al.,
1994a); magenta = semantic task on words—phonetic task on pseudo words (Binder et al., 1999). (See color
plate 11.)

additional activation reflects processing of these linguistic associations. On the other
hand, meaningful stimuli are likely to engage subjects' attention more effectively,
which could in itself alter activation levels. Several studies have demonstrated that
auditory cortex activation is modulated by attention to the stimuli (Grady et al., 1997;
O'Leary et al., 1996; Pugh et al., 1996). This factor may be particularly important
when a passive listening procedure is used that permits such variation in attention, but
use of an active task may not necessarily solve this problem. In one task commonly
employed in these studies, for example, subjects are required to repeat words they
hear (e.g., say "house" after hearing "house") but need recite only a single, prelearned
word in response to all nonword stimuli (e.g., say "crime" to any reversed-speech
stimulus) (Howard et al., 1992; Price, Wise, Warburton, et al., 1996). In this task,
then, the response in the word condition depends on perception of the stimulus, but
this is not true of the nonword condition. This difference could lead to differences
in attentional state and in the degree of top-down attentional influence exerted on
speech perceptual mechanisms.

Despite this ambiguity of interpretation, the consistent findings are (1) STG/STS
activation does not differ for meaningful and meaningless speech sounds, and (2)
nearby temporal and parietotemporal regions do show a dependence on stimulus
meaning. These findings make it unlikely that the STG or STS plays a prominent role
in processing lexical-semantic or syntactic information.

The model of temporal lobe speech processing that emerges from these data is based on a primarily dorsal-to-ventral hierarchical organization and includes at least three relatively distinct processing stages. In accord with anatomical and neurophysiological studies of the auditory cortex, the earliest stage comprises sensory processors located in primary and belt auditory regions on the superior temporal plane, including the PT, that respond to relatively simple aspects of auditory signals (Galaburda & Pandya, 1983; Mendelson & Cynader, 1985; Merzenich & Brugge, 1973; Morel et al., 1993; Phillips & Irvine, 1981; Rauschecker et al., 1997). Further ventrally, on the lateral surface of the STG and within the STS, are areas that appear to respond to more complex auditory phenomena, such as the frequency and amplitude modulations and spectral energy peaks that characterize speech sounds. This region might also conceivably be involved in encoding combinations of such temporal and spectral features as recognizable "forms" for phonetic perception, and in accessing stored phoneme representations to assist in this process. These representations might also be accessed during derivation of phonology from graphemic stimuli. Still further ventrally, beyond the STS, are large cortical regions that appear to process lexical and semantic (i.e., nonphysical) information associated with stimuli.

This model thus differs from the traditional view in placing much less emphasis on the STG and PT as "language centers." While these regions undoubtedly play a critical role in auditory perception, information processing of a specifically linguistic nature appears to depend primarily on cortical areas outside the STG. This model is in good agreement with lesion data, which suggest primarily auditory or phonemic perceptual deficits following isolated STG and STS injury (Barrett, 1910; Buchman et al., 1986; Henschen, 1918–1919; Tanaka et al., 1987), and naming and semantic deficits from temporal and parietal lesions located outside the STG (Alexander et al., 1989; H. Damasio et al., 1996; Henschen, 1920–1922; Warrington & Shallice, 1984). A large number of other PET and fMRI studies also demonstrate participation of these ventral temporal and inferior parietal regions in lexical-semantic processing (Bavelier et al., 1997; Binder et al., 1997, 1999; Bookheimer et al., 1995; Bottini et al., 1994; H. Damasio et al., 1996; Fiez, Raichle, et al., 1996; Frith et al., 1991a; Martin et al., 1996; Price, Moore, Humphreys, et al., 1996; Price et al., 1994; Price, Wise, & Frackowiak, 1996; Raichle et al., 1994; Smith et al., 1996; Vandenberghe et al., 1996; Warburton et al., 1996), as detailed in the section "Semantic Processing," below.

Visual Character Perception

Perceptual processing of written symbols has been studied using unfamiliar, letterlike characters ("false font"), single letters, unpronounceable letter strings, pronounceable pseudo words, words, and sentences. In contrast to the situation in the auditory system, the primary sensory and immediately adjacent association areas in the visual system have not traditionally been associated with language functions. Consequently, although the calcarine cortex and adjacent medial occipital extrastriate regions are activated by printed word stimuli in contrast to no visual stimuli, this activation has been interpreted as representing early visual information processing (Howard et al., 1992; Indefrey et al., 1997; Petersen et al., 1988; Price et al., 1994). Supporting this view is the observation that, in general, these visual areas are not differentially activated by words or pseudo words compared to other, less orthographically familiar character strings (Howard et al., 1992; Indefrey et al., 1997; Price et al., 1994). Using fMRI during presentation of pseudo words and false font strings, Indefrey et al. (1997) demonstrated that activation in medial occipital cortex—including calcarine sulcus, lingual gyrus, cuneus, and posterior fusiform gyrus—is strongly dependent on string length, but not on orthographic properties of stimuli.

Many imaging studies of word reading employed tasks in which subjects read stimuli aloud, thus activating both speech articulation and auditory perceptual processes in addition to visual letter and word processors (Bookheimer et al., 1995; Fiez & Petersen, 1998; Petersen et al., 1989; Rumsey et al., 1997). The following sections focus on studies incorporating controls for these sensory and motor processes, in which the aim was to isolate processing of graphemic, orthographic, and phonological knowledge associated with print stimuli.

Letters Contrasted with Other Visual Stimuli   Using fMRI, Puce et al. (1996) observed a lateral extrastriate visual region that showed preferential responses to letter strings. The letter stimuli, which consisted of unpronounceable consonant strings, were contrasted with faces and visual textures during a passive viewing paradigm. Images provided by Puce et al. suggest a locus for this letter-processing area in the posterolateral fusiform or inferior occipital gyrus. This letter-specific activation was strongly left-lateralized. Foci showing stronger responses to face and texture stimuli were also observed; these were medial to the letter focus and more bilateral. Unpronounceable letter strings have few or no semantic, lexical, or phonological associations. The focus observed by Puce et al. may thus represent a region specialized for processing purely visual features of letters. Whether these processes involve only visual features or also include grapheme-level representations could be investigated using contrasts between familiar letters and nonsense characters containing similar features. Studies incorporating such contrasts have yielded no clear consensus, with some showing activation differences in this region between letter strings and "false font" (Price, Wise, & Frackowiak, 1996; Pugh et al., 1996b) and others showing no differences (Howard et al., 1992; Indefrey et al., 1997; Petersen et al., 1990; Small et al., 1996).

Pronounceable Contrasted with Unpronounceable Letter Strings   Other brain regions have shown greater activation by orthographically familiar stimuli compared to non-orthographic strings, although some controversy persists concerning the location of these regions. Using PET, Petersen et al. (1990) measured activation during visual presentation of words (BOARD), pseudo words (TWEAL), unpronounceable consonant strings (NLPFZ), and false font. Both words and pseudo words produced activation in a left ventromedial extrastriate region located in approximately the posterior lingual gyrus or lingual-fusiform border (average Talairach & Tournoux [1988] x, y, z coordinates $= -23$, -68, $+3$), whereas false font and consonant strings did not activate this region.

Many subsequent similar comparisons, however, have not shown differential activation in this region by orthographic vs. nonorthographic stimuli (Howard et al., 1992; Indefrey et al., 1997; Price et al., 1994; Price, Wise, & Frackowiak, 1996). Herbster et al. (1994) reported activation of the left fusiform gyrus by words contrasted to consonant strings, but this differential activation did not occur using pronounceable pseudo words. The foci reported by Herbster et al. (average x, y, z coordinates $= -37$, -40, -24) were several centimeters anterior and inferior to the foci observed by Petersen et al. (1990). Although most of these studies used longer stimulus exposure durations than were used by Petersen et al., the failure by Price et al. (1994) to find differential activation in this region, using either long or short stimulus durations, suggests that this variable alone does not explain the discrepancy. The suggestion by Indefrey et al. (1997) that string length effects account for the differences observed by Petersen et al. also does not seem plausible in view of the fact that string length was matched across conditions in the Petersen et al. study.

Although the weight of this evidence suggests that medial occipital cortex is insensitive to the presence or absence of orthographic information, both PET and fMRI studies have demonstrated activation of the STS or neighboring posterior MTG in comparisons between orthographic and nonorthographic stimuli (Bavelier et al., 1997; Herbster et al., 1997; Howard et al., 1992; Indefrey et al., 1997; Price et al., 1994; Price, Wise, & Frackowiak, 1996; Small et al., 1996) (figure 7.7 and color plate 12). In most studies this activation was bilateral, but was always stronger and more extensive in the left hemisphere. STS activation in these studies was generally greatest in, or in some cases restricted to, the posterior aspect of the sulcus (Howard et al., 1992; Indefrey et al., 1997; Price et al., 1994; Small et al., 1996). This convergence of results is all the more striking given that the overt tasks used in these studies varied considerably, including passive viewing (Indefrey et al., 1997; Price et al., 1994), memorization for later recognition testing (Bavelier et al., 1997), reading aloud or saying a designated word repeatedly (Herbster et al., 1997; Howard et al., 1992;

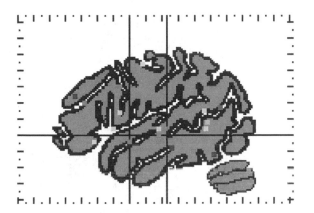

Figure 7.7
Left hemisphere foci of activation by orthographic greater than nonorthographic character strings. Magenta (Howard et al., 1992), red (Small et al., 1996), and green (Herbster et al., 1997) = reading words-saying same word to false font; yellow = passive words-false font (Price et al., 1994); blue = pseudo words-letters during a visual feature detection task (Price, Wise, & Frackowiak, 1996); cyan = words-letters, or words-false font, during a visual feature detection task (Price, Wise, & Frackowiak, 1996). (See color plate 12.)

Small et al., 1996), and nonlinguistic target detection (Price, Wise, & Frackowiak, 1996).

This STS activation could have several possible interpretations. As suggested by Petersen et al. (1990) for the left medial extrastriate activation, STS activation could reflect processing of visual word forms. This hypothesis is less plausible for the STS, a region in which lesions are more likely to produce phoneme processing deficits than specific reading impairments. Alternatively, STS activation in these studies might reflect activation of phonological information and/or phoneme representations associated with the pronounceable stimuli. This interpretation is in general agreement with the model of speech sound processing presented in the section "Spoken Speech Perception," and with the occurrence of speech sound-processing deficits following isolated STG/STS lesions (Barrett, 1910; Buchman et al., 1986; Henschen, 1918–1919; Tanaka et al., 1987). Severe reading disturbances may not occur in such cases because access to phonological information, although helpful and routine in the intact state (Van Orden, 1987), might not be crucial for reading comprehension or reading aloud (Beavois & Derouesne, 1979; Plaut et al., 1996). Damage to phoneme processors might also explain the frequent observation that patients with STG/STS lesions produce phonemic paraphasic errors in reading aloud and speaking, at least in the early period after occurrence of the lesion. A third possibility is that differential STS activation reflects processing of lexical or semantic information associated with the orthographic stimuli. Although the effect is observed with (supposedly meaningless) pseudo words as well as with words, there exists both behavioral evidence and theoretical support for the idea that pseudo word processing engages lexical (and thus, to some extent at least, semantic) representations (Baron, 1973; Glushko, 1979; McClelland & Rumelhart, 1981). This last interpretation seems less likely, however, given that the STS appears to be equally activated by meaningful and meaningless speech sounds (see the section "Spoken Speech Perception," above), and that other temporal and parietal regions have been more firmly implicated in lexical and semantic processing (see the section "Semantic Processing," below).

Frontal Lobe Activation by Orthographic Stimuli   Contrasts between orthographic and nonorthographic stimuli also occasionally result in left-lateralized frontal lobe activations despite controls for speech production and other motor requirements. Frontal activations have been observed particularly in the IFG (Bavelier et al., 1997; Herbster et al., 1997; Price et al., 1994; Price, Wise, & Frackowiak, 1996), inferior premotor cortex (Bavelier et al., 1997; Price, Wise, & Frackowiak, 1996), and mid-anterior cingulate gyrus (Herbster et al., 1997; Howard et al., 1992). In a PET study, Herbster et al. (1997) observed a dependence of left inferior frontal activation on spelling-to-sound regularity and lexicality. These investigators reported left IFG activation during reading aloud of midfrequency (average 28/million) irregular words (DEBT) and pseudo words but not of midfrequency (average 52/million) regular words (KITE).

Two other reading studies, in which reading aloud was contrasted with visual fixation, also resulted in regularity and lexicality effects in the inferior frontal region, although the findings were not entirely consistent. Like Herbster et al., Fiez and Petersen (1998) observed inferior frontal activation during reading of irregular low-frequency words and pseudo words, but not of regular words. Rumsey et al. (1997) found inferior frontal activation during reading of low-frequency irregular words but not of pseudo words. The activation peaks associated with pseudo-word and irregular-word reading in these studies were all in left anterior insula or neighboring left posterior frontal operculum, suggesting that this region may have a functional role distinct from other regions of the IFG (Fiez & Petersen, 1998). The absence of frontal activation by regular words in these studies is somewhat at odds with a number of studies that have shown such activation during word reading aloud or silently (Bavelier et al., 1997; Bookheimer et al., 1995; Petersen et al., 1990; Price et al., 1994; Price, Wise, & Frackowiak, 1996), although it could be argued that frontal activation in these studies may have been due to inclusion of irregular words among the stimuli. Activation in these other studies mainly occurred more dorsally and rostrally, in the inferior frontal sulcus and middle frontal gyrus (Bavelier et al., 1997; Petersen et al.,

1990; Price et al., 1994; Price, Wise, & Frackowiak, 1996), but also in the IFG (Bavelier et al., 1997; Bookheimer et al., 1995).

Stronger activation in the left anterior insula and frontal operculum by irregular words and pseudo words has been interpreted as indicating a specific role for this region in processing sublexical phonological knowledge (Fiez & Petersen, 1998; Herbster et al., 1997), based on interpretations of both dual-route and connectionist models of orthographic-to-phonologic translation (Humphreys & Evett, 1985; Seidenberg & McClelland, 1989). Greater activation by pseudo words is taken to reflect slower, less-efficient processing because of weaker tuning of the network to unfamiliar letter combinations (connectionist model) or greater dependence on sublexical assembly (dual-route model). Greater activation by irregular words is taken as evidence for additional sublexical phonological processing that must occur because of conflict between sublexical and lexical information (dual-route model) or statistical uncertainty resulting from a relatively small phonological neighborhood (connectionist model).

Although this connectionist account fits well with the frequency-by-regularity interaction observed on behavioral measures of low-frequency word recognition (Seidenberg et al., 1984), this account probably does not explain as well the large differences observed by Herbster et al. (1997) between regular and irregular medium-frequency words, since both of these categories would be expected to have fairly equivalent magnitude and time course of activation in phonological and hidden-unit layers of current connectionist models (Seidenberg & McClelland, 1989). Finally, because of the sublexical-lexical conflict envisioned by the dual-route model, this model could also be understood as predicting *less* activation of the assembled phonology pathway during irregular word processing, simply because inhibition of this pathway would be advantageous to performance. This last point raises yet another alternative interpretation of the regularity effect associated with left frontal opercular/insular activation: this region may play a higher, process-control role by selective enhancement vs. inhibition of phonological vs. orthographic inputs (connectionist model) or lexical vs. assembled routes (dual-route model) during irregular word processing, rather than a specific role in sublexical representation per se.

Phonological Tasks

"Phonological processing" refers to operations that involve the perception or production of speech sounds (phonemes). In the context of most speech tasks, phonological processing occurs effortlessly and without awareness. This is the case for both speech perception, when the phonemic content of heard speech is extracted from the acoustic input (see the section "Spoken Speech Perception"), and phonemic production, when the phonology associated with visually presented stimuli is generated (see the section "Visual Character Perception"). Once phonological content has been extracted, lexical and semantic processing can also proceed automatically and without awareness. The implication is that tasks involving phonological associations will also evoke lexical and semantic associations. This poses a problem for neuroimaging studies that are concerned with the localization of phonological perception or production. The difficulty rests in designing activation tasks that are purely phonological or reference tasks that engage lexical-semantic but not phonological processing.

To isolate the brain regions associated with phonological processing from those specialized for lexical-semantic processing, psychological tasks have been designed that focus attention on a particular characteristic of the stimulus. For example, Démonet et al. (1992, 1994a, 1994b) used tasks that required subjects to make an overt decision on the phonemic content of heard nonwords (e.g., detecting the presence of /d/ and /b/ in the nonword "redozabu") or the semantic content of real words. These tasks differentially weight phonemic and lexical-semantic processes, respectively, but in addition they require attention-demanding verbal strategies. For instance, one strategy for deciding whether the target sounds /d/ and /b/ are present in a heard nonword would entail (1) holding the target sounds in memory throughout the task, (2) attending to the auditory input, (3) featural analysis of the acoustic structure, (4) phonemic segmentation of sequential components (e.g., /r/ /e/ /d/ /o/ /z/ /a/ /b/ /u/), (5) holding the content and order of these components in short-term memory, (6) deciding whether the target phonemes are present, and (7) making a response. This might not be an exclusive strategy, and some subjects may adopt a different approach. One suggestion made by Démonet et al. (1994b), for example, is that the task can be performed by visualizing a graphemic representation of the stimuli. The point is that once an experiment introduces a task that requires an attention-demanding strategy, many psychological components will be called into play that do not necessarily relate to the speech perceptual processes that the experiment aims to isolate.

Such attention-demanding phonological strategies may vary slightly from subject to subject. They are also difficult to equate in the reference task. For instance, semantic decisions (e.g., deciding if a word is "positive" or denotes something "smaller than a chicken") require some but not all of the processes required for phonological decisions. Those in common include (1) memory for the targets, (2) attention to the auditory input, (3) featural analysis of the acoustic structure, (4) a decision on the presence of the target combination, and (5) a response. Differences between tasks include (1) the nature of the targets to be held in memory (sounds versus concepts), (2) the familiarity of the attended stimuli, (3) the type of attribute to be extracted (semantic versus phonological information), (4) the need to segment the stimulus into a sequence of components, (5) the demands placed on short-term memory (a sequence of segments for nonwords versus one familiar word), and (6) the demands placed on attention. In summary, attention-demanding phonological tasks differentially engage a number of distinct processes that are not directly related to the perception and production of speech sounds. If we are concerned with differences that can be attributed purely to such phonological processes, then we need to understand which activations are related to verbal short-term memory, phonological segmentation, and attention.

Inferior Frontal Activations   Below, we consider the role of the brain regions required for performing phonological awareness tasks (e.g., (Démonet et al., 1992, 1994a, 1994b; Fiez et al., 1995; Paulesu et al., 1993; Rumsey et al., 1997; Zatorre et al., 1992, 1996)). In each study, the active task required subjects to detect a phoneme or syllable target, and activation in the vicinity of the posterior left IFG (Broca's area) was recorded. The location of these activations varies, however, depending on the control task. Relative to simple visual fixation, Fiez et al. (1995) report activation in the frontal operculum (near Brodmann area 45 and the anterior insula) for the detection of target words, syllables, and tone sequences, but not for the detection of steady-state vowels. These findings suggest that the frontal operculum is concerned with the analysis of rapid temporal changes in the acoustic structure that are not present in steady-state vowels. However, in another experiment, activation of the left frontal operculum was also observed during detection of "long vowels" in visually presented words, precluding an explanation based solely on the analysis of acoustic input. An alternative hypothesis discussed by Fiez et al. (1995) is that this area relates to high-level articulatory coding, which may be required for phonemic discrimination tasks.

In the studies by Zatorre et al. (1992, 1996), phoneme discrimination on words or speech syllables was contrasted with passive listening to the same stimuli. Activation was not detected in the left frontal operculum but in a more posterior and dorsal region of the IFG, on the border with premotor cortex (BA 44/6). The authors argue that this region is concerned with phonemic segmentation because it was active for phoneme discrimination but not for pitch discrimination, a task that involves similar acoustic input, demands on memory, attention, decision making, and response execution. Démonet et al. also report activation in this posterior dorsal region of the IFG when phoneme detection on nonwords is contrasted to either pitch detection on tone sequences (1992) or semantic decisions on real words (1994a). However, a follow-up study by Démonet et al. (1994b) found that activation of BA 44/6 was observed only for the detection of two sequential phonemes /d/ and /b/ embedded in perceptually ambiguous stimuli. This region was less involved when perceptual ambiguity was reduced, and showed no activation (relative to pitch discrimination on tones) when the target was only one phoneme, even when the distracters were made perceptually ambiguous by using similar phonemes (e.g., /p/). Thus, activity in this posterior dorsal region of the IFG was maximum when the task involved sequential processing in a perceptually ambiguous context. Démonet et al. interpret this activity as sensorimotor transcoding of the phonemic stimuli, presumably used by subjects to rehearse and check the targets in the phonemic string. This explanation was derived from a study by Paulesu et al. (1993), who attributed activation of approximately the same region of Broca's area to "articulatory rehearsal" required for rhyming and verbal short-term memory tasks on single letters (but not for visual matching on unfamiliar Korean letters that do not have associated phonology).

In summary, there appear to be two distinct regions of the inferior frontal cortex that are involved in phoneme processing: the left frontal operculum (around the anterior insula and BA 45) and a more posterior dorsal region near the IFG/premotor boundary (BA 44/6). The left inferior frontal operculum is activated when phoneme detection tasks are contrasted to fixation. The same region (within the resolution of the PET scans) is also activated when phonetic judgments are made on visually presented words and when listening to words passively is contrasted to hearing reversed words (Price, Wise, Warburton, et al., 1996). Consistent with these findings, the left frontal operculum was not activated when phonetic judgment tasks were contrasted to passive listening (Zatorre et al., 1996), suggesting a fundamental role in phonemic perception. However, such an explanation does not show why activation is not always detected in the left frontal operculum for passive word listening relative to silence (Fiez et al., 1995; Price, Wise, Warburton, et al., 1996). One possibility is that during silent conditions, the left frontal operculum is engaged in inner speech and auditory verbal imagery (McGuire et al., 1996), thereby subtracting the activation seen when passive listening is contrasted to reversed words. The more posterior dorsal region of the inferior frontal cortex (BA 44/6) has been observed for phoneme processing relative to passive listening (Zatorre et al., 1996), relative to pitch decisions (Démonet et al., 1992; Zatorre et al., 1996), relative to semantic decisions (Démonet et al., 1994a), and relative to nonverbal visual tasks (Paulesu et al., 1993). It has also been observed during verbal short-term memory for a series of letters (Paulesu et al., 1993) and interpreted as reflecting inner speech, articulatory rehearsal, and phonetic segmentation.

Supramarginal Gyrus Activations Activation in temporoparietal regions during phoneme detection is less consistently reported. For instance, no temporoparietal activation was detected by Fiez et al. (1995) when contrasting phoneme detection on auditory or visual words to fixation. They suggest that temporoparietal activation might occur only when subjects are not focusing on phonological ambiguities and when there is a higher proportion of new words to repeated words. In contrast,

Zatorre et al. (1996) found activation of the left dorsal supramarginal gyrus (BA 40/7) for phoneme detection relative to passive listening, and activation of a more ventral region of the supramarginal gyrus (BA 40) was reported by Démonet et al. (1994a) for phoneme detection relative to semantic decision. The same ventral region was also activated during verbal short-term memory for letters relative to letter rhyming (Paulesu et al., 1993). The latter result led Paulesu et al. to suggest that this ventral region in the supramarginal gyrus is related to a short-term verbal store. If this is the case, we would expect the degree of activation to depend on the relative demands placed on verbal short-term storage. For instance, as described above, detecting the presence of a /d/ followed by a /b/ in an unfamiliar nonword requires short-term storage of the nonword while a phonological decision is made. There may be less supramarginal activation when the phonemic target is more easily detected because verbal short-term storage may not be required (e.g., in Fiez et al., 1995, the target was one of a set of five stimuli).

Other results are less consistent with the association of activation in the left supramarginal gyrus with verbal short-term storage. For instance, activation in the left supramarginal gyrus is not observed when phoneme detection on nonwords is contrasted with pitch detection on tone sequences that do not contain verbal material (Démonet et al., 1992, 1994b). Moreover, Binder et al. (1997) reported activation of the supramarginal gyrus bilaterally when pitch detection on tone sequences was contrasted to rest, and Démonet et al. (1994b) observed activation of the ventral supramarginal gyrus bilaterally when pitch detection on tone sequences was contrasted to phoneme processing. This suggests that the left supramarginal gyrus may be involved in nonverbal as well as verbal processes. Other evidence that stands against the association of the left supramarginal gyrus with a verbal short-term memory store comes from studies in which subjects were scanned during a condition that required them to retain ("store") previously presented words relative to fixation. Fiez, Raife, et al. (1996) failed to activate the supramarginal gyri under these conditions, while Jonides et al. (1998) found significant activation, but only in the right dorsal supramarginal gyrus.

Examination of other studies of short-term memory and phonological tasks suggests several different activation patterns in the supramarginal gyrus. First, as already mentioned, ventral activations occur that are probably distinct from dorsal activations. Second, supramarginal involvement during short-term memory tasks is often reported as bilateral (Jonides et al., 1998; Paulesu et al., 1993), while predominantly left-lateralized, ventral supramarginal activation is reported during phonological detection tasks (Démonet et al., 1994a) and when reading is contrasted to picture naming (Bookheimer et al., 1995; Menard et al., 1996; Moore & Price, 1999;

Vandenberghe et al., 1996). There is no reason to expect that reading requires short-term verbal storage, but there is a critical difference in the phonological processing required for reading and picture naming. That is, for reading, phonology can be generated sublexically via sequential letter processing, while for picture naming, phonology can be generated only at a lexical level.

Several studies have also demonstrated greater activation of the left supramarginal gyrus for pseudo words relative to real words (Price, Wise, & Frackowiak, 1986; Rumsey et al., 1997). One hypothesis that would account for many of these results is that the left supramarginal gyrus allows phonological information to be associated with nonlexical stimuli through a sublexical assembly process. This model would predict that an impairment in reading unfamiliar pseudo words relative to words, as occurs in the syndrome of phonological dyslexia (Coltheart et al., 1980), should result from damage in the left supramarginal gyrus. This prediction is indeed consistent with data from CT scans (Marin, 1980). However, this model still does not account for activation in this region during pitch discrimination on auditory tones (Binder et al., 1997; Démonet et al., 1994a). Other lesion studies have associated damage to the left supramarginal gyrus with deficits in spelling (Roeltgen & Heilman, 1984) and verbal short-term memory (Vallar & Shallice, 1990).

In summary, a ventral region of the left supramarginal gyrus is involved in some phoneme-processing tasks with both heard words and nonwords. The same region (within the limits of the spatial resolution of PET and fMRI) is also activated for pitch discrimination on tones, for reading visually presented words relative to picture naming, and for reading pseudo words relative to words. Explanations in terms of verbal short-term storage (Paulesu et al., 1993) and orthographic-to-phonological translation (Price, 1998) have been proposed, but neither explanation accounts for all of the available data. Clearly, as in the case of the frontal activations, many further studies are required to clarify these unresolved issues.

Semantic Processing

Semantic processes are those concerned with storing, retrieving, and using knowledge about the world, and are a key component of such ubiquitous behaviors as naming, comprehending and formulating language, problem solving, planning, and thinking. A consensus regarding the brain localization of such processes has begun to emerge from functional imaging and aphasia studies. The latter have made it increasingly clear that deficits involving naming and other acts of knowledge retrieval are associated with lesions in a variety of dominant hemisphere temporal and parietal locations (Alexander et al., 1989; H. Damasio et al., 1996; Hart & Gordon, 1990; Hillis & Caramazza, 1991; Warrington & Shallice, 1984). Recent functional imaging studies provide converging evidence, demonstrating that lexical-semantic processes engage a number of temporal, parietal, and prefrontal regions encompassing a large extent of the language-dominant hemisphere. Given the complexity and the sheer amount of semantic information learned by a typical person—including, for example, all defining characteristics of all conceptual categories and all category exemplars, all relationships between these entities, and all linguistic representations of these concepts and relationships—it is not surprising that a large proportion of the brain is devoted to managing this information.

Semantic tasks employed in functional imaging studies have included picture naming (Bookheimer et al., 1995; H. Damasio et al., 1996; Martin et al., 1996; Price, Moore, & Friston, 1996; Smith et al., 1996), semantic category decisions (e.g., large/small, concrete/abstract, living/nonliving, domestic/foreign) on single words (Binder et al., 1995; Demb et al., 1995; Démonet et al., 1992; Kapur et al., 1994; Petersen et al., 1989; Price, Moore, Humphreys, et al., 1997), semantic relatedness matching on word or picture pairs (Pugh et al., 1996b; Spitzer et al., 1996; Thompson-Schill et al., 1995; Vandenberghe et al., 1996; Wise et al., 1991), word generation using semantic relatedness criteria (Fiez, Raichle, et al., 1996; Frith et al., 1991a; Petersen et al., 1988; Raichle et al., 1994; Shaywitz, Pugh, et al., 1995; Thompson-Schill et al., 1997; Warburton et al., 1996; Wise et al., 1991), and sentence comprehension (Bottini et al., 1994; Nichelli et al., 1995). It is still somewhat unclear how differences in cognitive requirements among these semantic tasks affect the resulting activation patterns. It is generally agreed, however, that word generation and naming tasks introduce additional requirements for lexical search, selection, and speech output that are not as prominent in the other tasks (Démonet et al., 1993; Warburton et al., 1996). For this reason, and to simplify the following discussion, these word production tasks will be treated separately in the section "Word Production."

Also complicating matters is the fact that these different tasks have been used in combination with an array of different control conditions, including resting or passive stimulation (Wise et al., 1991), perceptual tasks on nonlinguistic stimuli (Binder et al., 1995; Démonet et al., 1992; Spitzer et al., 1996), perceptual tasks on linguistic stimuli (Demb et al., 1995; Kapur et al., 1994; Vandenberghe et al., 1996), phonological tasks on pseudo words (Binder et al., 1999; Démonet et al., 1992; Gabrieli et al., 1998; Pugh et al., 1996b), phonological tasks on words (Gabrieli et al., 1998; Price, Moore, Humphreys, et al., 1997), and lexical decision (Bottini et al., 1994). Given behavioral and functional imaging evidence for preattentive processing of linguistic stimuli (see figure 7.1), it is reasonable to expect activation patterns to depend on whether linguistic or nonlinguistic stimuli are used in the control task. The extent and the type of preattentive processing that occur may depend further on orthographic,

Table 7.1
PET and fMRI Semantic Studies

Study	IFG/S	SFG/S	STG/PT	STS	MTG/ITG	FG/PH	AG/TPO	PC	R-CBL	Other
Baseline = Perceptual Task on Nonlinguistic Stimuli										
Démonet et al. (1992)	+/−	+	−	+	+	+	+	−	na	L-aTh, Caud
Binder et al. (1997)	+	+	−	+	+	+	+	+	+	
Baseline = Perceptual Task on Word or Picture Stimuli										
Kapur et al. (1994)	+	−	−	−	−	−	−	−	na	—
Demb et al. (1995)	+	+	na	na	na	na	na	na	na	na
Vandenberghe et al. (1996)[1]	+	+	−	−	+	+	+	−	+	L-Hipp
Baseline = Phonological Task on Pseudo Word Stimuli										
Démonet et al. (1992, 1994a)	−	+	−	−	−[2]	+	+	+	na	R-AG
Pugh et al. (1996b)[1]	−	na	+(males)	+(males)	+(males)	+	na	na	na	R-STG, MTG
Gabrieli et al. (1998)	+	+	na	na	na	na	na	na	na	—
Binder et al. (1999)	+	+	na	−	−	+	+	+	−	—
Baseline = Phonological Task on Word Stimuli										
Price et al. (1997)	−	+/−	−	+/−	+/−	−	+	−	na	L-TP, Caud
Gabrieli et al. (1998)	+	+	na	na	na	na	na	na	na	—
Baseline = Lexical Decision										
Bottini et al. (1994)[3]	+	+	−	+	+	−	+	+	na	L-OF, TP

Baseline = "Rest"

Study	IFG/S	SFG/S	STG/PT	STS	MTG/ITG	FG/PH	AG/TPC	PC	R-CBL	Other
Wise et al. (1991)[1]	—	—	+	+	—	—	—	—	na	R-STG

Note: The semantic task procedure involved semantic word categorization unless otherwise specified. Region designations refer to the left hemisphere except in the case of the right cerebellum (R-CBL). Regions include the inferior frontal gyrus/sulcus (IFG/S), superior frontal gyrus/sulcus (SFG/S), superior temporal gyrus/planum temporale (STG/PT), superior temporal sulcus (STS), middle temporal gyrus (MTG), inferior temporal gyrus (ITG), fusiform and/or parahippocampal gyrus (FG/PH), angular gyrus and/or temporo-parietc-occipital junction (AG/TPO), posterior cingulate and/or ventral precuneus (PC), anterior thalamus (aTh), head of caudate (Caud), hippocampus (Hipp), temporal pole (TP), and orbital frontal region (OF); "na" indicates a region that was not assessed in the study.

[1] Task = semantic relatedness matching on word or picture pairs.

[2] Focus ascribed to MTG, located in deep white matter near junction of fusiform and parahippocampal gyri

[3] Task = sentence comprehension for literal meaning.

phonological, lexical, and semantic properties of the stimuli. Finally, these control conditions make differing demands on attentional resources, perhaps allowing different degrees of stimulus-unrelated processing to occur. For all of these reasons, the following discussion and table are organized according to the control task used in the various studies.

Semantic Tasks Contrasted with Nonlinguistic Tasks Functional imaging studies of semantic systems seek to distinguish brain areas involved in processing semantic knowledge about stimuli from sensory and attentional areas involved in processing physical aspects of the stimuli. A typical strategy for making this distinction is to contrast tasks that require knowledge retrieval (e.g., naming or categorization tasks) with tasks that do not (e.g., perceptual analysis tasks), using similar stimuli in both conditions to control for sensory processing. We first consider results obtained using perceptual tasks on nonlinguistic stimuli (see table 7.1). Assuming that linguistic stimuli (words and recognizable pictures) engage preattentive processing of associated lexical and semantic representations to some degree, control tasks involving nonlinguistic stimuli should provide the strongest contrast between activation and baseline states, and thus should have maximal sensitivity for identifying potential semantic processing areas. A problem with this design is that because the nonlinguistic control stimuli also lack orthographic and phonologic content, some of the resulting activation likely reflects processing of these aspects of the linguistic stimuli rather than semantic processing.

Démonet et al. (1992) performed the first such study. In the semantic condition, subjects heard word pairs consisting of an adjective and an animal name (e.g., kind horse) and were instructed to press a button with the right hand when the adjective was "positive" and was paired with an animal "smaller than a chicken." In the nonlinguistic task, subjects heard tone triplets and were instructed to respond when the third tone of the triplet was higher in pitch than the first two. Activation associated with the semantic task was strongly lateralized to the left hemisphere, involving STS (see figure 7.6), MTG, posterior ITG, middle part of the fusiform gyrus, angular gyrus (just anterior to the posterior ascending ramus of the STS), dorsal prefrontal cortex in the superior frontal gyrus (SFG), and a small part of the ventral IFG (pars orbitalis). This landmark study provided some of the first functional imaging evidence for participation of posterior association areas (MTG, ITG, angular gyrus) in tasks involving word meaning. Binder et al. (1997) used a similar task contrast during fMRI and recorded very similar results (figure 7.8 and color plate 13). An important aspect of this study is that reliability of the averaged activation maps was assessed by dividing the group of 30 subjects into two random samples and measuring the voxel-wise correlation between the resulting activation maps. Activation pat-

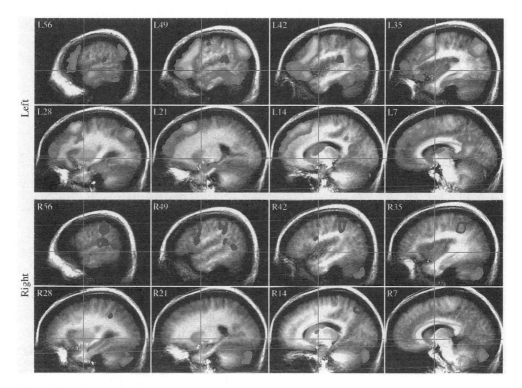

Figure 7.8
Serial sagittal sections showing significantly activated areas in the semantic processing study of Binder et al. Semantic processing areas, indicated in red-yellow, are strongly lateralized to the left cerebral hemisphere and right cerebellum. Blue shading indicates regions that were more active during the control (tone decision) task. Green lines indicate the standard stereotaxic *y* axis (AC-PC line) and *z* axis (vertical AC line). (Adapted with permission from Binder et al., 1997; copyright 1996, Society for Neuroscience.) (See color plate 13.)

terns were virtually identical in the two subgroups, showing a voxel-wise reliability coefficient of .92.

Although a number of large cortical regions in the left hemisphere are implicated in these studies, the results are also notable for the absence of activation in some areas traditionally associated with language processing. Most of the STG, for example, failed to show activation related to word processing. Moreover, the PT showed stronger activation by the tone task used as a control condition in these studies (Binder et al., 1996, 1997; Démonet et al., 1992). These results thus provide no evidence for specifically linguistic processes in this dorsal temporal region. Similarly, these studies show no activation related to the semantic tasks in supramarginal gyri or premotor cortices, arguing against a role for these regions in semantic processing.

Because of the considerable differences between the nonlinguistic and semantic stimuli employed in these studies, however, it remains unclear how much of the activation might be related to phonological, speech perceptual, or more general language processes rather than to semantic processing. Given the evidence discussed previously (see sections "Spoken Speech Perception" and "Visual Character Perception"), it seems likely that activation in the STS, for example, may be related to speech-sound processing requirements of the semantic tasks. Other areas, particularly in prefrontal cortex, may be involved in general processes engaged during language task performance, such as maintaining representations of task instructions and performance strategies, formulating relationships between this "task set" information and information acquired from task stimuli and/or long-term memory, or using these relationships to selectively attend to or retrieve only task-relevant information from a larger set of possible stimulus associations. These issues motivate studies, discussed below, contrasting semantic and perceptual tasks matched for stimulus characteristics, and contrasting semantic with other language tasks.

Perceptual Control Tasks Using Word or Picture Stimuli   Several investigators used comparisons between semantic and perceptual tasks in which the same stimuli were employed in both conditions, thereby obtaining an optimal match of stimulus information across conditions. In the semantic task of Kapur et al. (1994), subjects made a living/nonliving categorization of printed nouns, and in the perceptual condition monitored for the occurrence of a target letter in the same nouns. This baseline task introduces a complex set of issues related to task strategy, in that detection of a target letter in a word could theoretically be performed using purely visual information, or using additional phonological or word-level information. In addition there is the probability that some degree of preattentive processing of the orthographic, phonologic, lexical, and semantic information associated with the word stimuli took place during the control task (see figure 7.1). Perhaps not surprisingly, this semantic-perceptual task contrast produced no activation in posterior association areas, and the only significant activation difference favoring the semantic task was in the left IFG (probably pars orbitalis and pars triangularis). This finding reinforced previous evidence that the left IFG is active during semantic processing (Frith et al., 1991a; Petersen et al., 1988) and ruled out proposed explanations related to speech formulation or response selection (Frith et al., 1991a; Wise et al., 1991). Demb et al. (1995) subsequently used similar tasks during fMRI of the frontal lobes. Stronger activation during the semantic task was observed in both the left IFG and the left SFG.

In contrast to these studies, Vandenberghe et al. (1996) observed activation related to semantic processing in several posterior left hemisphere locations, using a perceptual baseline task with meaningful stimuli. Stimuli consisted of triplets (one sample and two match choices) of concrete nouns or pictures. In the semantic conditions, subjects selected one of the match choices based either on functional relatedness (PLIERS matches WRENCH better than SAW) or real-life size similarity (KEY matches PEN better than PITCHER). In the perceptual condition, subjects selected the match choice that was most similar in size as presented in the stimulus display. This baseline task proved rather difficult, as demonstrated by a significantly lower performance accuracy on both word and picture baseline conditions relative to semantic conditions. Relative to this baseline task, the semantic tasks activated left hemisphere and right cerebellar regions, including left IFG, left MTG and ITG, left fusiform gyrus, and left angular gyrus (temporo-parieto-occipital junction). Overall, this pattern of activation is very similar to that observed by Démonet et al. (1992) and Binder et al., (1997), except for a notable absence of activation in the SFG (table 7.1).

The striking differences between the Kapur et al. (1994) and Vandenberghe et al. (1996) results for posterior association cortices could have several explanations. The lack of posterior activations in the Kapur et al. study may relate simply to decreased sensitivity or statistical power, or to a more conservative threshold. The studies employed different semantic task procedures (category decision in the Kapur et al. study and similarity matching in the Vandenberghe et al. study). However, this factor in itself is unlikely to account for the observed differences in posterior cortical activation, in view of the fact that the studies of Démonet et al. (1992) and Binder et al. (1997) demonstrated such activation using category decision tasks. Alternatively, the greater difficulty of the baseline task used by Vandenberghe et al. may have more effectively precluded subjects from engaging in stimulus-unrelated language processing (section "Special Problems for Language Activation Imaging Studies"; see also section "Semantic Processing at Rest," below), providing a stronger contrast between baseline and semantic conditions. The control task used by Vandenberghe et al. may also have provided a stronger contrast by directing attention strongly to a physical feature of the stimulus (size), unlike the Kapur et al. task, which encouraged subjects to use letter name and word information.

Semantic Tasks Contrasted with Other Linguistic Tasks   In an effort to identify regions involved specifically in processing meaning, other investigators contrasted semantic tasks with tasks involving phonological or lexical processing. Démonet et al. (1992, 1994a) and Binder et al. (1999) contrasted auditory semantic categorization tasks with phoneme identification tasks on pseudo words. Results of these studies were strikingly similar (figure 7.2, table 7.1). The main areas in which activation was stronger during semantic processing included the SFG, left angular gyrus, left posterior cingulate, and left ventromedial temporal lobe. Stereotaxic coordinates for these foci were nearly identical in the two studies (Binder et al., 1999). Neither study found activation related to the semantic task in the IFG, STG, STS, or ITG. The lack of semantic-specific IFG activation calls into question the role of this region in semantic processing per se. Equivalent activation of the IFG during a phoneme discrimination task on pseudo words suggests that this region may play a more general role related to working memory or phoneme recognition. Equivalent activation of STG and STS is consistent with a proposed role for these regions in auditory and speech phoneme processing.

The lack of ITG or clear MTG activation in these studies is not entirely unexpected, given the evidence presented by Price, Wise, and Frackowiak (1996) that these regions are readily activated by pseudo words. This activation could indicate involvement of the MTG and ITG at the level of phonological word-form processing. Supporting evidence for such an account comes from lesion and functional imaging studies of name retrieval, which implicate the MTG and ITG as crucial sites for storage of phonological word representations (H. Damasio et al., 1996; Foundas et al., 1998; Martin et al., 1996; Mills & McConnell, 1895). Several investigators have also observed posterior ITG activation by auditory pseudo words, which could be explained by such an account (Démonet et al., 1992; Zatorre et al., 1992).

Two studies incorporated visually presented pseudo words in a phonological control task. Pugh et al. (1996b) studied a semantic relatedness matching task using visual word pairs. In the phonological control task, subjects judged whether two visual pseudo words rhymed. Consistent with the Démonet et al. (1992) and Binder et al. (1999) results, no differential activation by the semantic task was observed in the IFG. Greater activation by the semantic task was observed in a medial temporal region of interest that probably included fusiform and part of parahippocampal gyri, although this activation difference occurred bilaterally. Greater activation by the semantic task was also noted in STG and MTG regions of interest, although these differences also occurred bilaterally and only in males. Superior frontal, ITG, angular gyrus, and posterior cingulate regions were not assessed. In a study by Gabrieli et al. (1998), a semantic categorization task on visually presented words was contrasted with a task in which subjects judged whether visual pseudo words had two syllables or not. In contrast to the other semantic-phonological studies, this task combination produced stronger semantic task activation in the left IFG. Stronger semantic task activation was also found in the left SFG, consistent with the other studies. Posterior cortical areas were not assessed in this study.

Two semantic task studies employed visually presented words in a phonological control task. Price, Moore, Humphreys, et al. (1997) contrasted a semantic categorization (living/nonliving) task with a phonological task in which subjects judged the number of syllables in a presented word. Stronger semantic task activation was found in the left angular gyrus, left temporal pole (near amygdala), and head of left caudate nucleus. Marginally significant differences were observed in the left medial SFG (BA 9), left MTG, and left ITG. Consistent with most of the other semantic-phonologic studies, no differences occurred in the IFG. Using an almost identical task contrast, however, Gabrieli et al. (1998) did report stronger semantic task activation in the IFG. A large left SFG focus also showed stronger activation during the semantic task. Posterior cortical areas were not assessed in this study.

Finally, Bottini et al. (1994) reported a study in which semantic comprehension of sentences was contrasted with a lexical decision control task. In the semantic task, subjects saw sentences (e.g., "The bird watcher used binoculars as wings") and had to decide whether these were literally plausible in meaning. In the control task, subjects saw strings of eight to nine words (e.g., "Hot lamp into confusing after bencil entrance stick real") and had to decide whether the string contained a nonword. Relative to the lexical decision control task, the semantic task activated much of the left IFG and SFG, left MTG and ITG, left angular gyrus, and left posterior cingulate/precuneus. The pattern of activation is strikingly similar to that shown in figure 7.9 for semantic categorization contrasted with tone monitoring, despite the many apparent differences between the task contrasts used in these two studies.

These are interesting and informative results for several reasons. First, both tasks used word strings that would have evoked some degree of semantic processing, so the large magnitude, widespread activation differences between tasks are somewhat unexpected. This result confirms that task-induced "top-down" effects can have a large effect on activation levels. In this case, the explicit requirement to formulate a sentence-level representation and examine the semantic content of this more complex representation induced considerable additional left hemisphere activation. This finding is confounded, however, by the fact that formulation of a sentence-level representation also requires syntactic analysis, so some of the differences observed may have been due to this additional syntactic demand rather than to semantic processing per se. These results also suggest that lexical decision may engage semantic processes relatively little. Other evidence for this comes from a previous study in which lexical decision and reading tasks were both compared to a common control task involving feature detection on false font strings (Price et al., 1994). The reading task activated left SFG and left angular gyrus, the two areas most often associated with semantic tasks, while the lexical decision task failed to do so.

Summary of Areas Implicated in Semantic Processing   Together these studies implicate a number of regions in performance of tasks involving word meaning. It is worth noting that in all these studies, activation associated with such tasks has been strongly lateralized to the left hemisphere, in contrast to the much more symmetric activation typically seen in the STG in response to hearing speech sounds, and in the supramarginal gyri during verbal short-term memory and phonological tasks. The single most consistently activated region is the angular gyrus (Brodmann area 39), referring to the cortex surrounding the posterior parietal extension of the STS. Deriving its blood supply from the inferior trunk of the middle cerebral artery, this region is frequently damaged in cases of Wernicke's aphasia (H. Damasio, 1989; Kertesz et al., 1993; Metter et al., 1990; Naeser, 1981; Selnes et al., 1984). BA 39 is probably a phylogenetically recent and specifically human development (Geschwind, 1965) and is situated strategically between visual, auditory, and somatosensory centers, making it one of the more reasonable candidates for a multimodal "convergence area" involved in storing or processing very abstract representations of sensory experience and word meaning.

With only a few exceptions (Kapur et al., 1994; Vandenberghe et al., 1996), dorsal prefrontal cortex in the SFG was consistently activated in these studies. This region includes the medial aspect of BA 8 and 9, and lies rostral to both the supplementary motor area and pre-SMA (Pickard & Strick, 1996). Patients with lesions in this region typically demonstrate intact semantic knowledge in the presence of strongly directing cues (e.g., intact comprehension of words and intact naming of presented stimuli) but impaired access to this knowledge in the absence of constraining cues (e.g., impaired ability to generate lists of related words despite normal speech articulation and naming) (Alexander & Schmitt, 1980; Costello & Warrington, 1989; Freedman et al., 1984; Rapcsak & Rubens, 1994; Rubens, 1976; Stuss & Benson, 1986). Spontaneous speech is sparse or nonexistent, and phrase length in cued production tasks (e.g., description of pictures) is severely reduced. These deficits suggest an impairment involving self-initiation of language processes. We thus hypothesize that this brain region initiates (drives or motivates) the process of semantic information retrieval. That this area is activated by semantic relative to phonologic knowledge retrieval tasks indicates either a specific role in initiating retrieval from semantic stores or that semantic knowledge retrieval makes stronger demands on the initiation mechanism than does phonologic retrieval, possibly by virtue of the greater arbitrariness of the relations linking stimulus and stored knowledge in the case of semantic associations.

Activations in the ventral and lateral left temporal lobe are less consistent and appear to be more dependent on specific stimulus characteristics and task requirements. Semantic activation near the middle part of the fusiform gyrus or neighboring collateral sulcus (BA 20/36) is common. Activation in this region appears to depend on the lexical status of the control stimuli, since it occurred in all five studies involving nonword control stimuli but in only one of four involving word control stimuli.

This region has been implicated in lexical-semantic functions in a number of other functional imaging studies (Bookheimer et al., 1995; H. Damasio et al., 1996; Martin et al., 1996; Menard et al., 1996; Price, Moore, Humphreys, et al., 1996) and in studies using focal cortical stimulation and evoked potential recordings (Lüders et al., 1991; Nobre et al., 1994). As already discussed, the left MTG and ITG were associated with semantic processing in some, but not all, studies. The likelihood of detecting differential activation in these areas, using contrasts between semantic and phonological tasks, appears to depend partly on the modality of stimulus presentation. These regions were identified in four of five studies using visual stimuli, but in neither of two studies using auditory pseudo words. As mentioned earlier, these results may indicate a role for these regions in storing or processing sound-based representations of words. Such representations would likely be accessed in any task involving word or pseudo word processing (Van Orden, 1987), but perhaps more strongly when stimuli are presented in the auditory modality. Sound-based word representations must be accessed when naming objects, which may account for the activation of left MTG and ITG during such tasks (Bookheimer et al., 1995; H. Damasio et al., 1996; Martin et al., 1996; Price & Friston, 1997; Smith et al., 1996). The activation of MTG and ITG in comparisons between auditory word and reversed speech processing (figure 7.7) are also consistent with this model (Howard et al., 1992; Price, Wise, Warburton, et al., 1996), as is the finding that printed words and pseudo words activate this region relative to unpronounceable stimuli (figure 7.1).

By linking the left MTG and ITG with processing of sound-based word representations, we do not mean to imply that these functions are distinct from semantic processing or that concept-level representations are not also processed in these areas. Names represent concepts, and they become an integral part of the concepts they represent. Tasks used clinically to assess semantic knowledge also depend on knowledge of names and name-concept relationships. Thus, lesions affecting left MTG and ITG frequently disrupt performance on semantic tasks (Alexander et al., 1989; H. Damasio, 1981; Kertesz et al., 1982). Moreover, such patients sometimes show very selective knowledge deficits affecting only a particular semantic category or word class (A. Damasio & Tranel, 1993; H. Damasio et al., 1996; Hart & Gordon, 1990; Hillis & Caramazza, 1991; Warrington & Shallice, 1984). Functional imaging studies demonstrate that activation in this region depends partly on the semantic category associated with stimuli (H. Damasio et al., 1996; Martin et al., 1996; Mummery et al., 1996; Perani et al., 1995). (See chapter 6 in this volume for a detailed discussion of these findings.) This evidence of category-specific organization in the ventrolateral and ventral temporal lobe strongly suggests the presence of concept-level representations in this region. These data reinforce the view that names and the concepts they represent are intimately connected, interact during semantic tasks, and are very likely to have spatially overlapping representations in the brain.

Involvement of the left IFG in semantic processing has been a topic of considerable debate (Démonet et al., 1993; Frith et al., 1991a; Gabrieli et al., 1998; Kapur et al., 1994; Petersen et al., 1988; Thompson-Schill et al., 1997; Wise et al., 1991). This area is consistently activated during word production tasks (Frith et al., 1991a; Petersen et al., 1988; Warburton et al., 1996; Wise et al., 1991). Left IFG activation was also observed in five studies involving semantic (mostly word categorization) tasks contrasted with nonlinguistic perceptual control tasks (table 7.1), demonstrating that this activation is not specific to word generation tasks or the requirement for "willed action." In contrast, most of the studies employing phonological control tasks failed to show differential activation of the IFG. One explanation for these negative results is that the word and nonword stimuli used in these phonological control tasks may have inadvertently engaged the semantic system to some degree, causing obscuring of semantic-specific IFG activation. Although possible, this account does not explain why differential semantic activation occurred in other regions (angular gyrus, SFG, ventromedial temporal lobe) but not in the left IFG. Another possibility is that left IFG activation observed in some previous studies reflects phonological or verbal short-term memory demands of the word generation and comprehension tasks employed in these studies. This explanation applies particularly to posterior regions of the IFG, such as pars opercularis and adjacent premotor cortex, which have been repeatedly implicated in various aspects of phonological processing (Démonet et al., 1992; Fiez et al., 1995; Paulesu et al., 1993; Price, Moore, Humphreys, et al., 1997; Zatorre et al., 1992).

Another explanation for the IFG activation in some studies is that this activation reflects more general task demands related to linguistic knowledge retrieval. Thompson-Schill et al. (1997) have presented evidence that activation in left IFG, SMA, and anterior cingulate cortex is dependent on the requirement for selection of task-relevant information from a larger set of possible stimulus associations. Three semantic tasks using printed words or pictures were each contrasted with a non-semantic baseline task. Each semantic task type had two levels considered to have either low or high knowledge selection demands. In a verb generation task, selection demands were manipulated by varying the number of different verbs (i.e., different potential responses) associated with the stimulus noun. In a word-picture matching task, selection demands were manipulated by requiring a match to either a specific attribute of the object (high selection demand) or to the object name (low selection demand). In a similarity matching task, selection demands were manipulated by requiring either a match based on a specific attribute (high selection) or one based on global similarity (low selection). The findings support the hypothesis that selection demands modulate activity in the left IFG (primarily in BA 44) and also in other left hemisphere regions, including SMA, anterior cingulate, fusiform gyrus, ITG, and angular gyrus. This study thus provides evidence that general task performance requirements related to information retrieval and response selection can affect activation during semantic tasks and may partly explain left IFG activation during such tasks.

A final region implicated in several of these studies is the posterior cingulate and ventral precuneus. Although interpretation of this finding is unclear, part of this region coincides with retrosplenial cortex (Vogt, 1976), which has connections with hippocampus, parahippocampus (Mufson & Pandya, 1984; Suzuki & Amaral, 1994), and anterolaterodorsal thalamus (Sripanidkulchai & Wyss, 1986). This connectivity pattern suggests involvement of the posterior cingulate region in memory functions (Rudge & Warrington, 1991; Valenstein et al., 1987). Posterior cingulate activation may therefore be related to memory-encoding processes that accompany semantic task performance (Craik & Lockhart, 1972). This could also account for activation observed in some of these studies in left parahippocampus and hippocampus, structures closely tied to episodic memory encoding.

Semantic Processing at Rest   The constructs "semantic processing" and "thinking" share important functional features. In contrast to perceptual systems driven primarily by external sensory information, semantic processing and thinking rely on *internal* sources of information, such as episodic and semantic memory stores. Semantic processing and thinking both involve complex mechanisms for accessing task-relevant information from these stores and manipulating this information to reach an intended goal, such as planning an action or making a decision. To the extent that semantic processing is defined by these operations involving storage, retrieval, and manipulation of internal sources of information, the conscious "thinking" state could also be said to involve semantic processing.

In support of this view, Binder et al. (1999) presented evidence that many of the areas implicated in semantic processing are also active during a resting state compared to a nonsemantic task. A semantic-phonetic task contrast was used to identify areas specialized for semantic processing, including left angular gyrus, SFG, ventromedial temporal cortex, and posterior cingulate (see color plate 14 and figure 7.9A). To determine whether these areas are also active during rest, a resting state (subjects were instructed only to relax and remain still) was compared to a tone discrimination task. Areas that were more active during rest, illustrated in figure 7.9B, were nearly identical to those identified in the semantic-phonetic subtraction. Centers-of-mass in the two comparisons lay within 1 cm of each other for all four main activation areas.

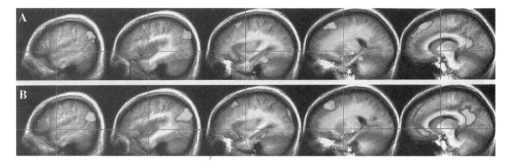

Figure 7.9
Left hemisphere areas associated with nonsensory semantic processing (Binder et al., 1999). Areas with higher signal during a semantic decision task compared to a phonemic decision task (*A*) are virtually identical to areas with higher signal during rest compared to a tone decision task (*B*). (Reproduced, with permission, from Binder, 1999.) (See color plate 14.)

Finally, when the resting state was compared to a semantic decision task, these areas showed little or no difference in activation, consistent with the hypothesis that these regions are engaged in semantic processing during both of these conditions. These cortical areas, which are relatively distant (as measured by cortico-cortical connections) from primary sensory areas (Felleman & Van Essen, 1991; Jones & Powell, 1970; Mesulam, 1985), thus appear to comprise a distributed network for storing, retrieving, and manipulating internal sources of information independent of external sensory input.

The hypothesis that stimulus-independent semantic processing occurs in these brain areas during rest accounts for several puzzling findings from functional activation studies. The first of these is that studies comparing semantic tasks to a resting or restlike (e.g., passive stimulation) baseline have not shown activation in these areas (Eulitz et al., 1994; Herholtz et al., 1994; Kawashima et al., 1993; Mazoyer et al., 1993; Tamas et al., 1993; Warburton et al., 1996; Wise et al., 1991; Yetkin et al., 1995), despite considerable evidence for their participation in semantic processing (see table 7.1). In contrast, comparisons between semantic tasks and attentionally demanding nonsemantic tasks typically show activation in some or all of these areas (Binder et al., 1997; Bottini et al., 1994; Démonet et al., 1992; Price, Moore, Humphreys, et al., 1997; Price, Wise, Watson et al., 1994; Vandenberge et al., 1996). Activation contrast in these areas may thus depend on the degree to which spontaneous semantic processing is suppressed during the baseline state, which may in turn depend on a number of task variables that determine attentional allocation, and on the amount of preattentive semantic processing elicited by control stimuli (Price, Wise, & Frackowiak, 1996).

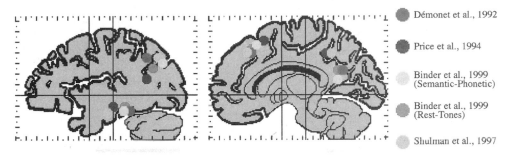

Figure 7.10
Convergence of results across four studies comparing either semantic to nonsemantic tasks (Binder et al., 1999; Démonet et al., 1992; Price et al., 1994) or resting to nonsemantic tasks (Binder et al., 1999; Shulman et al., 1997). (Reproduced with permission from Binder, 1999.) (See color plate 15.)

Spontaneous semantic processing during rest could also account for some instances of task-induced "deactivation" (Shulman et al., 1997). Interruption of spontaneous semantic processes by attentionally demanding, nonsemantic tasks would result in decreased neural activity in brain regions where these processes are localized. This account predicts that brain areas demonstrating "deactivation" during nonsemantic tasks relative to rest should be the same as those areas implicated in semantic processing. Evidence supporting this prediction was given in figure 7.9, in which areas demonstrating "deactivation" during the tones task were nearly identical to those identified with semantic processing in the semantic-phonetic task comparison. This convergence is also demonstrated by other studies of semantic processing and task-induced deactivation. For example, Démonet et al. (1992) and Price, Wise, Watson, et al. (1994) contrasted semantic tasks with attentionally demanding, nonsemantic tasks. Although different in many ways, these contrasts identified the same left hemisphere regions shown in figure 7.9. These four areas also consistently demonstrated task-induced deactivation across a variety of visual tasks in a meta-analysis by Shulman et al. (1997). This unusual convergence of results, illustrated in figure 7.10 (and color plate 15), is remarkable, given the considerable differences in methodology across the four studies. The hypothesis that task-induced deactivation in these brain areas results from interruption of spontaneous semantic processing provides one parsimonious explanation for this pattern of results.

Word Production

The production of words is a multicomponent operation involving, at a minimum, conceptual, lexical, phonetic, and articulatory processes (see Levelt, 1989). Word production can be either stimulus-driven from sensory stimuli (e.g., during reading and picture naming) or self-generated from inner thoughts, memories, and associations (e.g., during verbal fluency tasks). In the former case, processes involved in object or word recognition will be engaged in addition to word production processes. In the latter case, processes involved in willed action, lexical search, and sustained attention will be required. Isolating the neural correlates of the different components of word production with functional neuroimaging therefore depends on subtracting activation associated with sensory processing, willed action, and sustained attention.

Functional imaging studies of self-generated word production have focused on verbal fluency tasks. During these tasks, subjects are presented with an auditory or visual cue and asked to generate words associated with the cue (the word generation task). Tasks vary in (1) the type of cue used, which might be a word (Petersen et al., 1988; Raichle et al., 1994; Warburton et al., 1996; Wise et al., 1991), a letter (Frith et al., 1991b), or a word stem such as "GRE" (Buckner et al., 1995), and (2) the type of association required—for instance, retrieving semantically related verbs, category exemplars, synonyms, or rhymes (Klein et al., 1995; Shaywitz, Pugh, et al., 1995). Irrespective of the type of cue, type of association, or baseline used, self-generated word production results in activation of the left lateral frontal cortex, including the frontal operculum and IFG (BA 44–47), the posterior part of the middle frontal gyrus and inferior frontal sulcus, and the middorsal part of the precentral sulcus (BA 6, 8, 44). Some functional division of the different regions has been demonstrated by Buckner et al. (1995), who found that the left inferior prefrontal cortex (BA 44 and 45) was equally responsive to word stem completion ("GRE"—"green") and verb generation ("CAR"—"drive"), irrespective of baseline (visual fixation for word stem completion and reading for verb generation), but activation in the left anterior prefrontal cortex (near BA 10 or 46) was observed only for verb generation. Whether this difference in activation patterns is related to differences in the word generation tasks or in the baseline task is not yet clear.

The functional roles of these different prefrontal regions remains a topic of debate. For instance, Fiez (1997) demonstrated that different regions of the prefrontal cortex can be associated with semantic and phonological processes: the left ventral anterior frontal cortex (near BA 47) is activated for semantic decisions, whereas the more posterior regions (BA 44/6 and 45) are associated with phonological decisions (Démonet et al., 1992, 1994a; Fiez et al., 1995; Zatorre et al., 1992, 1996). Left-lateralized dorsolateral prefrontal activations (BA 46) have also been associated with encoding novel verbal information into episodic memory, such as when subjects memorize pairs of heard words relative to hearing the same words repeated continually (Fletcher et al., 1995; Tulving et al., 1994). In contrast, Frith et al. (1991b) observed activation in BA 46 in association with self-generated nonverbal actions. These authors suggested a more general nonverbal role for this region, perhaps in the exercise of "will" to perform a volitional act. The location of the peak activation associated with encoding into episodic memory (Fletcher et al., 1995) was 12 mm inferior to the peak activation associated with willed action in the Frith et al. study. These results may thus represent two functionally distinct activation foci or, alternatively, chance variability due to use of different subject samples and other random factors. Many further studies are required to correlate the different cytoarchitectural regions of the lateral prefrontal cortex with different functional roles. At this stage, one can only conclude that this general area is activated during self-generated word production, and that different regions appear to be involved in semantic and phonological processing, episodic memory encoding, and willed action.

Although the left lateral prefrontal cortex is robustly activated in self-generated word production, this activation is not as prominent when the task becomes more automated, as in the case of stimulus-driven word production. Indeed, Raichle et al. (1994) have demonstrated that activation in the left prefrontal cortex during self-generated word production decreases with practice on the same cue items. The reduced prefrontal activity as the task becomes more familiar is consistent with the association of the left prefrontal cortex with encoding novel stimuli into episodic memory (Fletcher et al., 1995; Tulving et al., 1994). It is also consistent with reduction of the demands placed on lexical-semantic search and response selection as the stimulus and response become more familiar.

Interestingly, the decreases in prefrontal activity with task familiarity reported by Raichle et al. (1994) were accompanied by increases in activation of the left insula. The relevance of this finding is that the left anterior insula and the surrounding left frontal operculum are almost universally activated during stimulus-driven naming tasks. For example, the left frontal operculum is activated for reading, picture naming, color naming, and letter naming relative to baseline tasks that attempt to control for visual and articulatory processing (Bookheimer et al., 1995; Price & Friston, 1997). It is also involved in repetition of heard words relative to passive word listening (Price, Wise, Warburton, et al., 1996), and when the demands on retrieving phonology are increased—for instance, during phonological detection tasks (Fiez et al., 1995) and for reading unfamiliar pseudo words (e.g., "latisam") relative to regularly spelled words (e.g., "market") or high-frequency irregular words (e.g., "pint") (Fiez & Petersen, 1998; Herbster et al., 1997; Price, Wise, & Frackowiak, 1996). Together, these findings suggest that activation of the left frontal operculum during self-generated and stimulus-driven word production can probably be related to the stage of lexical access in which the phonological form of a word is constructed (i.e., a role in encoding phonology prior to articulatory output). This conclusion is consistent with the data from lesion studies. The frontal operculum is in the vicinity of Broca's area, and isolated damage to this region particularly impairs the ability to transform word representations into corresponding articulatory sequences (A. Damasio & Geschwind, 1984; Mesulam, 1990; Mohr et al., 1978).

In addition to the left frontal operculum, word production during both self-generated and stimulus-driven paradigms usually results in activation of the left posterior ventral temporal lobe (BA 37) near the inferior temporal and fusiform gyri. For instance, this area is activated during naming tasks and reading relative to baselines that control for visual and articulatory processes (Bookheimer et al., 1995; Martin et al., 1996; Price & Friston, 1997). The same posterior ventral temporal region is also activated (along with the left frontal operculum) when blind subjects read Braille (Büechel et al., 1998) and when word generation to auditory words is contrasted with listening to words or semantic judgments on heard words (Warburton et al., 1996). (See figure 7.11 and color plate 17.) These findings suggest that the left frontal operculum and the left posterior ventral temporal region are involved in nam-

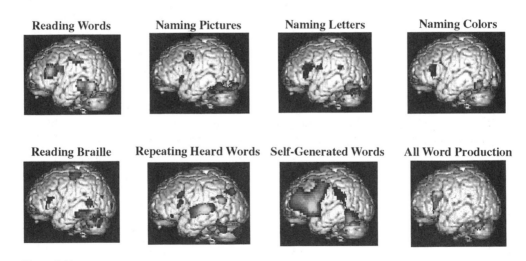

Figure 7.11
Areas of activation during a variety of word production tasks are rendered in red and yellow on a cartoon figure of the left hemisphere. Reading words (silently) was contrasted with viewing consonant letter strings (Price, Wise, & Frackowiak, 1996). Naming visual pictures was contrasted with viewing nonsense figures and saying "Okay" (Price, Moore, & Friston, 1997). Naming visual letters was contrasted with viewing single false font and saying "Okay." Naming the color of meaningless shapes was contrasted with viewing the same shapes and saying "Okay" (Price & Friston, 1997). Naming tactile words (reading braille) was contrasted with feeling consonant letter strings in braille (Büchel et al., 1998). Self-generated words were contrasted with auditory repetition (Frith et al., 1991a) and with repeating heard words. Regions of activation common to all types of word production were identified using conjunction analysis (Price, Moore, & Friston, 1997). (See color plate 17.)

ing, irrespective of the type of stimulus cue. The finding that the left posterior ventral temporal region is more active for word generation than for semantic decisions also suggests that this region plays a role in lexical retrieval over and above that involved in conceptual processing. Nevertheless, the left posterior ventral temporal region is in close proximity to an area that activates during conceptual processing, particularly tasks involving visual semantics. This semantic region lies medially and anteriorly in the fusiform gyrus (BA 20) relative to the area we are associating with lexical retrieval (BA 37). It has been observed during generation of color words relative to generation of action words, indicating a role in perceptual knowledge (Martin et al., 1995); for visual imagery of heard words relative to passive listening to words (D'Esposito et al., 1997); and for semantic decisions relative to phonological or perceptual decisions (Binder et al., 1997, 1999; Démonet et al., 1992; Vandenberghe et al., 1996). Responses in the medial and anterior region of the fusiform gyrus (BA 20) are therefore more concerned with conceptual than with phonological processing, whereas the lateral posterior ventral temporal cortex (BA 37) is more responsive to phonological than to semantic processing (Moore & Price, 1999).

Evidence from direct cortical stimulation and lesion studies also supports the role of the left ventral temporal lobe in lexical retrieval. For example, cortical stimulation of the ventral temporal region (including inferior temporal and fusiform gyri) in patients prior to surgery for epilepsy results in a transient failure to produce words (Burnstine et al., 1990; Lüders et al., 1986, 1991). Likewise, patients with lesions in the territory of the left posterior cerebral artery (usually occipital and inferior temporal lobe damage) show deficits in reading and in naming objects in response to visual presentation, tactile presentation, or verbal descriptions (De Renzi et al., 1987). A study by Foundas et al. (1998) demonstrated that a specific region in the left lateral posterior ventral temporal cortex resulted in a naming deficit in the absence of a recognition or semantic deficit. Together, the imaging and lesion data suggest that the left lateral posterior ventral temporal cortex may be concerned with retrieval of lexical entities from conceptual networks in more anterior and medial temporal cortex, while the left frontal operculum is concerned with translating the lexical entities into articulatory routines. Additional experiments are required to confirm the precise nature of the neuroanatomical structures that underlie these different stages of lexical access and word production.

Genetic and Developmental Influences on Language System Organization

The common practice of presenting averaged activation maps from a group of subjects (e.g., figure 7.8) obscures the fact that there is considerable variability among subjects in the precise spatial location, spatial extent, and magnitude of these activations (Bavelier et al., 1997; Binder, Rao, Hammeke, et al., 1994; Kim et al., 1997; Springer et al., 1997). This variation could conceivably arise from genetic or environmental sources, or from complex interactions between genome and environment. Two developmental factors that have received some attention in neuroimaging studies of language organization are the age of acquisition of languages learned by the subject (an almost purely environmental variable) and the sex of the subject (a genetic factor strongly associated with various environmental variables).

Studies of Bilingualism   Available evidence suggests that brain activation during a language task depends on the subject's proficiency with the language, which in turn depends roughly on the age at which the language was acquired. O. Yetkin et al. (1996) studied five adult multilingual subjects using fMRI. In the language activation condition, subjects were asked to silently generate words in their native language, a second fluent language, or a third nonfluent language known to the subject for less than five years. The baseline condition was a resting state in which subjects "refrained from thinking of words." Significantly more voxels in the frontal lobe showed activation in the nonfluent condition, while the native and second fluent languages produced equal activation. These results are consistent with the idea that, in general, tasks which are less practiced require more neural activity (Haier et al., 1992; Raichle et al., 1994). Because this extra neural activity could be related to attentional rather than linguistic processes, however, the data of Yetkin et al. do not address the issue of whether different languages are actually represented in different brain areas.

A report by Kim et al. (1997) provides some initial evidence on this question. The authors studied 12 adult bilingual subjects who acquired a second fluent language either simultaneously with a first ("early bilingual") or during young adulthood ("late bilingual"). In the language activation condition, subjects were asked to "mentally describe" events that had occurred the previous day, using a specified language. The baseline condition was a resting state in which subjects looked at a fixation point. In late bilinguals, the left inferior frontal activation foci associated with task performance in the native and second languages were spatially separated by an average distance of 6.4 mm (range 4.5 mm–9.0 mm). The relative locations of these native and second language foci were highly variable across subjects, with the native language focus lateral to the second language focus in some subjects and medial or posterior in other subjects. This fact alone could explain why a previous PET study (Klein et al., 1995) using averaged group activation maps showed no differences in cortical activation associated with native and second languages. Because Kim et al. did not report the relative language proficiency of their subjects or overall levels of activation as a function of language used, it is not clear whether the spatial separation of activation foci could be related to familiarity and attentional (i.e., workload) effects rather than to differences in the location of linguistic representations, although this seems unlikely, given the reported lack of spatial overlap between the native language and second language activation foci. Nevertheless, early bilinguals showed no differences in the location of activation foci associated with different languages, suggesting that when two languages are learned equally well early in life, these languages typically are represented in the same brain areas.

This conclusion may not apply, of course, to cases in which the languages in question differ greatly in terms of perceptual requirements or representational formats. Available evidence suggests, for example, that comprehension of American Sign Language (ASL) engages the right hemisphere (particularly the STS, angular gyrus, and IFG) much more than does comprehension of written English, even among subjects who learn both languages early in life and with equal competence (Neville et al., 1998). This difference almost certainly reflects the fact that the vocabulary and syntax of ASL are represented to a large extent by static and dynamic spatial relationships, which likely engage specialized right hemisphere mechanisms. Activation patterns related to ASL processing were virtually identical for bilingual and monolingual signers, indicating that the English-ASL differences observed in bilingual subjects are not related to bilingualism per se, but rather to the specific processing demands of ASL. This finding highlights a more general point concerning comparisons of activation during processing of different languages. Because different languages may make use of very different sensory distinctions, orthographic-to-phonologic mapping schemes, morphological systems, and syntactic representations, resulting differences in activation patterns could reflect any combination of these factors. Consequently, different studies will not necessarily produce consistent results for different language combinations or language tasks.

Sex Effects on Language Activation Patterns   Numerous studies report that women, on average, have slightly better verbal skills than men. Most of this evidence pertains to speech production tasks, whereas sex differences in higher-order language abilities like semantic processing are equivocal (see Halpern, 1992, for a review). Efforts to uncover the neurophysiological basis for these sex differences have so far met with limited success. Inferential techniques, such as deficit-lesion correlation, structural morphometry, and behavioral measures of lateralization (dichotic listening, divided visual field processing), have yielded very discrepant results (Frost et al., 1999). Compared to these other methods, functional imaging techniques provide a more direct measure of brain function, yet application of these methods has also generated inconsistent findings.

Using fMRI, Shaywitz, Shaywitz, et al. (1995) reported that frontal lobe activation is more left-lateralized in men than in women during a visual phonological task in which subjects judged whether two printed nonwords rhyme. In a later description of the same study (Pugh et al., 1996b), sex effects on functional lateralization were also reported during semantic processing (semantic categorization) of visually presented words. Compared with the phonological condition, the semantic task resulted in a larger volume of activation in men but not in women. This result was observed in the total area scanned, in medial extrastriate cortex, and in the middle and superior temporal gyri bilaterally. Based on this result, the authors suggested that there may be greater overlap between the semantic and phonological systems in women and, thus, more circumscribed representation of language processes in women. Activations in men were also significantly more left-lateralized than in women across the total area imaged, and in the inferior frontal gyrus during both phonologic and semantic tasks. No sex differences in *performance* were observed on these tasks; these data thus suggest that men and women carry out identical language processes with the same degree of proficiency, using very differently organized brain systems.

In contrast, several other functional imaging studies have not found significant sex differences during language processing. Price, Moore, and Friston (1996) used PET to examine activation during phonologic and semantic reading tasks that engaged many of the same processing components studied by Shaywitz, Shaywitz, et al. (1995). Large, statistically significant effects of task, task order, and type of baseline task were found, but sex effects were small and insignificant. In another PET study, Buckner et al. (1995) found no sex differences in activation during word stem completion and verb generation tasks, speech production measures similar to those on which men and women typically show subtle performance differences (Halpern, 1992). Thus, no significant sex differences in large-scale activation patterns were found even on tasks for which there is some evidence of sex-related differences in processing capacity. Finally, Frost et al. (1999) used fMRI to study a large subject cohort (50 women and 50 men) during performance of the semantic-tone task contrast developed by Binder et al. (1997). Men and women showed identical, strongly left-lateralized activation patterns (figure 7.12 and color plate 16). Voxel-wise comparisons between the male and female subjects showed no significantly different voxels. No sex differences in the degree of lateralization were observed for any region of interest, using both functionally defined regions and regions of interest identical to those employed in the Shaywitz, Shaywitz, et al. studies.

In summary, functional imaging research on developmental factors that influence language organization in the brain is still at a preliminary stage. Brain activation during language processing clearly depends on language proficiency, but whether this effect reflects changes in language organization as proficiency is acquired, or merely the additional effort associated with an unfamiliar task, is not yet clear. Available

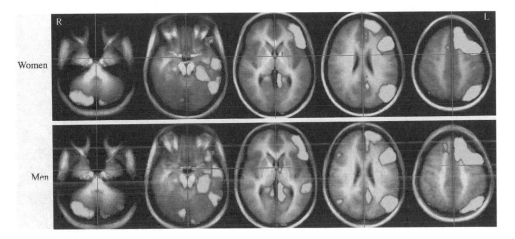

Figure 7.12
Serial axial sections showing average activation maps from 50 women and 50 men during a semantic word categorization task (Frost et al., 1999). Activation is strongly left-lateralized in both groups. There were no significant group differences at a voxel or regional level. (See color plate 16.)

data suggest that two similar languages learned equally well early in life typically are represented in the same brain areas (Kim et al., 1997). Although sex effects on language organization in the brain have been extensively investigated and debated, there remains considerable controversy on this topic. Functional imaging data have so far not resolved this issue, and more studies, using larger subject samples and a wider variety of task contrasts, are needed.

ISSUES

The past several years have witnessed an explosion of new data on functional imaging of language processes. Although it was not possible to review all of this material, some of which was appearing even as we were writing this chapter, it is apparent from the papers selected here that early consensus is beginning to emerge on several points. The following list summarizes some of these main points, presented in detail in earlier sections.

• As predicted by over a century of aphasia research, language-related processing is relatively lateralized to the left hemisphere. The degree of lateralization appears to be strongest for lexical-semantic areas, less for phonological and verbal working-memory areas, and still less for sensory cortex activations (e.g., auditory cortex in STG).

• Brain regions involved in language processing are widespread and include many areas other than the classical Broca area (posterior IFG) and Wernicke area (posterior superior temporal lobe).

• Activation of the dorsal STG (including planum temporale) is dependent on the amount of auditory stimulation but not on linguistic factors, linking this region more closely to auditory than to linguistic processes.

• Cortex in the STS (left > right) is activated more strongly by speech than by non-speech sounds, and more strongly by pronounceable than by unpronounceable print stimuli. These findings suggest that the STS may play a key role in processes involving phoneme representations.

• The left ventral temporal lobe is frequently activated by tasks emphasizing name retrieval, suggesting that this region may be a site for storage of names and/or name meanings. Responses in the medial and anterior region of the fusiform gyrus (BA 20) appear to be more concerned with processing conceptual than phonological representations of names and objects, whereas the lateral posterior ventral temporal cortex (BA 37) appears more responsive to phonological than to semantic task demands.

• The left angular gyrus (temporo-parieto-occipital junction), left dorsal prefrontal cortex (SFG), and left ventromedial temporal cortex (fusiform/parahippocampal junction) form a network of regions frequently activated in contrasts between semantic and nonsemantic tasks, and consistently "deactivated" by nonsemantic tasks relative to the conscious resting state. These regions may be involved in processing internal sources of information at the most abstract "conceptual" level, as occurs during semantic tasks and thinking states.

• The posterior IFG (BA 44, 45, 6) and supramarginal gyrus (BA 40) are often activated (often bilaterally) during tasks that require maintenance and manipulation of phonological information. These regions appear to be involved in various components of phonological task performance, including verbal short-term memory, phonological segmentation, and sublexical phonological access.

• The left IFG is activated across a variety of language tasks, including word retrieval, verbal working memory, reading, naming, and semantic tasks. Some of the computations provided by this region may be relatively general functions, in the sense of being common to a broad set of language processes or tasks. The inferior frontal opercular region, in particular, appears to be involved in any task using (word or nonword) phonological representations.

For each of these points of developing consensus, however, there remain many more unresolved questions. The following list includes a few general areas of inquiry in which there have been inconsistent results, conflicting interpretations, or relatively little investigation.

• How does the organization of different language subsystems vary as a function of handedness, sex, age, education, intelligence, and other subject variables? Is there subtle hemispheric specialization in areas that show relatively weak lateralization—such as the STG, supramarginal gyrus, and premotor cortex—that could be observed under appropriate task conditions? Are there identifiable relationships between functional and structural measures of hemispheric asymmetry?

• What are the computational roles played by some of the "nonclassical" regions identified in language activation studies? This question applies particularly to the unexpected activation in superior frontal gyrus and posterior cingulate cortex observed in some semantic studies, and to the right cerebellar activation seen in a variety of conditions.

• How and where do the complex processes involved in phoneme recognition and grapheme-to-phoneme conversion unfold? Are there functional subdivisions of the STS that can be distinguished, perhaps, on the basis of input modality, specialization for particular phonemic features, use of sublexical vs. lexical codes, or other variables?

• What organizational principles underlie semantic and lexical processing in the left inferolateral temporal lobe? Are there consistent patterns related to semantic category, word class, input modality, or type of semantic information (e.g., structural vs. functional) retrieved? How and where do the different processing stages involved in object recognition and name retrieval unfold?

• Under what task conditions are the regions involved in semantic processing and "thinking" inactive?

• What are the precise functions of the supramarginal region in phonological and verbal short-term memory tasks? Are there important functional subdivisions or areas with consistent hemispheric asymmetry in this region?

• What function(s) is(are) carried out by the IFG during language tasks? What are the important functional subdivisions of this region?

• How do the neural systems for language change with development, with exposure to a second language, and with brain lesions acquired at different ages?

Finally, with the current inundation of new information we recognize a parallel increase in the difficulty of assimilating the data in entirety and recognizing converging trends. This problem is compounded by several factors that have long complicated interpretation of functional imaging data. The most profound of these is the lack of a standard, meaningful nomenclature for describing the computational requirements of activation and control tasks. In some cases this problem manifests in the use of different terms for the same general process (as when, for example, semantic word categorization is referred to as both "semantic retrieval" and "semantic encoding"). More difficult are cases in which differences in terminology arise either from deep differences in underlying theoretical positions or from process distinctions recognized as relevant by some investigators but not by others. A few examples include the profound differences between sequential symbolic and parallel distributed processing accounts of cognition in general, the degree of theoretical distinction made between semantic and linguistic processes, differing theoretical conceptions of the "resting" state, and the extent to which "central executive" functions and other "cognitive modules" are decomposed into more elemental processes. Widespread agreement regarding the computational processes involved in activation tasks—and universal recognition that equal consideration must be given to the processes involved in "baseline" tasks—would appear to be a first prerequisite for agreement on the interpretation of results. Lacking such a standard theoretical background and well-defined terminology to represent elements of the theory, investigators using very different theoretical systems will continue to report apparently inconsistent or conflicting findings, forcing subsequent investigators to reinterpret the data in order to advance understanding.

A second factor complicating interpretation is the sometimes inconsistent or imprecise use of anatomical labels for describing the location of activation responses. Different authors not infrequently use different labels to describe activations in the same region or, in other cases, use the same label for activations in different regions. Particular problem areas in language studies involve distinctions between ventral premotor cortex and Broca's area (BA 6 vs. BA 44), IFG and "dorsolateral prefrontal cortex," superior and middle temporal gyri (BA 22 vs. BA 21), supramarginal and angular gyri (BA 40 vs. BA 39), and middle temporal and angular gyri. Causes for imprecision are probably many and could include (1) differential reliance on either anatomically visible landmarks, invisible (i.e., presumed) cytoarchitectonic boundaries, or general (i.e., poorly defined) regional labels (e.g., Broca's area, Wernicke's area, dorsolateral prefrontal cortex, "temporoparietal cortex") by different investigators; (2) differential reliance on the atlas of Talairach and Tournoux (1988), which is itself not entirely consistent across axial, sagittal, and coronal planes; and (3) a natural tendency to find activation foci where anticipated. Reporting locations in terms of the stereotaxic coordinates of peaks or centers-of-mass is a simple, objective alternative to anatomical labels. The limitation of this method used alone is that it usually fails to describe the full extent of the activated region and thus may cause apparent false negative results. An adequate solution to this problem will probably depend on the creation of a detailed, probabilistic, stereotaxic anatomical atlas and a fully standardized method for projecting data into the atlas space.

A final factor complicating interpretation is the lack of a standard method for reporting the reliability of observed activations. Reliability can be affected by many factors, including the degree of standardization of the task activation procedure, the within-subject measurement sample size and signal-to-noise ratio, the number of subjects and degree of intersubject variability, and the use of data-processing procedures like image registration, normalization, and spatial smoothing. A standard measure of overall reliability, such as a split-half correlation test (Binder et al., 1997), would allow different studies to be assigned relative weightings during meta-analysis, which might assist in identification of converging results by separation of true findings from spurious findings.

REFERENCES

Alexander, M. P., Hiltbrunner, B., & Fischer, R. S. (1989). Distributed anatomy of transcortical sensory aphasia. *Archives of Neurology* 46, 885–892.

Alexander, M. P., & Schmitt, M. A. (1980). The aphasia syndrome of stroke in the left anterior cerebral artery territory. *Archives of Neurology* 37, 97–100.

Antrobus, J. S., Singer, J. L., & Greenberg, S. (1966). Studies in the stream of consciousness: Experimental enhancement and suppression of spontaneous cognitive processes. *Perceptual and Motor Skills* 23, 399–417.

Aurell, C. G. (1979). Perception: A model comprising two modes of consciousness. *Perceptual and Motor Skills* 49, 431–444.

Bandettini, P. A., Jesmanowicz, A., VanKylen, J., Birn, R. M., & Hyde, J. S. (1997). Functional MRI of scanner acoustic noise induced brain activation. *NeuroImage* 5, S193.

Baron, J., & Thurston, I. (1973). An analysis of the word-superiority effect. *Cognitive Psychology* 4, 207–228.

Barrett, A. M. (1910). A case of pure word-deafness with autopsy. *Journal of Nervous and Mental Disease* 37, 73–92.

Bavelier, D., Corina, D., Jezzard, P., et al. (1997). Sentence reading: A functional MRI study at 4 tesla. *Journal of Cognitive Neuroscience* 9, 664–686.

Baylis, G. C., Rolls, E. T., & Leonard, C. M. (1987). Functional subdivisions of the temporal lobe neocortex. *Journal of Neuroscience* 7, 330–342.

Beauvois, M. F., & Derouesne, J. (1979). Phonological alexia: Three dissociations. *Journal of Neurology, Neurosurgery, and Psychiatry* 42, 1115–1124.

Binder, J. R. (1999). Functional MRI of the language system. In *Functional MRI*, C. T. W. Moonen & P. A. Bandettini, eds., 407–419. Berlin: Springer-Verlag.

Binder, J. R., Frost, J. A., Hammeke, T. A., Bellgowan, P. S. F., Rao, S. M., & Cox, R. W. (1999). Conceptual processing during the conscious resting state: A functional MRI study. *Journal of Cognitive Neuroscience* 11, 80–93.

Binder, J. R., Frost, J. A., Hammeke, T. A., Cox, R. W., Rao, S. M., & Prieto, T. (1997). Human brain language areas identified by functional magnetic resonance imaging. *Journal of Neuroscience* 17, 353–362.

Binder, J. R., Frost, J. A., Hammeke, T. A., Rao, S. M., & Cox, R. W. (1996). Function of the left planum temporale in auditory and linguistic processing. *Brain* 119, 1239–1247.

Binder, J. R., Rao, S. M., Hammeke, T. A., et al. (1994). Functional magnetic resonance imaging of human auditory cortex. *Annals of Neurology* 35, 662–672.

Binder, J. R., Rao, S. M., Hammeke, T. A., Frost, J. A., Bandettini, P. A., & Hyde, J. S. (1994). Effects of stimulus rate on signal response during functional magnetic resonance imaging of auditory cortex. *Cognitive Brain Research* 2, 31–38.

Binder, J. R., Rao, S. M., Hammeke, T. A., Frost, J. A., Bandettini, P. A., Jesmanowicz, A., & Hyde, J. S. (1995). Lateralized human brain language systems demonstrated by task subtraction functional magnetic resonance imaging. *Archives of Neurology* 52, 593–601.

Birn, R. M., Bandettini, P. A., Cox, R. W., Jesmanowicz, A., & Shaker, R. (1998). Magnetic field changes in the human brain due to swallowing or speaking. *Magnetic Resonance in Medicine* 40, 55–60.

Birn, R. M., Bandettini, P. A., Cox R. W., & Shaker, R. (1999). Event-related fMRI of tasks involving brief motion. *Human Brain Mapping* 7, 106–114.

Bogen, J. E., & Bogen, G. M. (1976). Wernicke's region—where is it? *Annals of the New York Academy of Sciences* 290, 834–843.

Bookheimer, S. Y., Zeffiro, T. A., Blaxton, T., Gaillard, W., & Theodore, W. (1995). Regional cerebral blood flow during object naming and word reading. *Human Brain Mapping* 3, 93–106.

Bottini, G., Corcoran, R., Sterzi, R., Paulesu, E., Schenone, P., Scarpa, P., Frackowiak, R. S., & Frith, C. D. (1994). The role of the right hemisphere in the interpretation of figurative aspects of language: A positron emission tomography study. *Brain* 117, 1241–1253.

Broca, P. (1861). Remarques sur le siége de la faculté du langage articulé; suivies d'une observation d'aphémie (perte de la parole). *Bulletin de la Société anatomique de Paris* 6, 330–357, 398–407.

Buchman, A. S., Garron, D. C., Trost-Cardamone, J. E., Wichter, M. D., & Schwartz, D. (1986). Word deafness: One hundred years later. *Journal of Neurology, Neurosurgery, and Psychiatry* 49, 489–499.

Buckner, R. L., Bandettini, P. A., O'Craven, K. M., Savoy, R. L., Petersen, S. E., Raichle, M. E., & Rosen, B. R. (1996). Detection of cortical activation during averaged single trials of a cognitive task using functional magnetic resonance imaging. *Proceedings of the National Academy of Sciences USA* 93, 14878–14883.

Buckner, R. L., Raichle, M. E., & Petersen, S. E. (1995). Dissociation of human prefrontal cortical areas across different speech production tasks and gender groups. *Journal of Neuroscience* 74, 2163–2173.

Büechel, C., Price, C. J., & Friston, K. J. (1998). A multimodal language area in the ventral visual pathway. *Nature* 394, 274–277.

Burnstine, T. H., Lesser, R. P., Hart, J. J., Uematsu, S., Zinreich, S. J., Drauss, G. L., et al. (1990). Characterization of the basal temporal language area in patients with left temporal lobe epilepsy. *Neurology* 40, 966–970.

Calvert, G. A., Bullmore, E. T., Brammer, M. J., et al. (1997). Activation of auditory cortex during silent lip-reading. *Science* 276, 593–596.

Carr, T. H., McCauley, C., Sperber, R. D., & Parmalee, C. M. (1982). Words, pictures, and priming: On semantic activation, conscious identification, and the automaticity of information processing. *Journal of Experimental Psychology: Human Perception and Performance* 8, 757–777.

Celesia, G. G. (1976). Organization of auditory cortical areas in man. *Brain* 99, 403–414.

Cohen, J. D., Perlstein, W. M., Braver, T. S., Nystrom, L. E., Noll, D. C., Jonides, J., & Smith, E. E. (1997). Temporal dynamics of brain activation during a working memory task. *Nature* 386, 604–607.

Coltheart, M., Patterson, K., & Marshall, J. (1980). *Deep Dyslexia*. London: Routledge and Kegan Paul.

Costello, A. L., & Warrington, E. K. (1989). Dynamic aphasia: The selective impairment of verbal planning. *Cortex* 25, 103–114.

Craik, F. I. M., & Lockhart, R. S. (1972). Levels of processing: A framework for memory research. *Journal of Verbal Learning and Verbal Behavior* 11, 671–684.

Creutzfeld, O., Ojemann, G., & Lettich, E. (1989). Neuronal activity in the human lateral temporal lobe. I. Responses to speech. *Experimental Brain Research* 77, 451–475.

Damasio, A., & Geschwind, N. (1984). The neural basis of language. *Annual Review Neuroscience* 7, 127–147.

Damasio, A. R., & Tranel, D. (1993). Nouns and verbs are retrieved with differently distributed neural systems. *Proceedings of the National Academy of Sciences USA* 90, 4957–4960.

Damasio, H. (1981). Cerebral localization of the aphasias. In Sarno MT (eds.) *Acquired Aphasia*, M. T. Sarno, ed., 27–50. Orlando, FL: Academic Press.

Damasio, H. (1989). Neuroimaging contributions to the understanding of aphasia. In *Handbook of neuropsychology*, F. Boller & J. Grafman, eds., 3–46. Amsterdam: Elsevier.

Damasio, H., Grabowski, T. J., Tranel, D., Hichwa, R. D., & Damasio, A. R. (1996). A neural basis for lexical retrieval. *Nature* 380, 499–505.

Dehaene, S., Dupoux, E., Mehler, J., et al. (1997). Anatomical variability in the cortical representation of first and second language. *NeuroReport* 8, 3809–3815.

Demb, J. B., Desmond, J. E., Wagner, A. D., Vaidya, C. J., Glover, G. H., & Gabrieli, J. D. E. (1995). Semantic encoding and retrieval in the left inferior prefrontal cortex: A functional MRI study of task difficulty and process specificity. *Journal of Neuroscience* 15, 5870–5878.

Démonet, J.-F., Chollet, F., Ramsay, S., et al. (1992). The anatomy of phonological and semantic processing in normal subjects. *Brain* 115, 1753–1768.

Démonet, J.-F., Price, C., Wise, R., & Frackowiak, R. S. J. (1994a). Differential activation of right and left posterior sylvian regions by semantic and phonological tasks: A positron emission tomography study in normal human subjects. *Neuroscience Letters* 182, 25–28.

Démonet, J.-F., Price, C. J., Wise, R., & Frackowiak, R. S. J. (1994b). A PET study of cognitive strategies in normal subjects during language tasks: Influence of phonetic ambiguity and sequence processing on phoneme monitoring. *Brain* 117, 671–682.

Démonet, J.-F., Wise, R., & Frackowiak R. S. J. (1993). Language functions explored in normal subjects by positron emission tomography: A critical review. *Human Brain Mapping* 1, 39–47.

De Renzi, E., Zambolin, A., & Crisi, G. (1987). The pattern of neuropsychological impairment associated with left posterior cerebral infarcts. *Brain* 110, 1099–1116.

Desimone, R., & Gross, C. G. (1979). Visual areas in the temporal cortex of the macaque. *Brain Research* 178, 363–380.

D'Esposito, M., Detre, J. A., Aguirre, G. K., Stallcup, M., Alsop, D. C., Tippet, L. J., & Farah, M. J. (1997). A functional MRI study of mental image generation. *Neuropsychologia* 35, 725–730.

DeYoe, E. A., Neitz, J., Bandettini, P. A., Wong, E. C., & Hyde, J. S. (1992). Time course of event-related MR signal enhancement in visual and motor cortex. In *Book of Abstracts, 11th Annual Meeting, Society for Magnetic Resonance in Medicine*, Berlin, Berkeley, CA: Society for Magnetic Resonance in Medicine 1824.

Dhankhar, A., Wexler, B. E., Fulbright, R. K., Halwes, T., Blamire, A. M., & Shulman, R. G. (1997). Functional magnetic resonance imaging assessment of the human brain auditory cortex response to increasing word presentation rates. *Journal of Neurophysiology* 77, 476–483.

Eulitz, C., Elbert, T., Bartenstein, P., Weiller, C., Müller, S. P., & Pantev, C. (1994). Comparison of magnetic and metabolic brain activity during a verb generation task. *NeuroReport* 6, 97–100.

Felleman, D. J., & Van Essen, D. C. (1991). Distributed hierarchical processing in the primate cerebral cortex. *Cerebral Cortex* 1, 1–47.

Fiez, J. A. (1997). Phonology, semantics and the role of the left inferior prefrontal cortex. *Human Brain Mapping* 5, 79–83.

Fiez, J. A., & Petersen, S. E. (1998). Neuroimaging studies of word reading. *Proceedings of the National Academy of Sciences of the United States of America* 95, 914–921.

Fiez, J. A., Raichle, M. E., Balota, D. A., Tallal, P., & Petersen, S. E. (1996). PET activation of posterior temporal regions during auditory word presentation and verb generation. *Cerebral Cortex* 6, 1–10.

Fiez, J. A., Raichle, M. E., Miezin, F. M., Petersen, S. E., Tallal, P., & Katz, W. F. (1995). PET studies of auditory and phonological processing: Effects of stimulus characteristics and task demands. *Journal of Cognitive Neuroscience* 7, 357–375.

Fiez, J. A., Raife, E. A., Balota, D. A., Schwarz, J. P., Raichle, M. E., & Petersen, S. E. (1996). A positron emission tomography study of short term maintenance of verbal information. *Journal of Neuroscience* 16, 808–822.

Filler, M. S., & Giambra, L. M. (1973). Daydreaming as a function of cueing and task difficulty. *Perceptual and Motor Skills* 37, 503–509.

Flechsig, P. (1908). Bemerkungen über die Hörsphäre des menschlichen Gehirns. *Neurologische Zentralblatt* 27, 2–7.

Fletcher, P. C., Frith, C. D., Grasby, P. M., Shallice, T, Frackowiak, R. S. J., & Dolan, R. J. (1995). Brain systems for encoding and retrieval of auditory-verbal memory. An in vivo study in humans. *Brain* 118, 401–416.

Foundas, A. L., Daniels, S. K., & Vasterling, J. J. (1998). Anomia: Case studies with lesion localisation. *Neurocase* 4, 35–43.

Foundas, A. L., Leonard, C. M., Gilmore, R., Fennell, E., & Heilman, K. M. (1994). Planum temporale asymmetry and language dominance. *Neuropsychologia* 32, 1225–1231.

Freedman, M., Alexander, M. P., & Naeser, M. A. (1984). Anatomic basis of transcortical motor aphasia. *Neurology* 40, 409–417.

Frith, C. D., Friston, K. J., Liddle, P. F., & Frackowiak, R. S. J. (1991a). A PET study of word finding. *Neuropsychologia* 29, 1137–1148.

Frith, C. D., Friston, K. J., Liddle, P. F., & Frackowiak, R. S. J. (1991b). Willed action and the prefrontal cortex in man: A study with PET. *Proceedings of the Royal Society of London* B244, 241–246.

Frost, J. A., Binder, J. R., Springer, J. A., Hammeke, T. A., Bellgowan, P. S. F., Rao, S. M., & Cox, R. W. (1999). Language processing is strongly left lateralized in both sexes: Evidence from MRI. *Brain* 122, 199–208.

Gabrieli, J. D. E., Poldrack, R. A., & Desmond, J. E. (1998). The role of left prefrontal cortex in language and memory. *Proceedings of the National Academy of Sciences USA* 95, 906–913.

Galaburda, A. M., LeMay, M., Kemper, T., & Geschwind, N. (1978). Right-left asymmetries in the brain: Structural differences between the hemispheres may underlie cerebral dominance. *Science* 199, 852–856.

Galaburda, A. M., & Pandya, D. N. (1983). The intrinsic architectonic and connectional organization of the superior temporal region of the rhesus monkey. *Journal of Comparative Neurology* 221, 169–184.

Ganong, W. F. (1980). Phonetic categorization in auditory word perception. *Journal of Experimental Psychology: Human Perception and Performance* 6, 110–115.

Geschwind, N. (1965). Disconnection syndromes in animals and man. *Brain* 88, 237–294, 585–644.

Geschwind, N. (1971). Aphasia. *New England Journal of Medicine* 284, 654–656.

Geschwind, N., & Levitsky, W. (1968). Human brain: Left-right asymmetries in temporal speech region. *Science* 161, 186–187.

Glushko, R. J. (1979). The organization and activation of orthographic knowledge in reading aloud. *Journal of Experimental Psychology: Human Perception and Performance* 5, 674–691.

Goldstein, K. (1948). *Language and Language Disturbances*. New York: Grune & Stratton.

Grady, C. L., Van Meter, J. W., Maisog, J. M., Pietrini, P., Krasuski, J., & Rauschecker, J. P. (1997). Attention-related modulation of activity in primary and secondary auditory cortex. *NeuroReport* 8, 2511–2516.

Hackett, T. A., Stepniewska, I., & Kaas, J. H. (1998). Subdivisions of auditory cortex and ipsilateral cortical connections of the parabelt auditory cortex in macaque monkeys. *Journal of Comparative Neurology* 394, 475–495.

Haier, R. G., Siegel, B. V., MacLachlan, A., et al. (1992). Regional glucose metabolic changes after learning a complex visuospatial/motor task: A positron emission tomographic study. *Brain Research* 570, 134–143.

Hajnal, J. V., Myers, R., Oatridge, A., Schwieso, J. E., Young, I. R., & Bydder, G. M. (1994). Artifacts due to stimulus correlated motion in functional imaging of the brain. *Magnetic Resonance in Medicine* 31, 283–291.

Halpern, D. F. (1992). *Sex Differences in Cognitive Abilities*, 2nd ed. Hillsdale, NJ: Lawrence Erlbaum.

Hart, J., & Gordon, B. (1990). Delineation of single-word semantic comprehension deficits in aphasia, with anatomic correlation. *Annals of Neurology* 27, 226–231.

Hebb, D. O. (1954). The problem of consciousness and introspection. In: *Brain Mechanisms and Consciousness: A Symposium*, E. D. Adrian, F. Bremer, & J. H. Jasper, eds., 402–421. Springfield, IL: Charles C. Thomas.

Henschen, S. E. (1918–1919). On the hearing sphere. *Acta Oto-laryngologica* 1, 423–486.

Henschen, S. E. (1920–1922). *Klinische und Anatomische Beiträge zur Pathologie des Gehirns*. Stockholm: Nordiska Bokhandeln. Vols. 5–7.

Herbster, A. N., Mintun, M. A., Nebes, R. D., & Becker, J. T. (1997). Regional cerebral blood flow during word and nonword reading. *Human Brain Mapping* 5, 84–92.

Herholz, K., Peitrzyk, U., Karbe, H., Würker, M., Wienhard, K., & Heiss, W.-D. (1994). Individual metabolic anatomy of repeating words demonstrated by MRI-guided positron emission tomography. *Neuroscience Letters* 182, 47–50.

Hikosawa, K., Iwai, E., Saito, H.-A., & Tanaka, K. (1988). Polysensory properties of neurons in the anterior bank of the caudal superior temporal sulcus of the macaque monkey. *Journal of Neurophysiology* 60, 1615–1637.

Hillis, A. E., & Caramazza, A. (1991). Category-specific naming and comprehension impairment: A double dissociation. *Brain* 114, 2081–2094.

Hirano, S., Naito, Y., Okazawa, H., et al. (1997). Cortical activation by monaural speech sound stimulation demonstrated by positron emission tomography. *Experimental Brain Research* 113, 75–80.

Howard, D., Patterson, K., Wise, R., Brown, W. D., Friston, K., Weiller, C., & Frackowiak, R. (1992). The cortical localization of the lexicons: The cortical localization of lexicons. *Brain* 115, 1769–1782.

Humphreys, G. W., & Evett, L. J. (1985). Are there independent lexical and nonlexical routes in word processing? An evaluation of the dual-route theory of reading. *Behavioral and Brain Sciences* 8, 689–740.

Indefrey, P., Kleinschmidt, A., Merboldt, K.-D., Krüger, G., Brown, C., Hagoort, P., & Frahm, J. (1997). Equivalent responses to lexical and nonlexical visual stimuli in occipital cortex: A functional magnetic resonance imaging study. *NeuroImage* 5, 78–81.

James, W. (1950). *Principles of Psychology*, vol. 1. New York: Dover.

Jäncke, L., Shah, N. J., Posse, S., Grosse-Ryuken, M., & Müller-Gärtner, H.-W. (1998). Intensity coding of auditory stimuli: An fMRI study. *Neuropsychologia* 36, 875–883.

Jones, E. G., & Burton, H. (1976). Areal differences in the laminar distribution of thalamic afferents in cortical fields of the insular, parietal and temporal regions of primates. *Journal of Comparative Neurology* 168, 197–247.

Jones, E. G., & Powell, T. S. P. (1970). An anatomical study of converging sensory pathways within the cerebral cortex of the monkey. *Brain* 93, 793–820.

Jonides, J., Schumacher, E. H., Smith, E. E., et al. (1998). The role of the parietal cortex in verbal working memory. *Journal of Neuroscience* 18, 5026–5034.

Kadah, Y. M., & Hu, X. (1997). Simulated phase evolution rewinding (SPHERE): A technique for reducing B0 inhomogeneity effects in MR images. *Magnetic Resonance in Medicine* 38, 615–627.

Kapur, S., Rose, R., Liddle, P. F., et al. (1994). The role of the left prefrontal cortex in verbal processing: Semantic processing or willed action? *NeuroReport* 5, 2193–2196.

Karmiloff-Smith, A. (1992). *Beyond Modularity: A Developmental Perspective on Cognitive Science.* Cambridge, MA: MIT Press.

Kawashima, R., Itoh, M., Hatazawa, J., Miyazawa, H., Yamada, K., Matsuzawa, T., & Fukuda, H. (1993). Changes of regional cerebral blood flow during listening to an unfamiliar spoken language. *Neuroscience Letters* 161, 69–72.

Kertesz, A., Lau, W. K., & Polk, M. (1993). The structural determinants of recovery in Wernicke's aphasia. *Brain and Language* 44, 153–164.

Kertesz, A., Sheppard, A., & MacKenzie, R. (1982). Localization in transcortical sensory aphasia. *Archives of Neurology* 39, 475–478.

Kim, K. H. S., Relkin, N. R., Lee, K.-M., & Hirsch, J. (1997). Distinct cortical areas associated with native and second languages. *Nature* 388, 171–174.

Klein, D., Milner, B., Zatorre, R. J., et al. (1995). The neural substrates underlying word generation: A bilingual functional imaging study. *Proceedings of the National Academy of Sciences USA* 92, 2899–2903.

Kraut, M. A., Marenco, S., Soher, B. J., Wong, D. F., & Bryan, R. N. (1995). Comparison of functional MR and H2 15O positron emission tomography in stimulation of the primary visual cortex. *American Journal of Neuroradiology* 16, 2101–2107.

Leinonen, L., Hyvärinen, J., & Sovijärvi, A. R. A. (1980). Functional properties of neurons in the temporo-parietal association cortex of awake monkey. *Experimental Brain Research* 39, 203–215.

Levelt, W. J. M. (1989). *Speaking: From Intention to Articulation.* Cambridge, MA: MIT Press.

Lichtheim, L. (1885). On aphasia. *Brain* 7, 433–484.

Lüders, H., Lesser, R. P., Hahn, J., Dinner, D. S., Morris, H., Resor, S., et al. (1986). Basal temporal language areas demonstrated by electrical stimulation. *Neurology* 36, 505–510.

Lüders, H., Lesser, R. P., Hahn, J., Dinner, D. S., Morris, H. H., Wyllie, E., & Godoy, J. (1991). Basal temporal language area. *Brain* 114, 743–754.

Luria, A. R. (1966). *Higher Cortical Functions in Man* B. Haigh, trans. New York: Basic Books Plenum Press.

Macleod, C. M. (1991). Half a century of research on the Stroop effect: An integrative review. *Psychological Bulletin* 109, 163–203.

Marcel, A. J. (1983). Conscious and unconscious perception: Experiments on visual masking and word recognition. *Cognitive Psychology* 15, 197–237.

Marin, O. S. M. (1980). Appendix 1: CAT scans of five deep dyslexic patients. In *Deep Dyslexia*, M. Coltheart, K. Patterson, & J. Marshall, eds., 407–433. London: Routledge and Kegan Paul.

Marslen-Wilson, W. D., & Tyler, L. K. (1981). Central processes in speech understanding. *Philosophical Transactions of the Royal Society of London* B295, 317–332.

Martin, A., Haxby, J. V., Lalonde, F. M., Wiggs, C. L., & Ungerleider, L. G. (1995). Discrete cortical regions associated with knowledge of color and knowledge of action. *Science* 270, 102–105.

Martin, A., Wiggs, C. L., Ungerleider, L. G., & Haxby, J. V. (1996). Neural correlates of category-specific knowledge. *Nature* 379, 649–652.

Mazoyer, B. M., Tzourio, N., Frak, V., et al. (1993). The cortical representation of speech. *Journal of Cognitive Neuroscience* 5, 467–479.

McClelland, J. L., & Kawamoto, A. H. (1986). Mechanisms of sentence processing: Assigning roles to constituents of sentences. In *Parallel Distributed Processing*, vol. 2, *Psychological and Biological Models*, J. L. McClelland & D. E. Rumelhart, eds., 272–325. Cambridge MA: MIT Press.

McClelland, J. L., & Rumelhart, D. E. (1981). An interactive activation model of context effects in letter perception: Part 1. An account of basic findings. *Psychological Review* 88, 375–407.

McGuire, P., Silberswieg, D. A., Murray, R. M., David, A. S., Frackowiak, R. S. J., & Frith, C. D. (1996). The functional anatomy of inner speech and auditory verbal imagery. *Psychological Medicine* 26, 29–38.

McGurk, H., & MacDonald, J. (1976). Hearing lips and seeing voices. *Nature* 264, 746–748.

Menard, M. T., Kosslyn, S. M., Thompson, W. L., Alpert, N. M., & Rauch, S. L. (1996). Encoding words and pictures: A positron emission tomography study. *Neuropsychologia* 34, 185–194.

Mendelson, J. R., & Cynader, M. S. (1985). Sensitivity of cat primary auditory cortex (AI) to the direction and rate of frequency modulation. *Brain Research* 327, 331–335.

Merzenich, M. M., & Brugge, J. F. (1973). Representation of the cochlear partition on the superior temporal plane of the macaque monkey. *Brain Research* 50, 275–296.

Mesulam, M. (1985). Patterns in behavioral neuroanatomy: Association areas, the limbic system, and hemispheric specialization. In *Principles of Behavioral Neurology*, M. Mesulam, ed., 1–70. Philadelphia: F. A. Davis.

Mesulam, M.-M. (1990). Large-scale neurocognitive networks and distributed processing for attention, language, and memory. *Annals of Neurology* 28, 597–613.

Mesulam, M.-M., & Pandya, D. N. (1973). The projections of the medial geniculate complex within the Sylvian fissure of the rhesus monkey. *Brain Research* 60, 315–333.

Metter, E. J., Hanson, W. R., Jackson, C. A., Kempler, D., van Lancker, D., Mazziotta, J. C., & Phelps, M. E. (1990). Temporoparietal cortex in aphasia: Evidence from positron emission tomography. *Archives of Neurology* 47, 1235–1238.

Miller, G. A., Galanter, E., & Pribram, K. (1960). *Plans and the Structure of Behavior*. New York: Holt.

Miller, G. A., & Isard, S. (1963). Some perceptual consequences of linguistic rules. *Journal of Verbal Learning and Verbal Behavior* 2, 217–228.

Mills, C. K., & McConnell, J. W. (1895). The naming centre, with the report of a case indicating its location in the temporal lobe. *Journal of Nervous and Mental Disease* 22, 1–7.

Mohr, J. P., Pessin, M. S., Finkelstein, S., Funkenstein, H. H., Duncan, G. W., & Davis, K. R. (1978). Broca aphasia: Pathologic and clinical. *Neurology* 28, 311–324.

Moore, C. J., & Price, C. J. (1999). Three distinct ventral occipitotemporal regions for reading and object naming. *Neuroimage*, 10(2), 181–192.

Morel, A., Garraghty, P. E., & Kaas, J. H. (1993). Tonotopic organization, architectonic fields, and connections of auditory cortex in Macaque monkeys. *Journal of Comparative Neurology* 335, 437–459.

Morel, A., & Kaas, J. H. (1992). Subdivisions and connections of auditory cortex in owl monkeys. *Journal of Comparative Neurology* 318, 27–63.

Mufson, E. J., & Pandya, D. N. (1984). Some observations on the course and composition of the cingulum bundle in the rhesus monkey. *Journal of Comparative Neurology* 225, 31–43.

Müller, R. A., Rothermell, R. D., Behen, M. E., Muzik, O., Mangner, T. J., & Chugani, H. T. (1997). Receptive and expressive language activations for sentences: A PET study. *NeuroReport* 8, 3767–3770.

Mummery, C. J., Patterson, K., Hodges, J. R., & Wise, R. J. S. (1996). Generating "tiger" as an animal name or a word beginning with T: Differences in brain activation. *Proceedings of the Royal Society of London* B263, 989–995.

Naeser, M., Hayward, R. W., Laughlin, S. A., & Zatz, L. M. (1981). Quantitative CT scan studies of aphasia. I. Infarct size and CT numbers. *Brain and Language* 12, 140–164.

Neville, H. J., Bavelier, D., Corina, D., et al. (1998). Cerebral organization for language in deaf and hearing subjects: Biological constraints and effects of experience. *Proceedings of the National Academy of Sciences USA* 95, 922–929.

Nichelli, P., Grafman, J., Pietrini, P., Clark, K., Lee, K. Y., & Miletich, R. (1995). Where the brain appreciates the moral of a story. *NeuroReport* 6, 2309–2313.

Nielsen, J. M. (1946). *Agnosia, Apraxia, Aphasia: Their Value in Cerebral Localization.* New York: Paul B. Hoeber.

Nobre, A. C., Allison, T., & McCarthy, G. (1994). Word recognition in the human inferior temporal lobe. *Nature* 372, 260–263.

O'Leary, D. S., Andreasen, N. C., Hurtig, R. R., et al. (1996). A positron emission tomography study of binaurally and dichotically presented stimuli: Effects of level of language and directed attention. *Brain and Language* 53, 20–39.

Paulesu, E., Frith, C. D., & Frackowiak, R. S. J. (1993). The neural correlates of the verbal component of working memory. *Nature* 362, 342–345.

Penfield, W., & Roberts, L. (1959). *Speech and Brain-Mechanisms.* New York: Atheneum.

Perani, D., Cappa, S. F., Bettinardi, V., Bressi, S., Gorno-Tempini, M., Matarrese, M., & Fazio, F. (1995). Different neural systems for the recognition of animals and man-made tools. *NeuroReport* 6, 1637–1641.

Perani, D., Dehaene, S., Grassi, F., et al. (1996). Brain processing of native and foreign languages. *NeuroReport* 7, 2439–2444.

Petersen, S. E., Fox, P. T., Posner, M. I., Mintun, M. A., & Raichle, M. E. (1988). Positron emission tomographic studies of the cortical anatomy of single-word processing. *Nature* 331, 585–589.

Petersen, S. E., Fox, P. T., Posner, M. I., Mintun, M., & Raichle, M. E. (1989). Positron emission tomographic studies of the processing of single words. *Journal of Cognitive Neuroscience* 1, 153–170.

Petersen, S. E., Fox, P. T., Snyder, A. Z., & Raichle, M. E. (1990). Activation of extrastriate and frontal cortical areas by visual words and word-like stimuli. *Science* 249, 1041–1044.

Phillips, D. P., & Irvine, D. R. F. (1981). Responses of single neurons in physiologically defined primary auditory cortex (AI) of the cat: Frequency tuning and responses to intensity. *Journal of Neurophysiology* 45, 48–58.

Picard, N., & Strick, P. L. (1996). Motor areas of the medial wall: A review of their location and functional activation. *Cerebral Cortex* 6, 342–353.

Picton, T. W., & Stuss, D. T. (1994). Neurobiology of conscious experience. *Current Opinion in Neurobiology* 4, 256–265.

Plaut, D. C., McClelland, J. L., Seidenberg, M. S., & Patterson, K. (1996). Understanding normal and impaired word reading: Computational principles in quasi-regular domains. *Psychological Review* 103, 45–115.

Poeppel, D. (1996). A critical review of PET studies of phonological processing. *Brain and Language* 55, 317–371.

Poline, J.-B., Vandenberghe, R., Holmes, A. P., Friston, K. J., & Frackowiak, R. S. J. (1996). Reproducibility of PET activation studies: Lessons from a multi-center European experiment. *NeuroImage* 4, 34–54.

Pope, K. S., & Singer, J. L. (1976). Regulation of the stream of consciousness: Toward a theory of ongoing thought. In *Consciousness and Self-Regulation*, G. E. Schwartz & D. Shapiro, eds., 101–135. New York: Plenum Press.

Price, C., Wise, R., Ramsay, S., Friston, K., Howard, D., Patterson, K., & Frackowiak, R. (1992). Regional response differences within the human auditory cortex when listening to words. *Neuroscience Letters* 146, 179–182.

Price, C. J. (1998). The functional anatomy of word comprehension and production. *Trends in Cognitive Sciences* 2, 281–288.

Price, C. J., & Friston, K. J. (1997). Cognitive conjunctions: A new approach to brain activation experiments. *NeuroImage* 5, 261–270.

Price, C. J., Moore, C. J., & Friston, K. J. (1996). Getting sex into perspective. *NeuroImage* 3, S586.

Price, C. J., Moore, C. J., & Friston, K. J. (1997). Subtractions, conjunctions, and interactions in experimental design of activation studies. *Human Brain Mapping* 5, 264–272.

Price, C. J., Moore, C. J., Humphreys, G. W., Frackowiak, R. S. J., & Friston, K. J. (1996). The neural regions sustaining object recognition and naming. *Proceedings of the Royal Society of London* B263, 1501–1507.

Price, C. J., Moore, C. J., Humphreys, G. W., & Wise, R. J. S. (1997). Segregating semantic from phonological processes during reading. *Journal of Cognitive Neuroscience* 9, 727–733.

Price, C. J., Wise, R. J. S., & Frackowiak, R. S. J. (1996). Demonstrating the implicit processing of visually presented words and pseudowords. *Cerebral Cortex* 6, 62–70.

Price, C. J., Wise, R. J. S., Warburton, E. A., et al. (1996). Hearing and saying: The functional neuroanatomy of auditory word processing. *Brain* 119, 919–931.

Price, C. J., Wise, R. J. S., Watson, J. D. G., Patterson, K., Howard, D., & Frackowiak, R. S. J. (1994). Brain activity during reading: The effects of exposure duration and task. *Brain* 117, 1255–1269.

Puce, A., Allison, T., Asgari, M., Gore, J. C., & McCarthy, G. (1996). Differential sensitivity of human visual cortex to faces, letter strings, and textures: A functional magnetic resonance imaging study. *Journal of Neuroscience* 16, 5205–5215.

Pugh, K. R., Shaywitz, B. A., Shaywitz, S. E., et al. (1996a). Auditory selective attention: An fMRI investigation. *NeuroImage* 4, 159–173.

Pugh, K. R., Shaywitz, B. A., Shaywitz, S. E., et al. (1996b). Cerebral organization of component processes in reading. *Brain* 119, 1221–1238.

Raichle, M. E., Fiez, J. A., Videen, T. O., MacLeod, A. M., Pardo, J. V., Fox, P. T., & Petersen, S. E. (1994). Practice-related changes in human brain functional anatomy during nonmotor learning. *Cerebral Cortex* 4, 8–26.

Ramsay, N. F., Kirkby, B. S., Van Gelderen, P., et al. (1996). Functional mapping of human sensorimotor cortex with 3D BOLD fMRI correlates highly with H2(15)O PET rCBF. *Journal of Cerebral Blood Flow and Metabolism* 17, 670–679.

Rapcsak, S. Z., & Rubens, A. B. (1994). Localization of lesions in transcortical aphasia. In *Localization and Neuroimaging in Neuropsychology*, A. Kertesz eds., 297–329. San Diego: Academic Press.

Rauschecker, J. P., Tian, B., Pons, T., & Mishkin, M. (1997). Serial and parallel processing in Rhesus monkey auditory cortex. *Journal of Comparative Neurology* 382, 89–103.

Reicher, G. M. (1969). Perceptual recognition as a function of meaningfulness of stimulus material. *Journal of Experimental Psychology* 81, 274–280.

Révész, G., ed. (1954). *Thinking and Speaking: A Symposium*. Amsterdam: North Holland.

Roeltgen, D. P., & Heilman, K. M. (1984). Lexical agraphia: Further support for the two-system hypothesis of linguistic agraphia. *Brain* 107, 811–827.

Rubens, A. B. (1976). Transcortical motor aphasia. In *Studies in Neurolinguistics*, H. Whitaker, ed., 293–306. New York: Academic Press.

Rudge, P., & Warrington, E. K. (1991). Selective impairment of memory and visual perception in splenial tumours. *Brain* 114, 349–360.

Rumsey, J. M., Horwitz, B., Donohue, B. C., Nace, K., Maisog, J. M., & Andreason, P. (1997). Phonological and orthographic components of word recognition: A PET-rCBF study. *Brain* 120, 739–759.

Segal, S. J., & Fusella, V. (1970). Influence of imaged pictures and sounds on detection of visual and auditory signals. *Journal of Experimental Psychology* 83, 458–464.

Seidenberg, M. S., & McClelland, J. L. (1989). A distributed, developmental model of word recognition and naming. *Psychological Review* 96, 523–568.

Seidenberg, M. S., Waters, G. S., Barnes, M. A., Tanenhaus, M. K. (1984). When does irregular spelling or pronunciation influence word recognition? *Journal of Verbal Learning and Verbal Behavior* 23, 383–404.

Selnes, O. A., Niccum, N., Knopman, D. S., & Rubens, A. B. (1984). Recovery of single word comprehension: CT-scan correlates. *Brain and Language* 21, 72–84.

Seltzer, B., & Pandya, D. N. (1994). Parietal, temporal, and occipital projections to cortex of the superior temporal sulcus in the rhesus monkey: A retrograde tracer study. *Journal of Comparative Neurology* 343, 445–463.

Shallice, T. (1988). *From Neuropsychology to Mental Structure*. Cambridge: Cambridge University Press.

Shaywitz, B. A., Pugh, K. R., & Constable, T., et al. (1995). Localization of semantic processing using functional magnetic resonance imaging. *Human Brain Mapping* 2, 149–158.

Shaywitz, B. A., Shaywitz, S. E., Pugh, K. R., et al. (1995). Sex differences in the functional organization of the brain for language. *Nature* 373, 607–609.

Shulman, G. L., Fiez, J. A., Corbetta, M., Buckner, R. L., Meizin, F. M., Raichle, M. E., & Petersen, S. E. (1997). Common blood flow changes across visual tasks: II. Decreases in cerebral cortex. *Journal of Cognitive Neuroscience* 9, 648–663.

Small, S. L., Noll, D. C., Perfetti, C. A., Hlustik, P., Wellington, R., & Schneider, W. (1996). Localizing the lexicon for reading aloud: Replication of a PET study using fMRI. *NeuroReport* 7, 961–965.

Smith, C. D., Andersen, A. H., Chen, Q., Blonder, L. X., Kirsch, J. E., & Avison, M. J. (1996). Cortical activation in confrontation naming. *NeuroReport* 7, 781–785.

Solomon, P., Kubzansky, P. E., Leiderman, P. H., Mendelson, J. H., Trumbull, R., & Wexler, D. (1961). *Sensory Deprivation*. Cambridge, MA: Harvard University Press.

Spitzer, M., Bellemann, M. E., Kammer, T., et al. (1996). Functional MR imaging of semantic information processing and learning-related effects using psychometrically controlled stimulation paradigms. *Cognitive Brain Research* 4, 149–161.

Springer, J. A., Binder, J. R., Hammeke, T. A., et al. (1997). Variability of language lateralization in normal controls and epilepsy patients: An MRI study. *NeuroImage* 5, S581.

Sripanidkulchai, K., & Wyss, J. M. (1986). Thalamic projections to retrosplenial cortex in the rat. *Journal of Comparative Neurology* 254, 143–165.

Steinmetz, H., Volkmann, J., Jäncke, L., & Freund, H.-J. (1991). Anatomical left-right asymmetry of language-related temporal cortex is different in left- and right-handers. *Annals of Neurology* 29, 315–319.

Stuss, D. T., & Benson, D. F. (1986). *The Frontal Lobes*. New York: Raven Press.

Suzuki, W. A., & Amaral, D. G. (1994). Perirhinal and parahippocampal cortices of the macaque monkey: Cortical afferents. *Journal of Comparative Neurology* 350, 497–533.

Talairach, J., & Tournoux, P. (1988). *Co-planar Stereotaxic Atlas of the Human Brain*. New York: Thieme Medical Publishers.

Tamas, L. B., Shibasaki, T., Horikoshi, S., & Ohye, C. (1993). General activation of cerebral metabolism with speech: A PET study. *International Journal of Psychophysiology* 14, 199–208.

Tanaka, Y., Yamadori, A., & Mori, E. (1987). Pure word deafness following bilateral lesions: A psychophysical analysis. *Brain* 110, 381–403.

Teasdale, J. D., Dritschel, B. H., Taylor, M. J., Proctor, L., Lloyd, C. A., Nimmo-Smith, I., & Baddeley, A. D. (1995). Stimulus-independent thought depends on central executive resources. *Memory and Cognition* 23, 551–559.

Teasdale, J. D., Proctor, L., Lloyd, C. A., & Baddeley, A. D. (1993). Working memory and stimulus-independent thought: Effects of memory load and presentation rate. *European Journal of Cognitive Psychology* 5, 417–433.

Thompson-Schill, S. L., D'Esposito, M., Aguirre, G. K., & Farah, M. J. (1997). Role of left inferior prefrontal cortex in retrieval of semantic knowledge: A reevaluation. *Proceedings of the National Academy of Sciences of the United States of America* 94, 14792–14797.

Tulving, E., & Gold, C. (1963). Stimulus information and contextual information as determinants of tachistoscopic recognition of words. *Journal of Experimental Psychology* 66, 319–327.

Tulving, E., Kapur, S., Craik, F. I. M., Moscovitch, M., & Houle, S. (1994). Hemispheric encoding/retrieval asymmetry in episodic memory: Positron emission tomography findings. *Proceedings of the National Academy of Sciences USA* 91, 2016–2020.

Valenstein, E., Bowers, D., Verfaellie, M., Heilman, K. M., Day, A., & Watson, R. T. (1987). Retrosplenial amnesia. *Brain* 110, 1631–1646.

Vallar, G., & Shallice, T. (1990). *Neuropsychological Impairments to Short Term Memory*. New York: Cambridge University Press.

Vandenberghe, R., Price, C. J., Wise. R., Josephs, O., & Frackowiak, R. S. (1996). Functional anatomy of a common semantic system for words and pictures. *Nature* 383, 254–256.

Van Orden, G. C. (1987). A ROWS is a ROSE: Spelling, sound, and reading. *Memory and Cognition* 15, 181–198.

Vogt, B. A. (1976). Retrosplenial cortex in the rhesus monkey: A cytoarchitectonic and Golgi study. *Journal of Comparative Neurology* 169, 63–97.

von Economo, C., & Horn, L. (1930). Über Windungsrelief, Maße und Rindenarchitektonik der Supratemporalfläche, ihre individuellen und ihre Seitenunterscheide. *Zeitschrift für Neurologie und Psychiatrie* 130, 678–757.

Vygotsky, L. S. (1962). *Thought and Language*. New York: Wiley.

Warburton, E., Wise, R. J., Price, C. J., Weiller, C., Hadar, U., Ramsay, S., & Frackowiak, R. S. (1996). Noun and verb retrieval by normal subjects: Studies with PET. *Brain* 119, 159–179.

Warren, R. M., & Obusek, C. J. (1971). Speech perception and phonemic restorations. *Perception & Psychophysics* 9, 358–362.

Warrington, E. K., & Shallice, T. (1984). Category specific semantic impairments. *Brain* 107, 829–854.

Weiskrantz, L., ed. (1988). *Thought Without Language*. Oxford: Clarendon Press.

Wernicke, C. (1874). *Der aphasische Symptomenkomplex*. Breslau: Cohn and Weigert.

Wise, R., Chollet, F., Hadar, U., Friston, K., Hoffner, E., & Frackowiak, R. (1991). Distribution of cortical neural networks involved in word comprehension and word retrieval. *Brain* 114, 1803–1817.

Yang, Q., Williams, G. D., Demeure, R. J., Mosher, T. J., & Smith, M. B. (1998). Removal of local field gradient artifacts in T2*-weighted images at high fields by gradient-echo slice excitation profile imaging. *Magnetic Resonance in Medicine* 39, 402–409.

Yetkin, F. Z., Hammeke, T. A., Swanson, S. J., Morris, G. L., Mueller, W. M., McAuliffe, T. L., & Haughton, V. M. (1995). A comparison of functional MR activation patterns during silent and audible language tasks. *American Journal of Neuroradiology* 16, 1087–1092.

Yetkin, O., Yetkin, F. Z., Haughton, V. M., & Cox, R. W. (1996). Use of functional MR to map language in multilingual volunteers. *American Journal of Neuroradiology* 17, 473–477.

Zatorre, R. J., Evans, A. C., Meyer, E., & Gjedde, A. (1992). Lateralization of phonetic and pitch discrimination in speech processing. *Science* 256, 846–849.

Zatorre, R. J., Meyer, E., Gjedde, A., & Evans, A. C. (1996). PET studies of phonetic processing of speech: Review, replication, and reanalysis. *Cerebral Cortex* 6, 21–30.

Zatorre, R. R., & Binder, J. R. (2000). The human auditory system. In *Brain Mapping: The Systems*, A. W. Toga, & J. C. Mazziotta, eds. San Diego: Academic Press, pp. 365–402.

8 Functional Neuroimaging of Episodic Memory

John D. E. Gabrieli

INTRODUCTION

People gain knowledge and skills through experiences that are recorded, retained, and retrieved by memory systems of the human brain. A memory system may defined as a specific mnemonic process that is mediated by a particular neural network. Memory systems vary in what they are used for, the kind of knowledge they acquire, the principles that govern their organization, and which parts of the brain are essential for their integrity (reviewed in Gabrieli, 1998).

Since the 1950s, insights into the psychological characteristics and neural underpinnings of multiple memory systems have been gained through experimental analyses of patients with memory deficits due to focal or degenerative brain injuries. Lesions have produced dramatic and often unexpected mnemonic deficits that provide clues about which brain regions are necessary for which memory processes. There are, however, some important limitations of lesion studies. The behavior of a memory-impaired patient with a brain lesion does not delineate what process is subserved by the injured tissue. Rather, the behavior reflects what uninjured brain regions can accomplish after the lesion. Further, naturally occurring lesions often impair multiple, adjacent brain structures, either by direct insult or by disconnection of interactive brain regions. It is, therefore, difficult to determine exact brain-behavior relations.

From the viewpoint of memory research, it is also problematic that memory is dynamic whereas lesions are static. Memory may be thought of as being comprised of three successive stages. Encoding (or learning) is the initial acquisition of new knowledge. Storage or consolidation processes maintain that knowledge in memory. Retrieval is the recovery of knowledge encoded in a previous time period. If a patient fails a test of memory due to a lesion, it is impossible to determine whether the failure reflects impaired encoding, impaired storage, or impaired retrieval (or some combination). A severe impairment at one or more stages would result in ultimate memory failure, but for different reasons altogether.

Over the 1990s, functional neuroimaging studies using positron emission tomography (PET) or functional magnetic resonance imaging (fMRI) have made possible the visualization of memory processes in the healthy brain. These techniques have their own limitations, such as limited temporal and spatial resolution. Nevertheless, functional neuroimaging has dramatically increased the range of studies aimed at delineating the functional neural architecture of human memory. Imaging studies allow for systematic and direct exploration of the brain organization of normal memory processes, instead of depending on the happenstance locations of lesions. Experiments can focus on particular brain regions and on particular stages of dynamic memory processes.

Lesion and imaging studies relate to one another in several important ways. First, the strengths and weaknesses of current functional neuroimaging techniques are only modestly understood, so lesion studies provide an important source of validation for functional neuroimaging studies. Second, lesion findings have provided rational and focused hypotheses for imaging studies. Third, lesion studies provide valuable constraints on interpreting activations seen in imaging studies. An activation may reflect processing in a brain region that is essential for a form of memory, or it may reflect a correlated process that does not mediate the form of memory under study. The correlated process may be a parallel learning circuit or some perceptual, attentional, motivational, or other nonmnemonic process that is engaged by the memory task. Such correlated processes are of interest, but they do not reflect the essential neural basis for a form of memory.

An illustration of how imaging evidence and lesion evidence can mutually constrain one another comes from studies of classical eyeblink delay conditioning that are further constrained by convergence of animal and human findings. In humans and rabbits, this kind of learning is abolished by cerebellar lesions (Daum et al., 1993; Thompson, 1990) and is associated with cerebellar activity: PET activations in humans (Blaxton, Zeffiro, et al., 1996; Logan & Grafton, 1995) and electrophysiological activity in rabbits (McCormick & Thompson, 1987). Thus, activation in the cerebellum reflects an essential neural basis for such learning. In addition, conditioning-correlated PET activation in humans and electrophysiological activity in rabbits occur concurrently in the medial temporal lobe (MTL) region (Blaxton, Zeffiro, et al., 1996; Disterhoft et al., 1986; Logan & Grafton, 1995). MTL lesions, however, have no effect on such learning in humans or rabbits (Gabrieli, et al., 1995; Schmaltz & Theios, 1972). MTL activation, therefore, likely reflects a correlated, parallel learning circuit that is not mediating the eyeblink delay conditioning. It is not yet clear how anything besides lesion evidence can indicate whether a task-related activation reflects a brain region that mediates part of the behavior of interest or a correlated, parallel process.

Episodic Memory

This chapter reviews functional neuroimaging studies of episodic memory—the mnemonic processes that record, retain, and retrieve autobiographical knowledge about experiences that occurred at a specific place and time (Tulving, 1983). Episodic memories may be contrasted on the basis of content with semantic memories, which represent generic knowledge, such as word meaning or widely known facts, and need not represent the spatial and temporal context in which they were learned. Episodic memories are declarative (Cohen & Squire, 1980) or explicit (Graf & Schacter, 1985), in that people can consciously and purposefully recollect specific experiences from their lives.

In the laboratory, episodic memory is measured by direct tests of free recall, cued recall, or recognition. Subjects typically are exposed to a set of materials in the study phase, such as words, sentences, or pictures. In the test phase, subjects are asked to recall or recognize what stimuli were seen or heard in that particular study phase. Thus, the study episode, an experience that occurred at a particular place and time, constitutes the spatial and temporal boundaries of the relevant experience.

Neural Substrates of Episodic Memory   The brain basis of episodic memory in humans has been deduced by interpretation of the effects of localized lesions upon episodic memory performance. In broad terms, it is likely that all parts of the brain make some sort of contribution to episodic memories. For example, in order to have episodic memories for visually presented words, the visual system must mediate the correct perception of the words and the language system must mediate the correct understanding of the words. Thus, particular domains of episodic memory will depend upon the integrity of relevant sensory and cognitive systems. Damage to these systems will result in domain-specific (visual but not auditory, or verbal but not visuospatial) episodic memory deficits. Among all the regions involved in creating an episodic memory, however, it is likely that only a subset will include the engram for that episode: the specific brain changes that constitute the biological basis of the memory for the episode.

MEDIAL TEMPORAL LOBES   There are brain regions that appear to play a global and essential role in all domains of episodic memory. These regions are injured bilaterally in patients who exhibit global amnesia, a selective deficit in episodic memory with sparing of short-term memory, remote or premorbid memories, and motor, perceptual, and cognitive capacities (Scoville & Milner, 1957; Cohen & Squire, 1980). All amnesic patients have an anterograde amnesia, an inability to gain new episodic memories after the onset of the amnesia. Most amnesic patients also have an inability to gain new semantic memories, such as learning the meanings of new words (e.g., Gabrieli et al., 1988). Amnesic patients vary in the severity and extent of their retrograde amnesia, a loss of information gained prior to the onset of the amnesia. Retrograde losses of memory in amnesia are usually temporally graded, in that they are most severe for time periods closest to amnesia onset.

Global amnesias result from bilateral lesions to regions of the medial temporal lobe (MTL), the diencephalon, or the basal forebrain. Among these brain regions, MTL lesions occur most often and have been most intensively studied, such as in the case of patient H.M. (Scoville & Milner, 1957). Also, functional neuroimaging studies have had far greater success in visualizing MTL activation than either diencephalic or basal forebrain activations. Finally, experiments with rats and monkeys provide convergent evidence about the essential role of MTL structures in mammalian episodic memory (reviewed in Squire, 1992). Therefore, the present review focuses on the MTL structures that play an essential role in episodic memory.

The MTL memory system consists of multiple structures, differing in their neural cytoarchitecture and connectivity, that may be classified as belonging to three major regions: (1) the parahippocampal region, (2) the hippocampal region, and (3) the amygdala. High-level unimodal and polymodal cortical regions provide convergent inputs to the parahippocampal region, which is comprised of parahippocampal and perirhinal cortices (Suzuki & Amaral, 1994). The parahippocampal region provides major inputs to the hippocampal region, which is composed of the subiculum, the CA fields, and the dentate gyrus. Entorhinal cortex is variably classified as belonging to either the hippocampal or the parahippocampal region. The amygdala is located in the MTL, but appears to have a specialized role in episodic memory that is discussed later.

It is likely that all of the hippocampal and parahippocampal component structures make unique contributions to declarative memory. In monkeys and rats, different components of the MTL memory system mediate separable memory processes, but there is not yet a consensus about how best to characterize the different, specific contributions of the hippocampal and parahippocampal structures to episodic memory. In humans, postmortem analysis of MTL damage in patients with well characterized amnesias shows that damage restricted to a small part of the hippocampal region, the CA1 field, is sufficient to produce a clinically significant anterograde amnesia. More extensive damage to additional MTL structures aggravates both the severity of the anterograde amnesia and the temporal extent of the retrograde amnesia. When lesions extend beyond the hippocampal region to entorhinal and perirhinal cortices, retrograde amnesias extend back one or two decades (Corkin et al., 1997; Rempel-Clower et al., 1996).

Unilateral MTL lesions can produce material-specific amnesias (Milner, 1971). Left MTL lesions can selectively impair verbal memory, and right MTL lesions can selectively impair nonverbal memory (e.g., faces, spatial positions, maze routes, nonverbal figures). These asymmetries are thought to reflect the primarily ipsilateral (or intrahemispheric) cortical inputs to the left and right MTL regions. Further, many of these lesions include damage to adjacent temporal lobe neocortex and may reflect damage both to the MTL and to some of its cortical inputs.

Lesion findings have illuminated the importance of the amygdala in emotional aspects of human memory (reviewed in Phelps & Anderson, 1997). Because the amygdala is near the hippocampal formation, amnesic patients, such as H.M., often have damage to both structures. It was, therefore, difficult to distinguish between the specific mnemonic roles of these adjacent limbic structures. However, a rare congenital dermatological disorder, Urbach-Weithe syndrome, leads to mineralization of the amygdala that spares the hippocampal formation. In addition, the amygdala is resected for treatment of pharmacologically intractable epilepsy, although the resection usually involves additional MTL structures. Studies with these patients have allowed for a more direct examination of the consequences of amygdala lesions in humans.

Injury to the amygdala does not result in a global memory impairment, but rather in a specific reduction in how emotion modulates episodic memory. Normal subjects show superior memory for emotionally disturbing, relative to emotionally neutral, stimuli. An Urbach-Weithe patient shows normal memory for neutral slides, but fails to show the normal additional memory for the emotionally salient slides (Cahill et al., 1995). Patients with amygdala lesions also show deficits on other aspects of emotional perception and learning, including impaired perception of fearful or angry facial expressions (Adolphs et al., 1994) or prosody (Scott et al., 1997), and impaired fear conditioning (a form of implicit memory that is intact in amnesic patients without amygdala lesions) (Bechara et al., 1995; LaBar et al., 1995). In combination, these studies suggest that the amygdala plays a particular role in emotion, and how emotion enhances episodic memory.

FRONTAL LOBES   Patients with lesions of the prefrontal cortex do not exhibit a severe or pervasive deficit in episodic memory (reviewed in Wheeler et al., 1995). Rather, they exhibit a specific and limited deficit on certain kinds of episodic memory tests. Episodic memory tasks differ in their strategic memory demands, that is, in how much retrieved memories must be evaluated, manipulated, or transformed. Recognition tests, in which studied items are re-presented along with novel distracter items, typically require the least amount of memory strategy or judgment because studied items can be identified relatively easily on the basis of stimulus familiarity. Patients with prefrontal lesions typically perform normally, or exhibit modest impairments, on recognition tests.

Other tests of episodic memory can require greater self-organization or greater detail for successful performance. Free recall tests require people to devise their own strategies for recollecting prior experiences. For example, one useful strategy for improving recall of a list of words is to subjectively reorganize the words from the order in which they were presented into sets of semantically related words (such as fruits or vehicles). Patients with frontal lobe lesions, despite intact recognition memory, are impaired on free recall (Janowsky, Shimamura, Kritchevsky, et al., 1989) and exhibit deficits in the subjective organization that aids recall (Gershberg & Shimamura, 1995; Stuss et al., 1994). Such patients are also impaired on other tasks with self-organizational demands, such as self-ordered pointing (Petrides & Milner, 1982).

Other strategic memory tests present the studied items to participants, but require the retrieval of detailed temporal or spatial information from the episodes in which the items were encountered. Such tests include memory for source (who presented the information, where it was presented, which list it was presented in), temporal order (which item was presented more recently), or frequency (which item was presented more often). Patients with frontal lobe lesions can be intact on recognition memory but impaired on tests of source (Janowsky, Shimamura, & Squire, 1989), temporal order or recency judgments (Butters et al., 1994; Milner, 1971; Milner et al., 1991; Shimamura et al., 1990), and frequency judgments (Angeles Juardo et al., 1997; Smith & Milner, 1988).

The episodic memory impairments in patients with frontal lobe lesions may be contrasted with those in patients with amnesia due to MTL lesions. The amnesic patients are severely impaired on both nonstrategic recognition tests and strategic memory tests (and their impairments on the strategic tests are typically much worse). Precise comparisons between MTL and frontal lobe deficits are, however, difficult because amnesic patients are usually selected on the basis of their behavioral syndrome, have bilateral lesions, and often have extensive damage to the MTL region. In contrast, most patients with frontal lobe lesions are selected on the basis of their lesion location, have unilateral lesions, and have less extensive, and probably more variable, damage to the large frontal lobe region. Laterality asymmetries are sometimes observed for verbal vs. nonverbal materials on strategic memory tests (e.g., Milner, 1971) in patients with frontal lobe lesions, but they are often not evident. There has not been any evidence that left or right prefrontal lesions produce fundamentally different kinds of memory failures.

Patients with frontal lobe lesions are also impaired on a variety of nonmnemonic thinking capacities, including problem solving, response inhibition, and following rules (e.g., Miller, 1985; Milner, 1964). The deficits in strategic memory may reflect an impairment in the application of thought to demanding episodic memory tasks that demand self-organization or subtle discriminations. Patients with frontal lobe lesions sometimes exhibit a propensity to make false alarms, that is, to endorse foil or baseline items as having been seen before (Schacter, Curran, et al., 1996). This, too, may be interpreted as a failure in judging what criterion should be used to distinguish between studied items and other items that are similar to the studied items.

FUNCTIONAL NEUROIMAGING OF EPISODIC MEMORY

This review focuses on fMRI and PET studies that examined activations associated with episodic memory. Because there is a substantial and convergent literature about the consequences of MTL and frontal lobe lesions for episodic memory, the present review focuses on those two brain regions. Many other regions have also been activated during episodic memory performance, including anterior cingulate regions, posterior midline regions (such as the cuneus and precuneus), temporal cortex, and the cerebellum (reviewed in Cabeza & Nyberg, 1997; Tulving et al., 1999).

As discussed above, functional neuroimaging studies have provided the first opportunity to distinguish between the neural bases of encoding and retrieval operations in the normal human brain. Therefore, the review is organized by studies that have focused on either the encoding or the retrieval of episodic memory. It would be of great interest to localize activations associated with consolidation and storage processes, but no experimental strategy has been devised so far to image what occurs between encoding and retrieval.

In any such review, a critical question concerns what degree of psychological resolution and anatomical resolution is appropriate. That is, what range of tasks and activation locations should be associated with each another or instead dissociated from each another? It is almost certainly the case that there are multiple encoding and retrieval processes. Further, encoding and retrieval activations are derived from comparison to one of many possible baseline or comparison conditions. Therefore, any given study will reveal activations associated with a particular set of encoding or retrieval processes and baseline comparisons. The goal of these studies, however, is to reveal processes that are likely used across a range of related tasks. Associating various studies may be useful in identifying processes that are used across multiple tasks.

Anatomical resolution refers to the precision of brain localization of activations associated with episodic memory performance. The precision of localization is limited in several ways. First, the hemodynamic basis of PET and fMRI probably warps the measured range of activation relative to the actual neural basis of encoding or retrieval. Second, most imaging studies of memory have used group averages that transform variable individual brain anatomies into a common space. Such transformation and averaging obscure anatomic precision. Third, it is unclear what level of anatomic precision is commensurate with present conceptual frameworks. The MTL is comprised of multiple structures (reviewed above). The frontal lobes are large regions that include multiple gyri, Brodmann cytoarchitectural areas (BA), and an unknown number of functional regions within those areas.

For the main review below, I have taken an integrative approach, emphasizing commonalities across diverse experimental paradigms and across relatively broad anatomical regions. In the long run, the goal of both behavioral and neuroscience research is the identification of specific encoding or retrieval processes that are mediated by specific neural networks. At present, however, conceptual frameworks in memory research are quite modest. There is little sense of how many encoding and retrieval processes there are, or how they differ from one another, or how they are specifically mediated by components of the MTL or frontal lobe regions.

Visualizing the Encoding of Episodic Memories in Functional Neuroimaging

Many paradigms aimed at identifying activations associated with encoding experiences into long-term episodic memory can be described in terms of five categories.

Rest Comparisons   Activation may be compared between an encoding condition in which stimuli are presented and a rest condition in which subjects do nothing. Such a comparison has the advantage that no psychological interpretation of the rest baseline is needed (or possible). There are, however, many processes that differentiate stimulus encoding from rest, including attention, perception, and motor control (eye movement); many of these processes may not be specifically related to episodic memory.

Processing Comparisons   These studies vary encoding tasks while holding constant the nature of the stimuli. Such comparisons control for many attentional and perceptual processes. Activations are compared between encoding tasks that yield later superior memory for stimuli versus tasks that yield later inferior memory for stimuli. Encoding tasks can vary greatly in terms of influencing subsequent accuracy of memory. For example, given identical stimuli, semantic (also called deep or elaborative) encoding (e.g., answering a question about the meaning of stimuli) typically yields better memory than nonsemantic (also called shallow or nonelaborative) encoding (e.g., answering question about the appearances or sound of a stimulus) (Craik & Lockhart, 1972; Craik & Tulving, 1975). Self-reference tasks, in which subjects judge whether adjectives (e.g., "kind" or "smart") apply to themselves, often yield the best later memory (Symons & Johnson, 1997), followed by generic semantic classifications, such as judging whether words refer to abstract or concrete entities or living or nonliving entities. Phonological tasks, such as rhyme judgments, yield intermediate levels of memory. Superficial judgments, such as judging whether a word is spoken by a male or a female voice or whether a word is shown in uppercase or lowercase, yield the worst memory. A number of imaging studies have used these sorts of task manipulations to identify brain regions that show greater activation in the condition which yields greater memory. Other encoding manipulations that enhance later memory are easy (relative to difficult) simultaneous distracter tasks, and intentional encoding (in which subjects study items for a later memory test), relative to more passive incidental encoding (in which subjects process items without intending to remember them).

Encoding tasks need to be interpreted not only in terms of their consequences upon subsequent episodic memory performance, but also in terms of the specific processes underlying specific encoding operations. Thus, semantic encoding tasks actually reveal neural circuits involved in the retrieval of semantic memory required to answer questions about stimulus meaning (relative to their baseline). Therefore, imaging studies that vary the degree of semantic processing for other purposes, such as the study of language, may be reinterpreted in terms of episodic memory encoding. For example, an influential study of language processing compared conditions in which subjects either read presented nouns or generated a verb related to the presented noun (Petersen et al., 1988). Generating a word in response to the meaning of a cue requires greater semantic processing than merely reading a presented word. Tulving, Kapur, Craik, et al. (1994) pointed out that this language manipulation resembles the "generation effect" in episodic memory encoding: the finding that people remember words they generate better than words they read (Slamecka & Graf, 1978). Thus, encoding tasks that promote or demote later memory actually reflect a broad range of specific semantic and other psychological processes.

Further, each encoding comparison reveals a particular kind of encoding process rather than some generalized encoding process. This point can be illustrated by a limitation of the depth-of-processing framework known as the principle of encoding specificity (Tulving & Thomson, 1973) or transfer-appropriate processing (Morris et al., 1977). This principle arises from the observation that superior memory performance results from congruence between processes engaged at encoding and at retrieval. Thus, if the test-phase recognition test requires subjects to remember information about the sound or appearance of study-phase stimuli, subjects perform better after shallow than after deep processing (e.g., Morris et al., 1977). Under typical circumstances, subjects recall and recognize on the basis of meaning, so that semantic encoding yields superior memory. Nevertheless, the fact that the nature of the memory test can reverse the advantages and disadvantages of semantic versus nonsemantic encoding indicates that there are multiple kinds of encoding processes.

Stimulus Comparisons A third approach to visualizing encoding-related processes is to compare activations between stimulus materials. In some studies, the tasks are held constant. For example, one study contrasted the encoding of meaningful actions with that of less memorable meaningless actions (Decety et al., 1997). In other studies, various kinds of stimuli (words, faces, drawings) have been compared against a minimal perceptual control, such as fixation or a noise field. These comparisons have the disadvantage that there are many differences in both stimulus properties and encoding tasks across conditions. For example, the processing of a series of words relative to fixation involves differences in the perceptual nature of the stimuli, the variety of the stimuli, the attention paid to the stimuli, and the meaningfulness of the stimuli. Activations could reflect any one or any combination of these differences. Stimulus manipulations thus vary both stimuli and the kinds of processes associated with the stimuli. Stimulus manipulations can be useful for contrasting encoding processes associated with different classes of stimuli, either by comparison to a common baseline (e.g., Kelley et al., 1998; Martin et al., 1997) or by direct comparison between different kinds of stimuli (e.g., Wagner, Poldrack, et al., 1998). These sorts of studies have been used to ask whether encoding processes differ for words, pictures, faces, and patterns.

Repetition Comparisons   A fourth approach to visualizing encoding processes has been comparison between novel stimuli, seen for the first time, and repeated stimuli that have become highly familiar due to prior presentations (e.g., Gabrieli, Brewer, et al., 1997; Stern et al., 1996; Tulving, Markowitsch, Kapur, et al., 1994). The logic underlying this comparison is that there is much more information to be encoded from a novel stimulus than from a familiar stimulus about which a great deal is already known. The advantage of this comparison is that it can hold both the encoding task and the stimulus class constant. This comparison, however, is not strictly one of encoding because appreciation of the familiarity of a previously presented stimulus depends upon the retrieval of memory gained in the prior presentations. Also, an activation could reflect a response to stimulus novelty per se that is not directly related to episodic encoding. Further, the comparisons of initial and repeated processing of a stimulus have been used to examine implicit memory in repetition priming (e.g., Demb et al., 1995; Gabrieli et al., 1996; Raichle et al., 1994; Wagner et al., 1997), a form of memory that is thought to be independent of episodic memory processes. Therefore, repetition-induced reductions in activation could signify either implicit or explicit memory processes.

Correlations with Subsequent Memory   Two more approaches have been based on correlations between activity during encoding and accuracy of subsequent performance on a test of memory. These approaches have two major appeals. First, they hold both encoding tasks and stimulus materials constant (without introducing stimulus repetition). Second, there is a more direct relation between the magnitude of encoding activation and the accuracy of subsequent episodic memory. These studies may constitute the most direct operationalization of episodic encoding.

Some studies have correlated activity across subjects, finding that subjects who show greater activation during encoding perform better on a later memory test (e.g., Cahill et al., 1996; Alkire et al., 1998). These studies cannot discern whether the between-subjects differences reflect state (e.g., subjects who are more alert) or trait (e.g., subjects who have superior memory) differences. Interpretation can be constrained, however, if the correlations are specific to a brain region or a stimulus category (e.g., Cahill et al., 1996; Alkire et al., 1998). Between-subject correlations will not reflect differences in the memorability of stimuli in a stimulus set because the stimuli are constant across subjects.

Other studies have correlated activity across items but within subjects by using event-related fMRI designs in which a separate activation is recorded during encoding for small sets of stimuli (e.g., Fenandez et al., 1998, 1999) or for each individual stimulus (e.g., Brewer et al., 1998; Wagner, Schacter, et al., 1998). Activations were compared between items that were encoded more successfully (i.e., were later remembered) or less successfully (i.e., were later forgotten). Because the critical comparisons are within subjects, activations are unlikely to reflect trait differences between subjects. Such activations could be driven by a particular stimulus dimension. For example, if half the stimuli in an event-related fMRI study were highly memorable and half were highly forgettable, then those stimulus properties would be expected to result in greater activation for the highly memorable stimuli (and to do so in a blocked design as well). That possibility can be evaluated by examining whether there is a great consistency in which stimuli are later remembered or forgotten. Even if there is considerable variability for which stimuli are remembered or forgotten, there must be some reasons why an individual finds various stimuli more or less memorable (i.e., interactions among subject traits, states, prior experience, and the stimuli).

For all of the above experimental designs, activations associated with superior encoding (between conditions, between subjects, or between trials) can reflect many sorts of processes, including attention, language, and motivation. Those processes may modulate the strength of encoding or be correlated, parallel processes that do not modulate episodic encoding.

Visualizing the Retrieval of Episodic Memories in Functional Neuroimaging

The constraints of functional neuroimaging have been more limiting for localizing activations associated with retrieval than with encoding. First, retrieval tests of free recall are difficult to administer in a controlled fashion because subjects vary widely in terms of the number of items recalled and the rate of recall. This uncontrolled variance also makes it difficult to design a suitable control condition. Thus, most imaging studies have involved either cued recall or recognition because these tests allow for a controlled rate of response. FMRI introduces another constraint, because overt speech introduces movement artifacts. Subjects can perform covert cued recall (silently recall), but the accuracy of such performance cannot be measured. Therefore, fMRI studies have focused primarily on recognition.

Second, all PET studies and most fMRI studies have employed blocked designs in which activation is averaged or integrated over many trials of one kind grouped together. Statistical comparisons are then made between blocks. This blocking of stimulus types is in direct contrast to the typical design of recognition tests, in which previously studied (old) and not studied (new) items are randomly mixed together and subjects must decide whether each item is old or new. Blocked-design functional neuroimaging studies have had to group blocks of old items and blocks of new items separately, so that activations can be contrasted between memory judgments for old items (for which subjects have a study-phase episodic memory) and new items (for which subjects lack such a memory). In PET studies, blocking occurs across separate scans; in fMRI studies the blocking occurs in alternating but continuous stimulus sets and may be less apparent. Such blocking raises the concern that subjects develop strategies built around the long runs of similar items and identical responses, and that the imaging may reflect these secondary strategies rather than memory retrieval per se. Some experiments have attempted to diminish such strategies by including a limited number of old items among new items (or vice versa) so that subjects cannot assume all items in a block are of a kind (e.g., Gabrieli, Brewer, et al., 1997; Rugg et al., 1996; Squire et al., 1992). This design trades off some loss of activation differences (by diminishing the contrast between blocks) in order to discourage subjects from assuming that all items in a block are old or new.

Many paradigms aimed at identifying activations associated with retrieving experiences from long-term episodic memory can be described in terms of six categories (some of which are similar to encoding paradigms). There are, however, limitations on how much encoding and retrieval can be dissociated. Every stimulus presentation on a retrieval task requires stimulus encoding. For example, subjects reencode old study-phase stimuli and newly encode new (foil) test-phase stimuli as they make test-phase episodic memory judgments.

Rest Comparisons   Some studies have compared activations between episodic retrieval and a rest condition in which subjects neither perceive stimuli nor perform any task. The limitations of such a comparison are reviewed above.

Processing Comparisons   Some studies have compared activations associated with episodic retrieval (cued recall or recognition of items from a prior study phase) with another kind of retrieval (most often semantic), holding the nature of the materials constant. For example, some studies have presented subjects with three-letter stems (e.g., STA). In one condition, the stems are the first three letters of a study-phase word (e.g., STAMP), and subjects attempt to recall the study-phase words. In the comparison condition, subjects complete other three-letter stems with the first word that comes to mind (silently, in an fMRI study). Other processing manipulations may compare episodic versus semantic retrieval to a cue (e.g., FRUIT), recognition versus semantic judgments, or recognition versus simple reading of words.

The logic of these comparisons is that stimulus class is held constant (e.g., stems or words) and activation is compared between episodic and nonepisodic retrieval. This comparison, however, involves two factors of interest: processes involved in making an episodic judgment and processes involved in retrieval of an actual episode. Both kinds of processes would be invoked when subjects make accurate judgments for previously seen stimuli, but only one kind would be invoked when subjects make episodic judgments about novel stimuli (in which case there are no episodic memories to be retrieved) or when subjects make incorrect judgments about previously seen stimuli (in which case episodic memories are not successfully retrieved).

Further, the memory status of stimuli (whether an item is old or new) may be held constant or varied between episodic and nonepisodic retrieval conditions. Prior presentation of a stimulus results in a number of brain changes related to multiple episodic and nonepisodic (implicit or procedural) memory mechanisms. Therefore, if one compares episodic judgments for old items to semantic judgments for new items, activations reflect both the differences in the kind of retrieval and all other consequences of prior presentation. The other consequences of prior presentation can be controlled by equating the ratios of new and old items shown for episodic and semantic judgments. This, however, raises the concern that incidental episodic retrieval will occur in the semantic condition as subjects note the re-presentation of studied stimuli. Thus, blocked processing manipulations vary both the nature of retrieval (episodic versus nonepisodic judgments) and the memory status (old or new) of stimuli in various ways that need to be considered for interpretation of a particular study.

Memory Status Comparisons   Other studies have held constant the goal of intentional episodic retrieval, but varied the memory status of the stimuli. Thus, some studies have compared retrieval activations for previously studied items versus new items, or for items likely to be well remembered versus items less well remembered due to encoding manipulations (such as semantic versus nonsemantic encoding). Such comparisons can dissociate processes invoked by episodic memory judgments (which are held constant) and processes related to memory retrieval of actual episodes.

Stimulus Comparisons Although stimulus manipulations have been common in encoding studies, to date they have been rare in retrieval studies (e.g., Wagner, Poldrack, et al., 1998; McDermott et al., 1999). In part, this may be due to concern that such a comparison would include differences due both to the encoding (processing) of different kinds of stimuli and to retrieval.

Correlations with Retrieval Performance Activations can be correlated with episodic retrieval accuracy across subjects or, in event-related designs, retrieval accuracy across items.

Retrieval Comparisons Some studies vary retrieval demands across different kinds of episodic memory tasks. These studies are motivated by the findings (reviewed above) that frontal lobe lesions have disproportionate effects upon strategic memory judgments (recall, temporal order, source) relative to nonstrategic recognition memory judgments. The designs of these studies pose some challenges. First, strategic memory tasks are typically more difficult than nonstrategic memory tasks (e.g., recall is typically far less accurate than recognition). Thus, differences between conditions may result from different levels of accuracy (i.e., the actual number of episodic retrievals) rather than different kinds of retrieval. One approach to this problem is to equate performance by providing extra study for the material to be recalled (e.g., Cabeza, Kapur, et al., 1997). The risk with this approach is that it may be the differential difficulty that accounts for the necessity of frontal involvement in strategic memory performance. If so, the training procedures involved in equating performance would actually eliminate the need for strategy at retrieval.

Second, recognition judgments typically require a discrimination between old and new items, whereas recency or source judgments require a discrimination between two old items (such as which was seen more recently or which was shown in the first list). Thus, an activation difference between recognition and more strategic memory judgments could reflect either the memory status of items (for example, a mixture of old and new items versus all old items) or the kind of retrieval. In blocked designs, this problem can be approached in several ways. For example, one can present three stimuli (two old and one new) and have subjects select the new one on recognition trials and the most recently seen one (or one from a particular source) on strategic retrieval trials.

An Overview of MTL and Frontal Lobe Activations Associated with Episodic Memory Encoding and Retrieval

On the basis of neuropsychological studies with patients, it would be expected that episodic memory tasks (encoding and/or retrieval) would consistently yield MTL activations (because MTL lesions result in global amnesia), whereas the same tasks would yield more subtle and variable frontal lobe activations (and perhaps none at all for recognition memory tests). In fact, the results have been the reverse: nearly all published studies report robust frontal lobe activations during episodic encoding or retrieval, and many studies fail to observe MTL activations even when frontal activations are obtained (e.g., Craik et al., 1999; S. Kapur et al., 1994; Shallice et al., 1994; Tulving, Kapur, Markowitsch, et al., 1994). If imaging findings had preceded lesion findings, we would have concluded that prefrontal cortex is essential for episodic memory and MTL structures play a limited role (the exact opposite of lesion consequences).

The frequent absence of MTL activations during episodic memory performance has been interpreted in a number of ways. First, imaging methods, especially fMRI, have modest power to detect signals relative to background noise. Even statistically reliable MTL activations reflect mean signal changes of around 1%. Measurement is weakened for structures that are deep in the brain (as opposed to surface cortex) and for structures near ventricles (as is the case for MTL structures adjacent to the posterior horn of the lateral ventricle). Also, the vascular organization of MTL regions may be disadvantageous for PET or fMRI measures. Therefore, the absence of MTL activation could reflect the weakness of functional imaging measurement. Alternatively, an absence of activation could reflect the actual nature of MTL neural processes. Some MTL structures may be constantly active, and therefore not show differences between experimental conditions. Alternatively, neural coding could be very fine-grained, below the spatial resolution of PET or fMRI. However, many studies have found MTL activations during encoding or retrieval of episodic memories, and these are reviewed below.

MTL Activations during Encoding of Episodic Memories

Rest Comparisons   MTL activations have been observed for the encoding, relative to rest, of visual patterns (Roland & Gulyas, 1995) and of faces (N. Kapur et al., 1995).

Processing Comparisons   Greater MTL activation is consistently associated with encoding conditions that enhance later memory. Greater MTL activation has been found for deep (semantic) than for shallow (nonsemantic) encoding tasks for words (Vandenberghe et al., 1996; Wagner, Schacter, et al., 1998) and for line drawings (Henke et al., 1997; Vandenberghe et al., 1996). Greater MTL activation has also been found for intentional memorization, relative to incidental processing, of words (S. Kapur et al., 1996; Kelley et al., 1998), faces (Haxby et al., 1996; Kelley et al., 1998), and figures (Schacter et al., 1995).

Stimulus Comparisons   Stimuli that are more memorable often elicit greater MTL activation at encoding than stimuli that are less memorable. There was greater MTL activation during the encoding of more memorable meaningful actions than of less memorable meaningless actions (Decety et al., 1997). MTL activations have occurred for the encoding of stimuli, relative to little or no encoding for fixation, noise fields, or false fonts. Such activations have been observed for words (Kelley et al., 1998; Martin et al., 1997; Price et al., 1994; Wagner, Schacter, et al., 1998), nonsense words (Martin et al., 1997), meaningful line drawings (Kelley et al., 1998; Martin et al., 1997; Wiggs et al., 1999), meaningless line drawings (Martin et al., 1996, 1997), and faces (Kelly et al., 1998). Asymmetrical activations are often noted, with greater left-lateralized activation during encoding of verbal stimuli (Kelley et al., 1998; Martin et al., 1997), and greater right-lateralized activation during encoding of nonverbal stimuli such as faces (Kelley et al., 1998) and nonsense objects (Martin et al., 1996, 1997).

Repetition Comparisons   MTL activations have occurred for novel stimuli relative to repeated stimuli that have become highly familiar due to prior presentations (i.e., when there is more novel information to be encoded). Such novelty-driven activations have been found for scenes (Gabrieli, Brewer, et al., 1997; Stern et al., 1996; Tulving et al., 1996), words (Kopelman et al., 1998), object-noun pairs (Rombouts et al., 1997), and word pairs (Dolan & Fletcher, 1997). The scene activations are typically bilateral, whereas the verbal activations are often left-lateralized.

Correlations with Subsequent Memory   Both between-subject and within-subject studies have found that greater MTL activation at encoding is associated with superior memory at retrieval. A PET study found a positive correlation between subjects' MTL activation while listening to unrelated words and free recall for the words 24 hours later (Alkire et al., 1998). Neuropsychological evidence (reviewed above) indicates that the amygdala has a particular role in emotional aspects of memory. Convergent PET studies have found that greater amygdala activation at encoding is correlated with superior recall for emotional, but not for neutral, film clips (Cahill et al. 1996), and with superior recognition for both negative and positive scenes (Hamann et al., 1999).

Two fMRI studies examined the correlation between MTL activity averaged across the encoding of small sets of six words and subsequent free recall or stem-cued recall for those sets of words (Fernandez et al., 1998, 1999). In both cases, there was a positive correlation between MTL activity during the encoding of sets of words and subsequent recall or cued recall for the sets.

Perhaps the most precise correlations between MTL activity and episodic encoding were found in two event-related fMRI studies that measured activations in response to individual scenes (Brewer et al., 1998) and to individual words (Wagner, Schacter, et al., 1998). After scanning, subjects in both studies received recognition tests in which they judged whether scenes or words were old or new. If a stimulus was judged as being old, subjects than classified their judgment as being more certain or less certain. Thus, each picture or word could have three mnemonic fates: to be well remembered, to be modestly remembered, or to be forgotten (items that subjects had seen at encoding but classified as new at test). Both studies found greater MTL activation during the encoding of individual words or scenes that were well remembered than of words or scenes that were subsequently forgotten. In addition, MTL activation for scenes modestly remembered was intermediate between that for well remembered scenes and forgotten scenes. Thus, the degree of MTL activation during study appears to reflect the success or failure of encoding episodes into long-term memory. These effects were bilateral for the scenes and left-lateralized for the words.

Summary   MTL activation is consistently associated, across many different paradigms, with superior encoding of episodic memories between conditions, between subjects, or between items. Material-specific effects are often observed with left-lateralized activations for verbal stimuli, right-lateralized activations for nonverbal stimuli, and bilateral activations for stimuli that are nonverbal but easily described by words, such as scenes or drawings of common objects.

MTL Activations during Retrieval of Episodic Memories

Rest Comparisons   MTL activations occur during episodic retrieval, relative to rest, for spatial information (Ghaem et al., 1997), words (Grasby et al., 1993), faces (N. Kapur et al., 1995), and visual patterns (Roland & Gulyas, 1995).

Processing Comparisons   MTL activations have occurred for episodic retrieval relative to matched nonepisodic lexical or semantic verbal retrieval tasks (e.g., Blaxton, Bookheimer, et al., 1996; Schacter, Alpert, et al., 1996; Schacter, Buckner, et al., 1997; Squire et al., 1992). MTL activations have also been found for episodic retrieval relative to simply viewing stimuli without performing any prescribed task; such activations have occurred for figural (Schacter et al., 1995; Schacter, Uecker, et al., 1997) and spatial (Maguire et al., 1996) materials. The laterality effects are less consistent than for the comparable encoding tasks.

Memory Status Comparisons   MTL retrieval activations also occur when subjects are constantly making episodic memory judgments, but the memory status of the stimuli varies across conditions. In some experiments, all the materials correspond to study-phase items, but accuracy is greater in one condition than in another due to study-phase encoding manipulations. In these studies, MTL activation is greater in the test-phase condition that yields superior memory performance for words (Rugg et al., 1997; Schacter, Alpert, et al., 1996). In other experiments, memory judgments are compared between studied items and new items (for new items, even when judgments are highly accurate, there is no relevant episodic memory that can be retrieved). These studies find greater MTL activation during episodic memory judgments for old than for new items, and this difference is evident for a wide range of verbal (Fujii et al., 1997; Gabrieli, Brewer, et al., 1997; Nyberg et al., 1995), figural (Gabrieli, Brewer, et al., 1997; Schacter et al., 1995; Schacter, Uecker, et al., 1997), and spatial (Maguire et al., 1998) materials. In many of these studies, subjects were accurate in identifying new items (correctly rejecting the items as not having been presented in the study phase). Therefore, the activations reflected actual retrieval of memory from a prior episode rather than the accuracy of the memory judgment.

Correlations with Retrieval Performance One PET study examined the relation between MTL activation and recognition memory accuracy for words (Nyberg, McIntosh, et al., 1996). Across subjects, greater left anterior MTL activation during retrieval correlated positively with greater recognition memory accuracy. An event-related fMRI study found greater posterior MTL activation for words well re-collected from a prior study phase than for new words correctly identified as not having been seen in the study phase (Henson et al., 1999).

Summary In combination, the above studies indicate that MTL activation is consistently associated with successful retrieval of episodic memories rather than with the attempt to retrieve memories, the re-presentation of study-phase stimuli, or the accuracy of memory judgments.

Frontal Lobe Activations during Encoding of Episodic Memories

Rest Comparisons Relative to rest, many different tasks that involve verbal encoding invoke activation of left prefrontal cortex, including word generation on the basis of semantic cues (Warburton et al., 1996; Wise et al., 1991) and word generation on the basis of lexical cues (Buckner et al., 1995).

Processing Comparisons When stimuli are held constant, greater left prefrontal activation commonly occurs for encoding tasks that promote subsequent episodic memory. Most such studies have involved verbal material. Generating words, relative to reading words, results in left prefrontal activations (Frith et al., 1991; Klein et al., 1995; Petersen et al., 1988; Raichle et al., 1994), as does generating the colors or uses of objects relative to the names of objects (Martin et al., 1995). Similar findings occur when intentional encoding of words is compared to incidental tasks, such as simply reading words (S. Kapur et al., 1996; Kelley et al., 1998). Intentional, relative to incidental, encoding of faces, however, results in greater right prefrontal activation (Kelley et al., 1998). Semantic tasks (such as abstract/concrete or living/nonliving judgments or self-reference judgments) yield left-lateralized prefrontal activations relative to nonsemantic tasks (such as orthographic or phonological judgments) (e.g., Craik et al., 1999; Demb et al., 1995; Desmond et al., 1995; Démonet et al., 1992; Gabrieli et al., 1996; S. Kapur et al., 1994; Poldrack et al., 1999; Wagner et al., 1997). Left prefrontal activations are apparent when attention to a study list is distracted by an easier secondary task relative to a more difficult secondary task (Shallice et al., 1994; Fletcher et al., 1995), and when subjects need to engage in more semantic organization of a study list (Fletcher et al., 1998). Phonological tasks yield more left prefrontal activation than orthographic tasks (Craik et al., 1999; Poldrack et al., 1999; Rumsey et al., 1997; Shaywitz et al., 1995).

These activations vary in their precise locations. Most activations include the left inferior frontal gyrus, but some occur in the middle frontal gyrus. Within the left inferior frontal gyrus, phonological processes tend to be associated with more posterior and dorsal activations (BA areas 44/45), and semantic processes with more anterior and ventral activations (BA areas 45/47) (reviewed by Fiez, 1997; Poldrack et al., 1999). Lesser right frontal activations are often observed, especially in fMRI studies.

In almost all of these studies, the condition that yields superior encoding also requires a longer response or processing time. For example, semantic judgments typically require more time than phonological or orthographic judgments. This raises the possibility that left prefrontal activations reflect the duration of encoding rather than the kind of encoding (with longer durations yielding greater activations). One study (Demb et al., 1995) compared semantic encoding to a nonsemantic encoding task that required a longer time for response. The semantic task still resulted in left prefrontal activation and in superior later memory. This result indicates that left prefrontal activations reflect differences in the kind of encoding brought to bear upon a stimulus, rather than simply the duration of encoding.

There are few processing comparisons involving nonverbal materials. One study compared the intentional encoding of faces to an incidental face-matching task, and found a left prefrontal activation (Haxby et al., 1996). The lateralization stands in marked contrast to the right-lateralized activations reported in stimulus comparison studies reviewed below. The findings, however, are not directly contradictory in several regards. First, the material-specific activations in stimulus comparison studies occur in a prefrontal location posterior to that reported in the processing comparison study. This suggests that different encoding processes are being localized in the stimulus versus processing comparisons. Second, the left-lateralized encoding activation for faces occurred in the same region that is often activated in the verbal processing comparisons reviewed above. This raises the possibility that the left-lateralized activation for face encoding reflects verbal processes being recruited to aid the encoding. This possibility is supported by another study from Haxby et al. (1995) that examined the retention of memory for unfamiliar faces for either a short (1 sec) or long (6 sec) duration. Short retention resulted in bilateral frontal activation, whereas long retention resulted in only left activation. The longer retention period may have promoted verbal encoding for the faces.

Three other studies have directly compared the intentional encoding and retrieval of episodic memories for nonverbal information. Such a comparison includes a stimulus-repetition comparison as items are encoded at study and then reencoded at test as a component of making an episodic memory judgment. In one study (Klingberg & Roland, 1998), there was greater right prefrontal activation (in the posterior BA 6/44 region) for encoding meaningless pairs of visual patterns and sounds relative to retrieval of those pairs. In a pair of related studies (Owen et al., 1996a, 1996b), there was greater left prefrontal activation for encoding than for retrieving both object locations and object features (e.g., one chair versus another, similar chair), and greater bilateral prefrontal activations for encoding than for retrieving spatial locations.

Stimulus Comparisons   Left prefrontal activations occur when verbal tasks are compared to fixation or other baseline tasks in which little information is likely to be encoded. Left prefrontal activations are seen for generation of words on the basis of lexical cues (Buckner et al., 1995), semantic decisions (Démonet et al., 1992), reading words (Herbster et al., 1997; Martin et al., 1996), lexical decisions (Price et al., 1994; Rumsey et al., 1997), phonetic discrimination (Zatorre et al., 1996), and passive viewing of words (Bookheimer et al., 1995; Menard et al., 1996; Petersen et al., 1990; Price et al., 1994). As reviewed above, there tends to be some segregation between semantic and phonological activations (Poldrack et al., 1999).

Stimulus comparison studies have examined hemispheric asymmetries for activations associated with verbal and nonverbal materials. Intentional encoding for words yielded left prefrontal activations relative to intentional encoding for textures (Wagner, Poldrack, et al., 1998), intentional encoding for faces (McDermott et al., 1999), and visual fixation (Kelley et al., 1998). Intentional encoding for faces yielded, conversely, right prefrontal activations relative to fixation (Kelley et al., 1998) and to intentional encoding for words (McDermott et al., 1999). Intentional encoding for textures, relative to words, also resulted in right prefrontal activation (Wagner, Poldrack, et al., 1998). Intentional encoding for famous faces and line drawings of common objects or animals yielded bilateral prefrontal activation relative to fixation

(Kelley et al., 1998, 1999). Thus, the intentional encoding of verbal material is associated with left prefrontal activation, the intentional encoding of nonverbal material (faces, textures) with right prefrontal activation, and the intentional encoding of material that is nonverbal but linked to verbal knowledge (the names of famous people or common objects) with bilateral prefrontal activation. The most consistent locus of material-specific encoding activations has been in a relatively posterior prefrontal region (BA 6/44).

Repetition Comparisons   One study (Gabrieli, Brewer, et al., 1997) has compared initial versus repeated encoding of stimuli in the context of episodic memory. For scenes, there was greater right prefrontal activation for novel than for repeated encoding (responses in anterior left prefrontal cortex were not measured). The multiple studies examining verbal repetition priming, however, may be conceptualized as repetition comparisons between initial and repeated encoding. In these studies, subjects encode and later reencode the same stimuli. The measure of priming is how much faster or how much more accurately the stimuli are reencoded relative to their initial encoding. Indeed, studies that include both a processing comparison of encoding and a repetition priming measure of reencoding show that the activations occur in the same left prefrontal locus (Gabrieli et al., 1996; Raichle et al., 1994). For all priming studies, there is greater left prefrontal activation for initial than for repeated encoding of stimuli, including repeated abstract/concrete judgments for words (Demb et al., 1995; Gabrieli et al., 1996), repeated verb generation (Raichle et al., 1994), and repeated living/nonliving judgments for words and for line drawings (Wagner et al., 1997).

Correlations with Subsequent Memory   Greater right prefrontal activation occurred for encoding scenes that would later be remembered than for scenes that would later be forgotten (Brewer et al., 1998). Greater left prefrontal activation occurred, both posteriorly in BA 6/44 and anteriorly in BA 45/47, during encoding for words that would later be well remembered than for words that would later be forgotten (Wagner, Schacter, et al., 1998). Greater left prefrontal activation also occurred for words that would later be distinctly recollected as having been seen in the study phase than for words that were classified as having been seen in the study phase but were not distinctly recollected (Henson et al., 1999).

Summary   Prefrontal cortex appears to play a consistent role in the modulation of episodic memory encoding. Left prefrontal activations, in several different regions, are consistently associated with superior encoding of episodic verbal memories between conditions and between items. Left prefrontal activations have also been associated with enhanced memory for nonverbal stimuli, namely faces; these activations may reflect verbal encoding processes being applied to nonverbal materials. There is prefrontal asymmetry for the encoding of verbal and nonverbal materials, with right-lateralized activations for the encoding of nonverbal materials (in a variety of comparisons) and greater right prefrontal activations for successfully encoded than unsuccessfully encoded scenes. There appears to be a more posterior set of bilateral encoding activations (BA 6/44) that are especially sensitive to the nature of the stimulus materials, and a more anterior, left-lateralized set of encoding activations (BA 45/47) that are sensitive to semantic processing.

Frontal Lobe Activations during Retrieval of Episodic Memories

Processing Comparisons   Right prefrontal activations occur consistently when subjects make episodic retrieval judgments for verbal materials relative to semantic tasks such as word generation (Buckner et al., 1995; Schacter et al., 1996; Shallice et al., 1994; Squire et al., 1992), word reading or repetition (Buckner et al., 1996; Fletcher et al., 1998; Nyberg et al., 1995; Petrides et al., 1995; Wagner, Desmond, et al., 1998), word fragment completion (Blaxton, Bookheimer, et al., 1996), word-pair reading (Cabeza, Kapur, et al., 1997), semantic judgments (S. Kapur et al., 1995; Tulving, Kapur, Markowitsch, et al., 1994), or a perceptual task (Rugg et al., 1996). Right prefrontal activations are also evident when subjects make episodic memory judgments for nonverbal materials, such as faces (relative to face matching, Haxby et al., 1993, 1996), and object identity or location (relative to object matching, Moscovitch et al., 1995; and relative to object-location encoding or location encoding, Owen et al., 1996a).

The right prefrontal activations in these studies, and the ones reviewed below, have clustered in two distinct regions: a posterior area (BA 9/46) and an anterior area (BA 10). Some studies obtain both activations, whereas others obtain one or the other. These activations likely reflect two different sets of processes related to episodic memory retrieval, but there is no strong evidence about what distinguishes the two processes. Also, many verbal episodic retrieval tasks report additional left prefrontal activations (e.g., Blaxton, Bookheimer, et al., 1996; Buckner et al., 1995; S. Kapur et al., 1995; Petrides et al., 1995; Rugg et al., 1996; Schacter, Alpert, et al., 1996; Tulving, Kapur, Markowitsch, et al., 1994).

Memory Status Comparisons   These studies aimed to characterize the contribution of prefrontal regions to episodic memory judgments by having subjects always make episodic memory judgments but varying the memory status of the stimuli across conditions. Some studies have compared activations between episodic judgments for old (studied) items and episodic judgments for new (baseline) items, or between well remembered versus poorly remembered study-phase items. Activation for well remembered study-phase items, relative to either new or poorly remembered items, would reflect processes associated with the actual retrieval of a relevant episodic memory. The term "retrieval success" has been used to denote such processes. In contrast, an absence of differences between conditions would suggest that prefrontal activations reflect processes related to making episodic judgments ("retrieval attempt" or "retrieval mode") regardless of whether items are old or new, well or poorly remembered.

Several studies have found greater right prefrontal activations associated with episodic judgments for old (studied) items than for episodic judgments for either new (not studied) items or old items that were poorly remembered due to encoding manipulations (Buckner, Koutstaal, Schacter, Wagner, et al., 1998; Rugg et al., 1996; Tulving, Kapur, Markowitsch, et al., 1994, Tulving et al., 1996). In contrast, other studies have found that right prefrontal activations are similar during episodic memory judgments for items well remembered, poorly remembered, or not previously studied (e.g., S. Kapur et al., 1995; Nyberg et al., 1995; Rugg et al., 1997; Wagner, Desmond, et al., 1998). Thus, results have been divided between the retrieval success and retrieval attempt hypotheses.

The conclusions of these studies appear to be in conflict, but closer examination of the findings suggests some resolutions (discussed in Rugg et al., 1996; Wagner, Desmond, et al., 1998). For example, some PET studies presented materials in scans that were either predominantly old or predominantly new (e.g., Tulving, Kapur, Markowitsch, et al., 1994; Tulving et al., 1996). Subjects were asked to identify the infrequent new among the old (or the infrequent old among the new) items, and thus were warned about the imbalance of old and new items in each set of stimuli. There was greater right prefrontal activation during the identification of the infrequent new items among the old items than of the infrequent old items among the new items. An fMRI study employed a similar design, but varied whether subjects were warned or not warned about the imbalance of new and old items (Wagner, Desmond, et al., 1998). There was greater right prefrontal activation for predominantly old than for new items only when subjects were warned about the imbalance (as in the PET studies). No difference was observed for predominantly old or new items when subjects were not warned about the imbalance. Thus, at least some of the PET findings of greater activation during episodic memory judgments for old versus new items may reflect the strategic use of knowledge about the imbalance of items rather than the memory status per se of old versus new items.

Stimulus Comparisons Three fMRI studies have compared activations for the retrieval of verbal versus nonverbal information. One study (Wagner, Desmond, et al.,

1998) compared activations during episodic judgments for words versus textures. There was predominantly left-lateralized prefrontal activation for episodic retrieval of words relative to textures, and predominantly right-lateralized prefrontal activation for episodic retrieval of textures relative to words. The exception was greater right anterior (BA 10) activation during recognition judgments of words relative to textures. One interpretation of this exception is that recognition judgments for words involve greater discrimination for the study-phase episode because all the words are familiar from many prior experiences. In contrast, novel stimuli, such as textures, do not require such episodic discrimination: if a texture seems familiar, it is likely to have been seen in the study phase.

Because this study compared episodic judgments for words relative to textures, it could not identify regions that were involved in both kinds of episodic judgments. A subsequent study (Gabrieli, Poldrack, & Wagner, 1998) included a fixation condition, and this study showed that right prefrontal areas were activated during episodic judgments for both words ands textures. Another study compared prefrontal activation for words versus novel faces (McDermott et al., 1999). Retrieval activations in the inferior frontal gyri (BA 6/44) were lateralized mainly by material: greater on the left for words and greater on the right for faces. Retrieval for both words and faces activated right anterior cortex (BA 10). In combination, these studies suggest that the posterior prefrontal activations may reflect material-specific retrieval processes, whereas the anterior activation (BA 10) may reflect processes more related to the recollection of a particular episode.

Correlations with Retrieval Performance   Two event-related fMRI studies have examined retrieval-related activations on an item-by-item basis. One study (Buckner, Koutstall, Schacter, Dale, et al., 1998) found both left posterior and right anterior prefrontal activations during episodic memory judgments for both old (studied) and new (not studied) word judgments. There were, however, no differences in the responses between old versus new words. This result is consistent with the retrieval attempt rather than the retrieval success interpretation of right prefrontal activations associated with episodic retrieval.

An unexpected finding, however, related to the time course of the hemodynamic responses to the single words. Most activations, including the one in left prefrontal cortex, exhibited the typical slow rise and fall in MR signal that peaked about 4 sec after word presentation and response. The right anterior activation, in contrast, exhibited a delayed rise that was sustained for 10 sec or more (similar to Schacter, Buckner, et al., 1997). This unusual response could reflect vascular rather than neural processes. More likely, it reflects a late-occurring psychological process. It may reflect metamemory verification or monitoring processes that evaluate the outcomes of retrieval searches in memory (Rugg et al., 1996). Alternatively, it may reflect processes constructing a retrieval mode in preparation for the next episodic memory judgment (Buckner, Koutstall, Schacter, Dale, et al., 1998).

The other event-related fMRI study (Henson et al., 1999) examined differences in activation during correct memory judgments for old and new words. For words classified as old, participants had to classify their subjective experience as one in which they had a distinct recollection of the episode in which the word had been presented ("remember" responses) or as one in which they thought the word had been presented but lacked any recollection of a specific episode ("know" responses). Left prefrontal activations, anterior and posterior, were observed for well remembered relative to new words, and, in a more superior left prefrontal locus, for "remember" relative to "know" responses. Neither comparison resulted in any right prefrontal activations. When "know" responses were compared to new responses, there were bilateral posterior prefrontal activations. This complex pattern of results does not favor the view that activation in right prefrontal regions reflects retrieval success, because the most successfully retrieved memories ("remember" responses) failed to activate right prefrontal cortex in any comparison. Rather, the results support the view that there are several distinct areas, in both left and right prefrontal cortices, that make different contributions to episodic retrieval.

Retrieval Manipulations   Several imaging studies have compared activation during episodic retrieval on strategic tasks (recall, temporal order, and source) that are often failed by patients with frontal lobe lesions versus nonstrategic recognition memory tasks that are rarely failed by such patients. One study (Cabeza, Kapur, et al., 1997) equated recall and recognition accuracy for word pairs by providing extra study of the pairs to be recalled, and compared activation for recall and recognition. Relative to reading unstudied words, both recall and recognition activated right prefrontal regions. Although many brain regions were more activated for recall relative to recognition or for recognition relative to recall, there were no differences in frontal activation. One possibility is that the additional study for the word pairs to be recalled eliminated the differential contribution of prefrontal cortex for recall (which is usually far less accurate than recognition when study is held constant).

A PET study contrasted item memory (judging which of two words had been seen in a study list) and temporal-order memory (judging which of two words, both from the study list, appeared later in the study list) (Cabeza, Kapur, et al., 1997). The critical findings were that temporal-order judgments, relative to item judgments, yielded greater bilateral prefrontal activations, whereas item judgments yielded greater bilateral medial temporal activations. These results parallel lesion evidence about the essential roles of MTL and frontal regions, respectively, in item and temporal-order memory.

An event-related fMRI study (Nolde, Johnson, & D'Esposito, 1998) contrasted item memory and source memory. Four subjects saw words and nameable objects (line drawings) in a study phase. At test, subjects saw only words (either the words seen before or the names of the objects) and made either old/new item recognition judgments or source judgments. For the source judgments, subjects had to determine whether test-phase words had been presented as a study-phase word, study-phase picture, or not at all (new). Item and source activations were compared against fixation. There was right prefrontal activation for both item and source judgments, but activation was similar for both judgments. In contrast, left prefrontal activations tended to be greater for the source than for the item judgments.

Nolde, Johnson, and Raye (1998) reviewed episodic retrieval activations in order to examine when left prefrontal activations were likely to occur in addition to the right prefrontal activations that occur ubiquitously for episodic retrieval. They noted that retrieval-related activations in the frontal lobes were typically right-lateralized in forced-choice (multiple-choice) recognition, and bilateral in single-item yes/no or old/new recognition. For cued recall tests, activations were right-lateralized when retrieval demands were relatively easy (e.g., there was a strong cue-target relation, the pairs had been very well learned, all the cues had been presented at study). Activations were bilateral when the cued recall was more complex or difficult (e.g., unstudied cues were also presented, pairs were less well learned). The studies reviewed by Nolde et al. varied in many ways, but it is clear that left prefrontal activations often occur during retrieval, and that these activations tend to occur as the retrieval demands become more challenging.

Summary Perhaps the most unexpected finding in the functional neuroimaging of episodic memory has been a consistent right prefrontal activation that occurs for all sorts of materials (verbal, nonverbal) and all sorts of memory tests (recall, recognition, etc.). Some studies suggest that the right prefrontal activations reflect successful retrieval, but other studies find that the activations are unrelated to successful retrieval and occur whenever subjects attempt to retrieve. The variability of the relation between right prefrontal activations and successful retrieval stands in sharp contrast to the consistency of that relation in MTL activation studies. The weak relation between right prefrontal activation and retrieval accuracy is, however, consistent with the minimal effect of prefrontal lesions on recognition memory accuracy. The observation that strategic memory judgments (temporal order, source) yield more extensive, bilateral frontal activations may be consistent with the consequences of pre-frontal lesions on these sorts of memory tasks.

Posterior prefrontal areas show material-specific activations during episodic retrieval: left-lateralized activations are associated with the retrieval of verbal materials, and right-lateralized activations are associated with the retrieval of nonverbal materials (faces, textures). Anterior prefrontal activations appear to be more related to material-independent retrieval processes associated with memory tests requiring greater temporal and spatial precision.

ISSUES

Current Issues and Questions

There are many unsettled issues and questions about how the brain encodes and retrieves episodic memories. One major issue concerns the characterization of the roles of brain regions other than the MTL or prefrontal cortex in episodic memory. Many activations have been noted during episodic encoding or retrieval in these other brain regions, but there have been few systematic studies aimed at elucidating the mnemonic processes signified by those activations. Because the above review has focused on the MTL and frontal regions, however, I will discuss a few current questions and issues pertaining to those brain regions.

Questions about the MTL and Episodic Memory   There is remarkable agreement among functional imaging studies in finding that MTL activations are associated with successful encoding and retrieval of episodic memories (although the frequent absence of MTL activations is not understood). The major current topic concerning MTL activations is the elucidation of more precise relations between specific MTL structures and specific episodic memory processes (besides the amygdala's specific role in the emotional modulation of memory). Most imaging studies have examined either episodic encoding or episodic retrieval. One fMRI study (Gabrieli, Brewer, et al., 1997) examined both encoding and retrieval in the same participants, and found evidence for a dissociation between MTL areas activated for episodic encoding versus episodic retrieval. That study observed an encoding activation for novel relative to repeated scenes in a posterior MTL region (parahippocampal cortex), and a retrieval activation for word-cued memory of line drawings in a more anterior MTL region (subiculum). There were many possible interpretations of these findings, but they indicated that functional imaging studies could go beyond merely noting the presence or absence of MTL activations. Rather, imaging studies could provide information on the organization of multiple episodic memory processes within anatomic components of the MTL system.

Reviews of functional imaging studies have shown that the anatomic organization of MTL episodic memory processes is much more complex than a simple anterior/posterior retrieval/encoding distinction. A review of 52 PET studies (Lepage et al., 1998), which included 22 encoding and 32 retrieval activations, noted the exact opposite pattern: 91% of encoding activations were predominantly anterior and 91% of retrieval activations were predominantly posterior in the MTL region. A subsequent review (Schacter & Wagner, 1999) included both fMRI studies and additional PET studies. The more extensive review of PET studies found that 58% of encoding activations occurred in anterior MTL and 80% of retrieval activations occurred in posterior MTL. PET and fMRI studies tended to differ in terms of the locus of MTL encoding activations, with fMRI studies consistently reporting posterior (parahippocampal cortex or caudal hippocampus) activations (e.g., Aguirre et al., 1996; Brewer et al., 1998; Fernandez et al., 1998; Kelley et al., 1998; Rombouts et al., 1997; Stern et al., 1996; Wagner, Schacter, et al., 1998).

The differences in the above studies and reviews may reflect several factors. One factor relates to the advantages and disadvantages of PET versus fMRI techniques. The MTL region, especially its anterior extent, is susceptible to artifacts for fMRI, but not for PET, measures. Some fMRI studies may be failing to identify anterior MTL encoding activations. On the other hand, as typically performed, fMRI may be more precise in its mapping of activations onto anatomy. Single-subject fMRI activations can be mapped relatively easily onto an individual's structural MRI. Most PET studies report only group averages and have to align activations across imaging modalities. Despite these methodological differences, PET and fMRI studies have yielded concordant findings in many brain regions. It may be that the difficulties of imaging MTL activations (noted earlier) reveal methodological limitations of one or both methods.

A more theoretically interesting factor is the possibility that there are multiple processes engaged during episodic encoding and during episodic retrieval. Most of the differences across studies, then, would not reflect imaging methodologies but instead the specific encoding and retrieval processes invoked by different tasks (or baseline comparisons). Thus, it may be an error to group together a variety of encoding or retrieval processes as if each were a unitary process. Instead, it may be useful to exploit the diversity of findings in order to discover the neural bases of multiple encoding and multiple retrieval processes. For example, Cohen and Eichenbaum (1993) have proposed that particular MTL components are involved in relational processing, and various encoding and retrieval tasks may vary in their demands upon relational versus nonrelational episodic processes mediated by the MTL.

As discussed above, it has been difficult for psychologists to define multiple, specific processes that mediate episodic encoding or retrieval. Most psychological debates have been over whether particular two-process recognition retrieval models are valid or not (e.g., Jacoby, 1991; Knowlton & Squire, 1995; Wagner & Gabrieli, 1998). Yet it is virtually certain that there are multiple encoding and retrieval processes which vary according to materials and to task demands. From this perspective, the variability in imaging findings suggests that future imaging studies may provide an impetus not only for more precise process-structure mappings but also for a new level of rigor and precision in understanding the psychological organization of episodic memory.

Questions about Frontal Lobes and Episodic Memory   In contrast to the MTL, interpretation of unexpectedly ubiquitous frontal lobe activations that occur during episodic encoding and retrieval has been filled with surprises and debates. One major surprise was the robust and consistent presence of such activations, given the limited and specific consequences of frontal lobe lesions on episodic memory. A second surprise was the frequent asymmetry of encoding and retrieval activations, because patients with unilateral frontal lobe lesions do not appear to exhibit a corresponding asymmetry in their deficits. The third surprise was the unexpected right prefrontal activation observed during verbal retrieval, an apparent violation of left-hemisphere specialization for verbal processes. Altogether, these findings motivated a dichotomy between left prefrontal activations associated with encoding and right prefrontal activations associated with retrieval, regardless of the materials involved or the tasks being performed (the hemispheric encoding/retrieval asymmetry or HERA model from Nyberg, Cabeza, et al., 1996; Tulving, Kapur, Craik, et al., 1994). Subsequent studies have also shown that there are material-specific encoding and retrieval processes, but that the prefrontal regions most sensitive to material-specific processing are posterior to the areas in which activations motivated the HERA proposal. Furthermore, strategic memory tests appear to activate bilateral anterior frontal areas.

One topic for further research will be disentangling material-dependent and material-independent activations. This will be challenging, because the material-dependent activations in frontal cortex actually reflect high-level processes associated with materials rather than simple perceptual analyses of the materials. Many apparent contradictions between material-dependent and material-independent processes may be resolved in targeted experiments. For example, most studies that inspired classification of left prefrontal cortex as mediating material-independent episodic encoding processes have varied encoding tasks (e.g., levels of processing) and held materials (usually words) constant. Most studies that have revealed material-dependent hemispheric asymmetries for verbal versus nonverbal encoding have varied materials (e.g., words versus faces) and held encoding tasks constant (usually intentional memorization). It remains to be determined whether there are right-hemisphere activations (in frontal cortex or elsewhere) that occur when encoding processes, which are not overtly verbal, modulate episodic encoding for nonverbal materials.

Another topic for future research will be achieving a better understanding of the nature of frontal lobe episodic memory processes, especially in relation to the limited and relatively symmetric consequences of left or right frontal lobe lesion on episodic memory performance. One strategy is to consider the episodic memory activations in terms of psychological abilities that are more powerfully associated with frontal lobe integrity. Good candidates are working memory and problem-solving capacities that are known to be dependent upon the integrity of primate frontal cortex. Thus, frontal lobe contributions to episodic memory may be viewed as processes that work with or solve problems about episodic memory encoding or retrieval.

Three examples may be cited of such attempts to conceptualize frontal lobe encoding or retrieval processes in terms of working-memory operations. As reviewed above, left prefrontal activations commonly occur for encoding tasks that promote later episodic memory. Two imaging studies (Desmond et al., 1998; Thompson-Schill et al., 1997) have examined prefrontal activations in which verbal tasks were held constant (verb generation to presented nouns or word-stem completion) and varied the number of possible response alternatives (nouns had few or many associated verbs; stems had few or many possible completions into words). In both cases, there was greater left prefrontal activation for items that had many possible responses than for items that had few possible responses, even though subjects had to generate only one response per item. These results may be interpreted as reflecting working-memory demands being greater when a single response must be selected from among many competing alternatives than from few competing alternatives. Thus, these studies suggest that left frontal lobe activations for verbal tasks, often interpreted as episodic memory activations, may be understood in terms of working-memory demands (Gabrieli et al., 1996).

Another study (Gabrieli, Rypma, et al., 1997) compared both episodic (long-term) and working (short-term) retrieval memory tasks to a common baseline. The episodic memory task required subjects to judge whether words had been shown in an earlier study phase. The working-memory task required subjects to judge whether the currently presented word was or was not identical to the word presented two trials (a few seconds) earlier. Thus, only working or short-term memory was relevant for this task. The baseline task required classification of words as being shown in uppercase or lowercase, a task that required neither long-term episodic memory nor short-term working memory. The episodic retrieval activations were a subset of the working-memory activations. These results suggest that the frontal lobe activations observed in this and other episodic memory studies may reflect working-memory (short-term memory) processes engaged in episodic test performance (such as response monitoring and evaluation).

Future Issues

Perhaps the greatest challenge in functional neuroimaging (important technical issues aside) is the lack of constraints on selecting the best among many plausible interpretations as to what psychological process is signified by a particular activation. Other conditions within an experiment, other imaging experiments, animal research (perhaps future functional imaging in animals), and human lesion findings offer sources of constraint. Coordinated studies with other imaging modalities offering superior temporal resolution, such as event-related potentials (ERPs) and magnetoencephalography (MEG), may provide important insights into when brain regions participate in episodic encoding or retrieval processes. These studies could provide temporal constraints on the interpretation of fMRI and PET findings. Also, functional imaging studies with amnesic patients (e.g., Gabrieli, Poldrack, & Desmond, 1998) or other groups with memory difficulties, such as older people (e.g., Cabeza, Grady, et al., 1997), may provide not only insights about the neural bases of the memory disorders, but also a more direct relation between imaging studies of the healthy brain and the consequences of lesions.

Finally, it is noteworthy that the current consensus is that the engram for an episode, the biological basis of memory for a specific event, resides neither in the frontal lobes (because frontal lobe lesions have such limited consequences for episodic memory) nor in the MTL region (because amnesic patients have intact remote memories, although this issue has been complicated by the finding that extensive MTL lesions result in decades-long retrograde amnesias). A strategy for imaging the engram for an episode would offer a successful conclusion to the search for one of the Holy Grails of memory research.

ACKNOWLEDGMENTS

I thank Heidi Sivers and Anthony Wagner for comments on a draft of this chapter, and Moriah Thomason for help in preparing the manuscript. Support was provided by NIH grants NIA AG11121 and AG12995.

REFERENCES

Adolphs, R., Tranel, D., Damasio, H., & Damasio, A. (1994). Impaired recognition of emotion in facial expressions following bilateral damage to the human amygdala. *Nature* 372, 669–672.

Aguirre, G. K., Detre, J. A., Alsop, D. C., D'Esposito, M. (1996). The parahippocampus subserves topographical learning in man. *Cerebral Cortex* 6, 823–829.

Alkire, M. T., Haier, R. J., Fallon, J. H., & Cahill, L. (1998). Hippocampal, but not amygdala, activity at encoding correlates with long-term, free recall of nonemotional information. *Proceedings of the National Academy of Sciences of the United States of America* 95, 14506–14510.

Angeles-Jurado, M., Junique, C., Pujol, J., Oliver, B., & Vendrell, P. (1997). Impaired estimation of word occurence frequency in frontal lobe patients. *Neuropsychologia* 35, 635–641.

Bechara, A., Tranel, D., Damasio, H., Adolphs, R., Rockland, C., & Damasio, A. (1995). Double-dissociation of conditioning and declarative knowledge relative to the amygdala and the hippocampus in humans. *Science* 269, 1115–1118.

Blaxton, T. A., Bookheimer, S. Y., Zeffiro, T. A., Figlozzi, C. M., William, D. G., & Theodore, W. H. (1996). Functional mapping of human memory using PET: Comparisons of conceptual and perceptual tasks. *Canadian Journal of Experimental Psychology* 50, 42–56.

Blaxton, T. A., Zeffiro, T. A., Gabrieli, J. D. E., Bookheimer, S. Y., Carrillo, M. C., Theodore, W. H., & Disterhoft, J. F. (1996). Functional mapping of human learning: A PET activation study of eyeblink conditioning. *Journal of Neuroscience* 16, 4032–4040.

Bookheimer, S. Y., Zeffiro, T. A., Blaxton, T., Gaillard, W., & Theodore, W. (1995). Regional cerebral blood flow during object naming and word reading. *Human Brain Mapping* 3, 93–106.

Brewer, J. B., Zhao, Z., Desmond, J. E., Glover, G. H., & Gabrieli, J. D. E. (1998). Making memories: Brain activity that predicts how well visual experience will be remembered. *Science* 281, 1185–1187.

Buckner, R. L., Bandettini, P. A., O'Craven, K. M., Savoy, R. L., Petersen, S. E., Raichle, M. E., & Rosen, B. R. (1996). Detection of cortical activation during averaged single trials of a cognitive task using functional magnetic resonance imaging. *Proceedings of the National Academy of Sciences USA* 93, 14878–14883.

Buckner, R. L., Koutstaal, W., Schacter, D. L., Dale, A. M., Rotte, M. R., & Rosen, B. R. (1998). Functional-anatomic study of episodic retrieval: II. Selective averaging of event-related fMRI trials to test the retrieval success hypothesis. *NeurOimage* 7, 163–175.

Buckner, R. L., Koutstaal, W., Schacter, D. L., Wagner, A. D., & Rosen, B. R. (1998). Functional-anatomic study of episodic retrieval using fMRI: I. Retrieval effort versus retrieval success. *NeuroImage* 7, 151–162.

Buckner, R. L., Petersen, S. E., Ojemann, J. G., Miezin, F. M., Squire, L. R., & Raichle, M. E. (1995). Functional anatomical studies of explicit and implicit memory retrieval tasks. *Journal of Neuroscience* 15, 12–29.

Butters, M. A., Kaszniak, A. W., Glisky, E. L., Eslinger, P. J., & Schacter, D. L. (1994). Recency discrimination deficits in frontal lobe patients. *Neuropsychology* 8, 343–353.

Cabeza, R., Grady, C. L., Nyberg, L., McIntosh, A. R., Tulving, E., Kapur, S., Jennings, J. M., Houle, S., & Craik, F. I. M. (1997). Age-related differences in neural activity during memory encoding and retrieval: A positron emission tomography study. *Journal of Neuroscience* 17, 391–400.

Cabeza, R., Kapur, S., Craik, F. I. M., & McIntosh, A. R. (1997). Functional neuroanatomy of recall and recognition: A PET study of episodic memory. *Journal of Cognitive Neuroscience* 9, 254–256.

Cabeza, R., & Nyberg, L. (1997). Imaging cognition: An empirical review of PET studies with normal subjects. *Journal of Cognitive Neuroscience* 9, 1–26.

Cahill, L., Babinsky, R., Markowitsch, H., & McGaugh, J. (1995). The amygdala and emotional memory. *Nature* 377, 295–296.

Cahill, L., Haier, R., Fallon, J., Alkire, M., Tang, C., Keator, D., Wu, J., & McGaugh, J. (1996). Amygdala activity at encoding correlated with long-term, free recall of emotional memory. *Proceedings of the National Academy of Sciences of the United States of America* 93, 8016–8021.

Cohen, N. J., & Eichenbaum, H. (1993). *Memory, Amnesia and the Hippocampal System.* Cambridge, MA: MIT Press.

Cohen, N. J., & Squire, L. R. (1980). Preserved learning and retention of pattern-analyzing skill in amnesia: Dissociation of knowing how and knowing that. *Science* 210, 207–210.

Corkin, S., Amaral, D., Gonzalez, R., Johnson, K., & Hyman, B. (1997). H.M.'s medial temporal-lobe lesion: Findings from MRI. *Journal of Neuroscience* 17, 3964–3979.

Craik, F. I. M., & Lockhart, R. S. (1972). Levels of processing: A framework for memory research. *Journal of Verbal Learning and Verbal Behavior* 11, 671–684.

Craik, F. I. M., Moroz, T. M., Moscovitch, M., Stuss, D. T., Winocur, G., Tulving, E., & Kapur, S. (1999). In search of the self: A positron emission tomography study. *Psychological Science* 10, 26–34.

Craik, F. I. M., & Tulving, E. (1975). Depth of processing and the retention of words in episodic memory. *Journal of Experimental Psychology: General* 104, 268–294.

Daum, I., Ackermann, H., Schugens, M. M., Reimold, C., Dichgans, J., & Birbaumer, N. (1993). The cerebellum and cognitive functions in humans. *Behavioral Neuroscience* 117, 411–419.

Decety, J., Grezes, J., Costes, N., Perani, D., Jeannerod, M., Procyk, E., Grassi, F., & Fazio, F. (1997). Brain activity during observation of actions: Influence of action content and subject's strategy. *Brain* 120, 1763–1777.

Demb, J. B., Desmond, J. E., Wagner, A. D., Vaidya, C. J., Glover, G. H., & Gabrieli, J. D. E. (1995). Semantic encoding and retrieval in the left inferior cortex: A functional MRI study of task difficulty and process specificity. *Journal of Neuroscience* 15, 5870–5878.

Démonet, J. F., Chollet, F., Ramsay, S., Cardebat, D., Nespoulos, J. L., Wise, R., Rascol, A., & Frackowiak, R. (1992). The anatomy of phonological and semantic processing in normal subjects. *Brain* 115, 1753–1768.

Desmond, J. E., Gabrieli, J. D. E., & Glover, G. H. (1998). Dissociation of frontal and cerebellar activity in a cognitive task: Evidence for a distinction between selection and search. *NeuroImage* 7, 368–376.

Desmond, J. E., Sum, J. M., Wagner, A. D., Demb, J. B., Shear, P. K., Glover, G. H., Gabrieli, J. D. E., & Morell, M. J. (1995). Functional MRI measurement of language lateralization in Wada-tested patients. *Brain* 118, 1411–1419.

Disterhoft, J. F., Coulter, D. A., & Alkon, D. L. (1986). Conditioning-specific membrane changes of rabbit hippocampal neurons measured in vitro. *Proceedings of the National Academy of Sciences of the United States of America* 83, 2733–2737.

Dolan, R., & Fletcher, P. (1997). Dissociating prefrontal and hippocampal function in episodic memory encoding. *Nature* 388, 582–585.

Fernandez, G., Brewer, J. B., Zhao, Z., Glover, G. H., & Gabrieli, J. D. E. (1999). Level of sustained entorhinal activity at study correlates with subsequent cued-recall performance: A functional magnetic resonance imaging study with high acquisition rate. *Hippocampus* 9, 35–44.

Fernandez, G., Weyerts, H., Schrader-Bolsche, M., Tendolkar, I., Smid, H. G. O. M., Tempelmann, C., Hinrichs, H., Scheich, H., Elger, C. E., Mangun, G. R., & Heinze, H. J. (1998). Successful verbal encoding into episodic memory engages the posterior hippocampus: A parametrically analyzed functional magnetic resonance imaging study. *Journal of Neuroscience* 18, 1841–1847.

Fiez, J. A. (1997). Phonology, semantics, and the role of the left inferior prefrontal cortex. *Human Brain Mapping* 5, 79–83.

Fletcher, P. C., Frith, C. D., Grasby, P. M., Shallice, T., Frackowiak, R. S. J., & Dolan, R. J. (1995). Brain systems for encoding and retrieval of auditory-verbal memory: An in vivo study in humans. *Brain* 118, 401–416.

Fletcher, P. C., Shallice, T., & Dolan, R. J. (1998). The functional roles of prefrontal cortex in episodic memory. *Brain* 121, 1239–1248.

Frith, C. D., Friston, K. J., Liddle, P. F., & Frackowiak, R. S. J. (1991). A PET study of word finding. *Neuropsychologia* 29, 1137–1148.

Fujii, T., Okuda, J., Kawashima, R., Yamadori, A., Fukatsu, R., Suzuki, K., Ito, M., Goto, R., & Fukuda, H. (1997). Different roles of the left and right parahippocampal regions in verbal recognition: A PET study. *NeuroReport* 8, 1113–1117.

Gabrieli, J. D. E. (1998). Cognitive neuroscience of human memory. *Annual Review of Psychology* 49, 87–115.

Gabrieli, J. D. E., Brewer, J. B., Desmond, J. E., & Glover, G. H. (1997). Separate neural bases of two fundamental memory processes in the human medial temporal lobe. *Science* 276, 264–266.

Gabrieli, J. D. E., Cohen, N. J., & Corkin, S. (1988). The impaired learning of semantic knowledge following bilateral medial temporal-lobe resection. *Brain and Cognition* 7, 525–539.

Gabrieli, J. D. E., Desmond, J. E., Demb, J. B., Wagner, A. D., Stone, M. V., Vaidya, C. J., & Glover, G. H. (1996). Functional magnetic resonance imaging of semantic memory processes in the frontal lobes. *Psychological Science* 7, 278–283.

Gabrieli, J. D. E., McGlinchey-Berroth, R., Carillo, M. C., Gluck, M. A., Cermak, L. S., & Disterhoft, J. F. (1995). Intact delay-eyeblink classical conditioning in amnesia. *Behavioral Neuroscience* 109, 819–827.

Gabrieli, J. D. E., Poldrack, R., & Desmond, J. E. (1998). The role of left prefrontal cortex in language and memory. *Proceedings of the National Academy of Sciences USA* 95, 906–913.

Gabrieli, J. D. E., Poldrack, R. A., & Wagner, A. D. (1998). Material specific and nonspecific prefrontal activations associated with encoding and retrieval of episodic memories. *Society for Neuroscience Abstracts* 24, 761.

Gabrieli, J. D. E., Rypma, B., Prabhakaran, V., Wagner, J. E., Desmond, J. E., & Glover, G. H. (1997). Common right prefrontal processes involved in episodic retrieval, working memory, and reasoning. *Society for Neuroscience Abstracts* 23, 1679.

Gershberg, F. B., & Shimamura, A. P. (1995). Impaired use of organizational strategies in free recall following frontal lobe damage. *Neuropsychologia* 33, 1305–1333.

Ghaem, O., Mellet, E., Crivello, F., Tzourio, N., Mazoyer, B., Berthoz, A., & Denis, M. (1997). Mental navigation along memorized routes activates the hippocampus, precuneus, and insula. *NeuroReport* 8, 739–744.

Graf, P., & Schacter, D. L. (1985). Implicit and explicit memory for new associations in normal and amnesic subjects. *Journal of Experimental Psychology: Learning, Memory, and Cognition* 11, 501–518.

Grasby, P. M., Frith, C. D., Friston, K. J., Bench, C., Frackowiak, R. S. J., & Dolan, R. J. (1993). Functional mapping of brain areas implicated in auditory-verbal memory function. *Brain* 116, 1–20.

Hamann, S. B., Ely, T. D., Grafton, S. T., & Kilts, C. D. (1999). Amygdala activity related to enhanced memory for pleasant and aversive stimuli. *Nature Neuroscience* 2, 289–293.

Haxby, J. V., Horwitz, B., Maisog, J. M., Ungerleider, L. G., Mishkin, M., Schapiro, M. B., Rapoport, S. I., & Grady, C. L. (1993). Frontal and temporal participation in long-term recognition memory for faces: A PET-rCBF activation study. *Journal of Cerebral Blood Flow and Metabolism* 13(supp. 1), 499.

Haxby, J. V., Ungerleider, L. G., Horwitz, B., Maisog, J. M., Rapoport, S. I., & Grady, C. L. (1996). Face encoding and recognition in the human brain. *Proceedings of the National Academy of Sciences USA* 93, 922–927.

Haxby, J. V., Ungerleider, L. G., Horwitz, B., Rapoport, S. I., & Grady, C. L. (1995). Hemispheric differences in neural systems for face working memory: A PET rCBF study. *Human Brain Mapping* 3, 68–82.

Henke, K., Buck, A., Weber, B., & Wieser, H. G. (1997). Human hippocampus establishes associations in memory. *Hippocampus* 7, 249–256.

Henson, R. N. A., Rugg, M. D., Shallice, T., Josephs, O., & Dolan, R. J. (1999). Recollection and familiarity in recognition memory: An event-related functional magnetic resonance imaging study. *Journal of Neuroscience* 19, 3962–3972.

Herbster, A. N., Mintun, M. A., Nebes, R. D., & Becker, J. T. (1997). Regional cerebral blood flow during word and nonword reading. *Human Brain Mapping* 5, 84–92.

Jacoby, L. L. (1991). A process dissociation framework: Separating automatic from intentional uses of memory. *Journal of Memory and Language* 30, 513–541.

Janowsky, J. S., Shimamura, A. P., Kritchevsky, M., & Squire, L. R. (1989). Cognitive impairment following frontal lobe damage and its relevance to human amnesia. *Behavioral Neuroscience* 103, 548–560.

Janowsky, J. S., Shimamura, A. P., & Squire, L. R. (1989). Source memory impairment in patients with frontal lobe lesions. *Neuropsychologia* 8, 1043–1056.

Kapur, N., Friston, K. J., Young, A., Frith, C. D., & Frackowiak, R. S. J. (1995). Activation of human hippocampal formation during memory for faces: A PET study. *Cortex* 31, 99–108.

Kapur, S., Craik, F. I. M., Jones, C., Brown, G. M., Houle, S., & Tulving, E. (1995). Functional role of the prefrontal cortex in memory retrieval: A PET study. *NeuroReport* 6, 1880–1884.

Kapur, S., Craik, F. I. M., Tulving, E., Wilson, A. A., Houle, S. H., & Brown, G. M. (1994). Neuroanatomical correlates of encoding in episodic memory: Levels of processing effects. *Proceedings of the National Academy of Sciences of the United States of America* 91, 2008–2011.

Kapur, S., Tulving, E., Cabeza, R., McIntosh, A. R., Houle, S., & Craik, F. I. M. (1996). The neural correlates of intentional learning of verbal materials: A PET study in humans. *Cognitive Brain Research* 4, 243–249.

Kelley, W. M., Buckner, R. L., Miezin, F. M., Cohen, N. J., Ollinger, J. M., Sanders, A. L., Ryan, J., & Petersen, S. E. (2000). Brain areas active during memorization of famous faces and names support multiple-code models of human memory. Submitted for publication.

Kelley, W. M., Miezin, F. M., McDermott, K. B., Buckner, R. L., Raichle, M. E., Cohen, N. J., Ollinger, J. M., Akbudak, E., Conturo, T. E., Snyder, A. Z., & Peterson, S. E. (1998). Hemispheric specialization in human dorsal frontal cortex and medial temporal lobe for verbal and nonverbal memory encoding. *Neuron* 20, 927–936.

Klein, D., Milner, B., Zatorre, R. J., Meyer, E., & Evans, A. (1995). The neural substrates underlying word generation: A bilingual functional-imaging study. *Proceedings of the National Academy of Sciences USA* 92, 2899–2903.

Klingberg, T., & Roland, P. E. (1998). Right prefrontal activation during encoding, but not during retrieval, in a non-verbal paired associates task. *Cerebral Cortex* 8, 73–79.

Knowlton, B. J., & Squire, L. R. (1995). Remembering and knowing: Two different expressions of declarative memory. *Journal of Experimental Psychology: Learning, Memory, and Cognition* 21, 699–710.

Kopelman, M., Stevens, T., Foli, S., & Grasby, P. (1998). PET activation of the medial temporal lobe in learning. *Brain* 121, 875–887.

LaBar, K., Ledoux, J., Spencer, D., & Phelps, E. (1995). Impaired fear conditioning following unilateral temporal lobectomy in humans. *Journal of Neuroscience* 15, 6846–6855.

Lepage, M., Habib, R., & Tulving, E. (1998). Hippocampal PET activation of memory encoding and retrieval: The HIPER model. *Hippocampus* 8, 313–322.

Logan, C. G., & Grafton, S. T. (1995). Functional anatomy of human eyeblink conditioning determined with regional cerebral glucose metabolism and position-emission tomography. *Proceedings of the National Academy of Sciences USA* 92, 7500–7504.

Maguire, E. A., Burgess, N., Donnett, J. G., Frackowiak, R. S. J., Frith, C. D., & O'Keefe, J. (1998). Knowing where and getting there: A human navigation network. *Science* 280, 921–924.

Maguire, E. A., Frackowiak, R. S. J., & Frith, C. D. (1996). Learning to find your way: A role for the human hippocampal formation. *Proceedings of the Royal Society of London* B263, 1745–1750.

Martin, A., Haxby, J. V., Lalonde, F. M., Wiggs, C. L., & Ungerleider, L. G. (1995). Discrete cortical regions associated with knowledge of color and knowledge of action. *Science* 270, 102–105.

Martin, A., Wiggs, C. L., Ungerleider, L. G., & Haxby, J. V. (1996). Neural correlates of category-specific knowledge. *Nature* 379, 649–652.

Martin, A., Wiggs, C. L., & Weisberg, J. (1997). Modulation of human medial temporal lobe activity by form, meaning, and experience. *Hippocampus* 7, 587–593.

McCormick, D. A., & Thompson, R. F. (1987). Neuronal responses of the rabbit cerebellum during acquisition and performance of a classically conditioned NM-eyelid response. *Journal of Neuroscience* 4, 2811–2822.

McDermott, K. B., Buckner, R. L., Petersen, S. E., Kelley, W. M., & Sanders, A. L. (1999). Set-specific and code-specific activation in frontal cortex: An fMRI study of encoding and retrieval of faces and words. *Journal of Cognitive Neuroscience* 11, 631–640.

Menard, M., Kosslyn, S. M., Thomson, W. L., Albert, N. M., & Rauch, S. L. (1996). Encoding words and pictures: A position emission tomography study. *Neuropsychologia* 34, 185–194.

Miller, L. (1985). Cognitive risk taking after frontal or temporal lobectomy. I. The synthesis of fragmental visual information. *Neuropsychologia* 23, 359–369.

Milner, B. (1964). Some effects of frontal lobectomy in man. In J. M. Warren & K. Akert, eds., *The Frontal Granular Cortex and Behavior*. New York: McGraw-Hill.

Milner, B. (1971). Interhemispheric differences in the localization of psychological processes in man. *British Medical Journal* 27, 272–277.

Milner, B., Corsi, P., & Leonard, G. (1991). Frontal-lobe contribution to recency judgements. *Neuropsychologia* 29, 601–618.

Morris, D. C., Bransford, J. D., & Franks, J. J. (1977). Levels of processing versus transfer appropiate processing. *Journal of Verbal Learning and Verbal Behavior* 16, 519–533.

Moscovitch, M., Kapur, S., Kohler, S., & Houle, S. (1995). Distinct neural correlates of visual long-term memory for spatial location and object identity: A positron emission tomography (PET) study in humans. *Proceedings of the National Academy of Sciences USA* 92, 3721–3725.

Nolde, S. F., Johnson, M. K., & D'Esposito, M. (1998). Left prefrontal activation during episodic remembering: An event-related fMRI study. *NeuroReport* 9, 3509–3514.

Nolde, S. F., Johnson, M. K., & Raye, C. L. (1998). The role of the prefrontal cortex during tests of episodic memory. *Trends in Cognitive Sciences* 2, 399–406.

Nyberg, L., Cabeza, R., & Tulving, E. (1996). PET studies of encoding and retrieval: The HERA model. *Psychonomic Bulletin & Review* 3, 135–148.

Nyberg, L., McIntosh, A. R., Houle, S., Nilsson, L., & Tulving, E. (1996). Activation of medial temporal structures during episodic memory retrieval. *Nature* 380, 715–717.

Nyberg, L., Tulving, E., Habib, R., Nilsson, L., Kapur, S., Houle, S., Cabeza, R., & McIntosh, A. R. (1995). Functional brain maps of retrieval mode and recovery of episodic information. *NeuroReport* 7, 249–252.

Owen, A. M., Milner, B., Petrides, M., & Evans, A. C. (1996a). Memory for object features versus memory for object location: A positron-emission tomography study of encoding and retrieval processes. *Proceedings of the National Academy of Sciences USA* 93, 9212–9217.

Owen, A. M., Milner, B., Petrides, M., & Evans, A. C. (1996b). A specific role for the right parahippocampal gyrus in the retrieval of object location: A positron emission tomography study. *Journal of Cognitive Neuroscience* 8, 588–602.

Petersen, S. E., Fox, P. T., Posner, M. I., Mintun, M., & Raichle, M. E. (1988). Positron emission tomographic studies of the cortical anatomy of single-word processing. *Nature* 331, 585–589.

Petersen, S. E., Fox, P. T., Snyder, A. Z., & Raichle, M. E. (1990). Activation of extrastriate and frontal cortical areas by visual words and word-like stimuli. *Science* 249, 1041–1044.

Petrides, M., Alivisatos, B., & Evans, A. C. (1995). Functional activation of the human ventrolateral frontal cortex during mnemonic retrieval of verbal information. *Proceedings of the National Academy of Sciences USA* 92, 5803–5807.

Petrides, M., & Milner, B. (1982). Deficits on subject-ordered tasks after frontal and temporal lobe lesions in man. *Neuropsychologia* 20, 601–614.

Phelps, E. A., & Anderson, A. K. (1997). Emotional memory: What does the amygdala do? *Current Opinion in Biology* 7, 11–13.

Poldrack, R. A., Wagner, A. D., Prull, M. W., Desmond, J. E., Glover, G. H., & Gabrieli, J. D. E. (1999). Functional specialization for semantic and phonological processing in the left inferior prefrontal cortex. *NeuroImage* 10, 15–35.

Price, C. J., Wise, R. J. S., Watson, J. D. G., Patterson, K., Howard, D., & Frackowiak, R. S. J. (1994). Brain activity during reading: The effects of exposure duration and task. *Brain* 117, 1255–1269.

Raichle, M. E., Fiez, J. A., Videen, T. O., MacLeod, A. M., Pardo, J. V., Fox, P. T., & Petersen, S. E. (1994). Practice-related changes in human brain functional anatomy during nonmotor learning. *Cerebral Cortex* 4, 8–26.

Rempel-Clower, N., Zola, S., Squire, L., & Amaral, D. (1996). Three cases of enduring memory impairment after bilateral damage limited to the hippocampal formation. *Journal of Neuroscience* 16, 5233–5255.

Roland, P., & Gulyas, B. (1995). Visual memory, visual imagery, and visual recognition of large field patterns by the human brain: Functional anatomy by positron emission tomography. *Cerebral Cortex* 1, 79–93.

Rombouts, S., Machielsen, W., Witter, M., Barkhof, F., Lindeboom, J., & Scheltens, P. (1997). Visual association encoding activates the medial temporal lobe: A functional magnetic resonance imaging study. *Hippocampus* 7, 594–601.

Rugg, M. D., Fletcher, P. C., Frith, C. D., Frackowiak, R. S. J., & Dolan, R. J. (1996). Differential activation of the prefrontal cortex in successful and unsuccessful memory retrieval. *Brain* 119, 2073–2083.

Rugg, M. D., Fletcher, P. C., Frith, C. D., Frackowiak, R. S. J., & Dolan, R. J. (1997). Brain regions supporting intentional and incidental memory: A PET study. *NeuroReport* 8, 1283–1287.

Rumsey, J. M., Horwitz, B., Donohue, B. C., Nace, K., Maisog, J. M., & Andreason, P. (1997). Phonological and orthographic components of word recognition: A PET-rCBF study. *Brain* 120, 739–759.

Schacter, D. L., Alpert, N. M., Savage, C. R., Rauch, S. L., & Albert, M. S. (1996). Conscious recollection and the human hippocampal formation: Evidence from positron emission tomography. *Proceedings of the National Academy of Sciences USA* 93, 321–325.

Schacter, D. L., Buckner, R. L., Koutstaal, W., Dale, A. M., & Rosen, B. R. (1997). Late onset of anterior prefrontal activity during true and false recognition: An event-related fMRI study. *NeuroImage* 6, 259–269.

Schacter, D. L., Curran, T., Galluccio, L., Milberg, W. P., & Bates, J. F. (1996). False recognition and the right frontal lobe: A case study. *Neuropsychologia* 34, 793–808.

Schacter, D. L., Reiman, E., Uecker, A., Polster, M. R., Yung, L. S., & Cooper, L. A. (1995). Brain regions associated with retrieval of structurally coherent visual information. *Nature* 368, 633–635.

Schacter, D. L., Uecker, A., Reiman, E., Yun, L. S., Brandy, D., Chen, K., Cooper, L. A., & Curran, T. (1997). Effects of size and orientation change on hippocampal activation during episodic recognition: A PET study. *NeuroReport* 8, 3993–3998.

Schacter, D. L., & Wagner, A. D. (1999). Medial temporal lobe activations in fMRI and PET studies of episodic encoding and retrieval. *Hippocampus* 9, 7–24.

Schmaltz, L. W., & Theios, J. (1972). Acquisition and extinction of a classically conditioned response in hippocampectomized rabbits (*Oryctolagus cuniculus*). *Journal of Comparative and Physiological Psychology* 79, 328–333.

Scott, S. K., Young, A. W., Calder, A. J., Hellawell, D. J., Aggleton, J. P., & Johnson, M. (1997). Impaired auditory recognition of fear and anger following bilateral amygdala lesions. *Nature* 385, 254–257.

Scoville, W. B., & Milner, B. (1957). Loss of recent memory after bilateral hippocampal lesions. *Journal of Neurology, Neurosurgery, and Psychiatry* 20, 11–21.

Shallice, T., Fletcher, P., Frith, C. D., Grasby, P., Frackowiak, R. S. J., & Dolan, R. J. (1994). Brain regions associated with acquisition and retrieval of verbal episodic memory. *Nature* 368, 633–635.

Shaywitz, B. A., Pugh, K. R., Constable, R. T., Shaywitz, S. E., Bronen, R. A., Fulbright, R. K., Shankweiler, D. P., Katz, L., Fletcher, J. M. S. E., Skudlarski, P., & Gore, J. C. (1995). Localization of semantic processing using functional magnetic resonance imaging. *Human Brain Mapping* 2, 149–158.

Shimamura, A. P., Janowsky, J. S., & Squire, L. R. (1990). Memory for the temporal order of events in patients with frontal lobe lesions and amnesic patients. *Neuropsychologia* 28, 803–813.

Slamecka, N. J., & Graf, P. (1978). The generation effect: Delineation of a phenomemon. *Journal of Experimental Psychology: Human Learning and Memory* 4, 492–604.

Smith, M. L., & Milner, B. (1988). Estimation of frequency of occurrence of abstract designs after frontal or temporal lobectomy. *Neuropsychologia* 26, 297–306.

Squire, L. R. (1992). Memory and the hippocampus: A synthesis from findings with rats, monkeys, and humans. *Psychological Review* 99, 195–231.

Squire, L. R., Ojemann, J. G., Miezin, F. M., Petersen, S. E., Videen, T. O., & Raichle, M. E. (1992). Activation of the hippocampus in normal humans: A functional anatomical study of memory. *Proceedings of the National Academy of Sciences of the United States of America* 89, 1837–1841.

Stern, C., Corkin, S., Gonzalez, R., Guimares, A., Baker, J., Jennings, P., Carr, C., Sugiura, R., Vedantham, V., & Rosen, B. (1996). The hippocampal formation participates in novel picture encoding: Evidence from functional magnetic resonance imaging. *Proceedings of the National Academy of Sciences USA* 93, 8660–8665.

Stuss, D. T., Alexander, M. P., Palumbo, C. L., Buckle, L., Sayer, L., & Pogue, J. (1994). Organizational strategies of patients with unilateral or bilateral frontal lobe damage. *Neuropsychology* 8, 355–373.

Suzuki, W. A., & Amaral, D. G. (1994). Perirhinal and parahippocampal cortices of the macaque monkey: Cortical afferents. *Journal of Comparative Neurology* 350, 497–533.

Symons, C. S., & Johnson, B. T. (1997). The self-reference effect in memory: A meta-analysis. *Psychological Bulletin* 121, 371–394.

Thompson, R. F. (1990). Neural mechanisms of classical conditioning in mammals. *Philosophical Transactions of the Royal Society of London* B329, 161–170.

Thompson-Schill, S. L., D'Esposito, M., Aguirre, G. K., & Farah, M. J. (1997). Role of the left inferior prefrontal cortex in retrieval of semantic knowledge: A reevaluation. *Proceedings of the National Academy of Sciences USA* 94, 14792–14797.

Tulving, E. (1983). *Elements of Episodic Memory*. New York: Oxford University Press.

Tulving, E., Habib, R., Nyberg, L., Lepage, M., & McIntosh, A. R. (1999). Positron emission tomography correlations in and beyond medial temporal lobes. *Hippocampus* 9, 71–82.

Tulving, E., Kapur, S., Craik, F. I. M., Moscovitch, M., & Houle, S. (1994). Hemispheric encoding/ retrieval asymmetry in episodic memory: Positron emission tomography findings. *Proceedings of the National Academy of Sciences USA* 91, 2016–2020.

Tulving, E., Kapur, S., Markowitsch, H. J., Craik, F. I., Habib, R., & Houle, S. (1994). Neuroanatomical correlates of retrieval in episodic memory: Auditory sentence recognition. *Proceedings of the National Academy of Sciences USA* 91, 2012–2015.

Tulving, E., Markowitsch, H. J., Craik, F. I. M., Habib, R., & Houle, S. (1996). Novelty and familiarity activations in PET studies of memory encoding and retrieval. *Cerebral Cortex* 6, 71–79.

Tulving, E., Markowitsch, H. J., Kapur, S., Habib, R., & Houle, S. (1994). Novelty encoding networks in the human brain: Positron emission tomography data. *NeuroReport* 5, 2525–2528.

Tulving, E., & Thompson, D. M. (1973). Encoding specificity and retrieval processes in episodic memory. *Psychological Review* 80, 352–373.

Vandenberghe, R., Price, C., Wise, R., Josephs, O., & Frackowiak, R. S. J. (1996). Functional anatomy of a common semantic system for words and pictures. *Nature* 383, 254–256.

Wagner, A. D., Desmond, J. E., Demb, J. B., Glover, G. H., & Gabrieli, J. D. E. (1997). Semantic repetition priming for verbal and pictorial knowledge: A functional MRI study of left inferior prefrontal cortex. *Journal of Cognitive Neuroscience* 9, 714–726.

Wagner, A. D., Desmond, J. E., Glover, G. H., & Gabrieli, J. D. E. (1998). Prefrontal cortex and recognition memory: fMRI evidence for context-dependent retrieval processes. *Brain* 121, 1985–2002.

Wagner, A. D., & Gabrieli, J. D. E. (1998). On the relationship between recognition familiarity and perceptual fluency: Evidence for distinct mnemonic processes. *Acta Psychologica* 98, 211–230.

Wagner, A. D., Poldrack, R. A., Eldridge, L. E., Desmond, J. E., Glover, G. H., & Gabrieli, J. D. E. (1998). Material-specific lateralization of prefrontal activation during episodic encoding and retrieval. *NeuroReport* 9, 3711–3717.

Wagner, A. D., Schacter, D. L., Rotte, M., Koutstaal, W., Maril, A., Dale, A. M., Rosen, B. R., & Buckner, R. L. (1998). Building memories: Remembering and forgetting verbal experiences as predicted by brain activity. *Science* 281, 1188–1191.

Warburton, E., Wise, R. J., Price, C. J., Weiller, C., Hadar, U., Ramsay, S., & Frackowiak, R. S. (1996). Noun and verb retrieval by normal subjects: Studies with PET. *Brain* 119, 159–179.

Wheeler, M. A., Stuss, D. T., & Tulving, E. (1995). Frontal lobe damage produces episodic memory impairment. *Journal of the International Neuropsychological Society* 1, 525–536.

Wiggs, C. L., Weisberg, J. M., & Martin, A. (1999). Neural correlates of semantic and episodic memory retrieval. *Neuropsychologia* 37(1), 103–118.

Wise, R., Chollet, F., Hadar, U., Friston, K., Hoffner, E., & Frackowiak, R. (1991). Distribution of cortical neural networks involved in word comprehension and word retrieval. *Brain* 114, 1803–1817.

Zatorre, R. J., Meyer, E., Gjedde, A., & Evans, A. C. (1996). PET studies of phonetic processing of speech: Review, replication, and reanalysis. *Cerbral Cortex* 6, 21–30.

9 Functional Neuroimaging of Working Memory

Mark D'Esposito

INTRODUCTION

Working memory is an evolving concept that refers to the short-term storage of information which is not accessible in the environment, and the set of processes that keep this information active for later use in behavior. It is a system that is critically important in cognition and seems necessary in the course of performing many other cognitive functions, such as reasoning, language comprehension, planning, and spatial processing. Animal studies initially provided important evidence for the neural basis of working memory (for review, see Fuster, 1997). For example, electrophysiological studies of awake behaving monkeys have used delayed-response tasks to study working memory. In these tasks, the monkey must keep "in mind," or actively maintain, a stimulus over a short delay. During such tasks, neurons within the prefrontal cortex (PFC) are found to be persistently activated during the delay period of a delayed-response task, when the monkey is maintaining information in memory prior to a making a motor response (Funahashi et al., 1989; Fuster & Alexander, 1971). The necessity of this region for active maintenance of information over short delays has been demonstrated in monkey studies which have shown that lesions of the lateral PFC impair performance on these tasks (Bauer & Fuster, 1976; Funahashi et al., 1993).

From a psychological point of view, working memory has been conceptualized as comprising multiple components that support executive control processes as well as active maintenance of information. For example, Baddeley (1986) has proposed the existence of a "central executive system" that, based on behavioral studies of normal subjects, is a system which actively regulates the distribution of limited attentional resources and coordinates information within limited-capacity verbal and spatial memory storage buffers. The central executive system, based on the analogous supervisory attentional system introduced by Norman and Shallice (1986), is proposed to take *control* over cognitive processing when novel tasks are engaged and/or when existing behavioral routines have to be overridden. Both Baddeley and Shallice originally argued that an executive controller is a distinct cognitive module which is supported by the PFC, and that damage to this module, or system, accurately describes some of the behavior of patients with PFC damage. More recently, however, Baddeley has postulated that the central executive does not function as a single module and can be fractionated into subcomponents (Baddeley, 1998).

Although the concept of a "central executive" has influenced our thinking about the function of the PFC, other researchers have proposed that the PFC does not house an "executive controller," but instead serves processes that are simpler and more fundamental. For example, Cohen and Servan-Schreiber (1992, p. 46) have proposed a neural network model of the underlying cognitive and linguistic impairments in schizophrenia, which, they hypothesize, results from impaired function of the PFC. Their model proposes "a degradation in the ability to construct and maintain an internal representation of context, [by which] we mean information held in mind in such a form that it can be used to mediate an appropriate behavioral response." In their model, disordered performance is seen as a consequence of a change to a single low-level parameter. This simple change allows them to account for performance on a variety of tasks thought to be dependent on PFC function. In this way, it serves as a model case in understanding how behaviors that appear outwardly different may have their roots in similar fundamental processes.

Kimberg and Farah (1993) have also attempted to provide a parsimonious account of the computations underlying the diverse cognitive processes, considered to be "executive" in nature, that are impaired following damage to the PFC. Their model suggests that executive dysfunction can be interpreted in terms of damage to simple working memory components, and demonstrates how disparate impairments that follow PFC damage can be due to a common underlying mechanism. In this model, the term "working memory" refers to the functions and properties of the human cognitive system that allow representations to have levels of activation appropriate to the current task. It is a memory system in that the levels of activation reflect recent events, but it is not simply the capacity to remember. Items are not "in" working memory, but they do have levels of activation that can be higher or lower. Thus, performance on a task requiring working memory is determined by levels of activation of relevant representations, and the discriminability between activation levels of relevant and irrelevant representations. In selecting among competing responses, the model contains no "central executive" but simply considers the sum of the sources of activation contributing to each potential response. Specifically, their account of PFC dysfunction postulates that damage weakens the associative contribution to the activation of working-memory representations, achieved in the simulation by attenuating the strengths of these associations. Thus, the pattern of deficits following damage to this component of working memory would reflect an inability to coactivate mutually relevant, or associated, representations. A simple implementation of this model did indeed reproduce characteristic patterns of behavior on four disparate "executive" tasks, such as the Wisconsin Card Sorting Test and the Stroop Task.

Fuster (1997) has proposed that the PFC is critically important in tasks which require the temporal integration of information. Drawing on evidence from both animal and human research, Fuster has proposed three distinct PFC functions: active, or working, memory; preparatory task set, or the ability to prepared for future action; and inhibitory control. He also has argued explicitly against the executive interpretation of PFC function, writing that "the PFC would not superimpose a steering or directing function on the remainder of the nervous system, but rather, by expanding the temporal perspectives of the system, would allow it to integrate longer, newer, and more complex structures of behavior" (Fuster, 1995 p. 172). Thus, based on the interpretation of empirical evidence from animal studies, a notion similar to that derived from computation models arises, that is, executive control is an emergent property that arises from lower-level memory functions which serve to integrate behavior.

Goldman-Rakic (1987) has also proposed a working-memory account of PFC function, according to which lateral PFC instantiates a form of working memory that she terms "representational memory." Based on evidence from both electrophysiological studies and studies of lesions of monkeys, as referenced above, Goldman-Rakic concluded that the ability to keep information in mind across short intervals depends critically on the lateral PFC. She has also suggested that this framework could be extended to explain a range of human cognitive impairments following focal frontal lesions, as well as nonfocal pathologies affecting lateral PFC (e.g. schizophrenia, Huntington's and Parkinson's diseases). Moreover, like Fuster, she has explicitly stated that "based on anatomical, physiological, and lesion evidence in both monkeys and humans, 'a central-executive' in the form of an all-purpose polymodal processor may not exist, and to the contrary, a strong case can be made for the view that the substrates of cognition reside in the parallelism of the brain's modularized information processing systems" (Goldman-Rakic, 1996).

In summary, working memory is not a unitary system and can be viewed as a set of properties that characterize how this cognitive system makes use of temporarily activated representations to guide behavior. These properties may be behaviorally and neurally dissociable. Many methods exist to examine the neural basis of working memory in humans. The lesion method, for example, has been helpful in establishing the necessity of PFC in working-memory function (e.g., Ptito et al., 1995; Verin et al., 1993). However, since injury to PFC in humans is rarely restricted in its location, using lesion studies in humans to test ideas about the necessity of a specific region of PFC for specific components of working memory is difficult. Functional neuroimaging, such as positron emission tomography (PET) or functional MRI (fMRI), provides another means of testing such ideas and will be reviewed in the next section.

It is important to realize however, that unlike lesion studies, imaging studies only support inferences about the *engagement* of a particular brain system by a cognitive process, but not about the system's *necessity* to the process (Sarter et al., 1996). That is, neuroimaging studies cannot, alone, tell us whether the function of a neural system represents a neural substrate of that function, or is a nonessential process associated with that function. Moreover, this observation applies equally to all methods of physiological measurement, such as single-unit and multiunit electrophysiology, EEG, or MEG. Thus, data derived from neuroimaging studies provide one piece of converging evidence that is being accumulated to determine the neural basis of working memory.

FUNCTIONAL NEUROIMAGING OF WORKING MEMORY

Active Maintenance Processes

There is now a critical mass of studies (more than 30) using functional neuroimaging in humans which have demonstrated that the PFC is engaged during working-memory tasks (for review, see D'Esposito et al., 1998). Review of the details of each of these studies is beyond the scope of this chapter, but those studies which highlight the critical advancement of our understanding of the neural basis of working memory will be considered. For example, Jonides and colleagues (1993) performed the first imaging study, using PET, to show that PFC was activated during performance of a spatial working-memory task analogous to the one used in the monkey studies. In this study, subjects were presented with two types of trials (left side of figure 9.1 and color plate 18). In the memory condition, subjects were required to maintain the spatial location of three dots appearing on a visual display across a 3 sec delay. After this delay, a probe for location memory consisted of a single outline circle that either surrounded the location of one of the previous dots or did not. In the perception condition, the three dots were again presented on a visual display, but immediately following their presentation, a probe circle appeared simultaneously with the dots, and the subject merely made a perceptual judgment as to whether or not the probe encircled a dot.

The rationale of this study was that "subtraction" of images obtained during the perceptual condition from images obtained from the memory condition would reveal brain regions which require the storage of spatial information during the retention interval, and not sensorimotor components of the task. Comparison of the block of trials with a delay period to a block of trials without a delay period produced activation within PFC (right side of figure 9.1) as well as in occipital, parietal, and premotor cortices. The location of the PFC activation in this study was within right Brodmann's area 47 (inferior frontal gyrus), which is inferior to proposed homologous regions to the principal sulcus (area 46), the site of spatial working memory in monkeys (Funahashi et al., 1989, 1993). Nevertheless, this study was an important

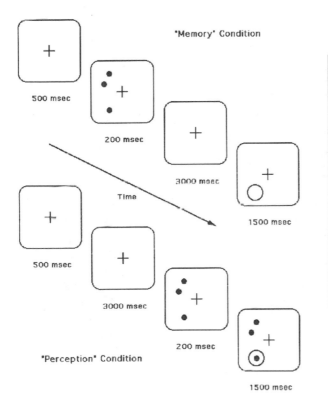 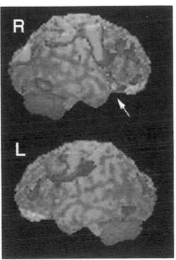

Figure 9.1
(Left) The spatial working-memory task used in the Jonides et al. (1993) PET study. (Right) A surface rendering of the activated regions. White arrow points to significant activation in right ventral prefrontal cortex, Brodmann's area 47. (See color plate 18.)

demonstration that human PFC, like monkey PFC, may be critical for maintaining internal representations across time. Subsequently, numerous other imaging studies have utilized delayed-response tasks with requirements for storage of spatial (e.g., Anderson et al., 1994; Baker et al., 1996; Goldberg et al., 1996; O'Sullivan et al., 1995; Smith et al., 1995; Sweeney et al., 1996) as well as nonspatial (i.e., letters, words, faces, objects) information (e.g., Baker et al., 1996; Becker et al., 1994; Paulesu et al., 1993; Salmon et al., 1996; Smith et al., 1995, 1996; Swartz et al., 1995). Also, many studies have been performed using more complex types of working-memory tasks, such as n-back tasks (e.g., Cohen et al., 1994; McCarthy et al., 1994; Owen et al., 1996; Petrides, Alivisatos, Evans, et al., 1993; Petrides, Alivisatos, Meyer, et al., 1993; Salmon et al., 1996; Smith et al., 1996). Consistent across these studies is the demonstration of lateral PFC activation in a comparison between blocks of trials designed to have greater memory requirements than a matched control task.

A potential problem in interpretation of an imaging study such as that of Jonides et al. (1993), or the many others that were subsequently reported, is that each relies on the assumptions of the method of cognitive subtraction. Cognitive subtraction attempts to correlate brain activity with specific processes by pairing two tasks that are assumed to be matched perfectly for every sensory, motor, and cognitive process except the process of interest (Posner et al., 1988). For example, Jonides et al. assumed that the only difference between the two experimental conditions was the delay period and, therefore, the process of memory storage. Although the application of cognitive subtraction to imaging was a major innovation when originally introduced (Petersen et al., 1988), it has become clear that it is a potentially flawed methodology which may lead to erroneous interpretation of imaging data.

The assumptions that must be relied upon for cognitive subtraction methodology can be faulty for at least two reasons. First, it involves the assumption of *additivity* (or *pure insertion*), the idea that a cognitive process can be added to a preexisting set of cognitive processes without affecting them (Sternberg, 1969). For example, the delayed-response paradigm typically used to study working memory (see figure 9.1) is comprised of a memory-requiring delay period between a "perceptual" process (the presentation of the item[s] to be stored) and a "choice" process (a required decision based upon the item[s] stored). It is proposed that the neural substrates of the memory process are revealed by a subtraction of the integrated (i.e., averaged, summed, or totaled) functional hemodynamic signal during a no-delay condition (i.e., a block of trials without a delay period) from the signal during a delay condition (i.e., a block of trials with a delay period). In this example, failure to meet the assumptions of cognitive subtraction will occur if the insertion of a delay period between the "perceptual" and "choice" processes interacts with the other behavioral processes in the task. For example, the nonmemory processes may be different in delay trials compared to no-delay trials.

A second reason that cognitive subtraction methodology can be faulty is that in neuroimaging, an additional requirement must be met in order for cognitive subtractive methodology to yield nonartifactual results: the transform between the neural signal and the neuroimaging signal must be linear. In two studies using functional MRI (fMRI), some nonlinearities have been observed in this system (Boynton et al., 1996; Vazquez & Noll, 1998). In our example of a delayed-response paradigm, failure will occur if the sum of the transform of neural activity to hemodynamic signal for the "perceptual" and "choice" processes differs when a delay is inserted as compared to when it is not present. In this example, artifacts of cognitive subtraction might lead to the inference that a region displayed delay-correlated increases in neural activity when in actuality it did not.

To overcome these potential problems, a new class of designs called "event-related" fMRI have been developed that do not rely on cognitive subtraction (for review, see D'Esposito, Zarahn, et al., 1998; Rosen et al., 1998). These designs allow one to detect changes in fMRI signal evoked by neural events associated with single behavioral trials as opposed to blocks of such trials. Event-related fMRI designs are some-what analogous to designs employed in event-related potential (ERP) studies, in that the functional responses occurring during different temporal portions within the trial can be analyzed.

As mentioned, spatial delayed-response tasks typically have a stimulus presentation period, an ensuing delay (of a few seconds), and a choice period. Changes in single-unit neural activity have been observed during each of these task components in elec-trophysiological studies of nonhuman primates. For example, Fuster and colleagues (1982), using a visual delayed-response task, observed that responses of single PFC neurons to the initial stimulus presentation ended within a few hundred millisec-onds of stimulus offset. They also observed changes in firing rate in single neurons in lateral PFC during the delay period that were sustained for several seconds. If these results also characterize human PFC function, it should be possible with an event-related fMRI design to resolve temporally functional changes correlated with the delay period from those correlated with the stimulus presentation/early delay period.

The logic of one implementation of an event-related fMRI design (Zarahn et al., 1997) is illustrated in figure 9.2. A single behavioral trial may be hypothesized to be associated with one brief neural event, or with several brief neural events that are sub-component processes engaged within a trial (i.e., encoding or retrieval in a delayed-response task). A neural event will cause a brief fMRI signal change, which is called the hemodynamic response. If we wish to detect and differentiate the fMRI signal evoked by a series of sequential neural events (such as the presentation of the stimulus and, seconds later, the execution of the response), one method would be to statis-tically model the evoked fMRI signal, using a pair of hemodynamic responses as covariates, each shifted to the time period where the event of interest is thought to occur. Importantly, a combination of hemodynamic responses could theoretically be used to model any neural event, even if the event is sustained, such as delay-period activity.

Analyzing in the manner described above, during the performance of a spatial delayed-response task we observed that several brain regions, including PFC, consis-tently displayed activity which correlated with the delay period across subjects (Zarahn et al., 1996, 1999). This finding suggests that these regions may be involved

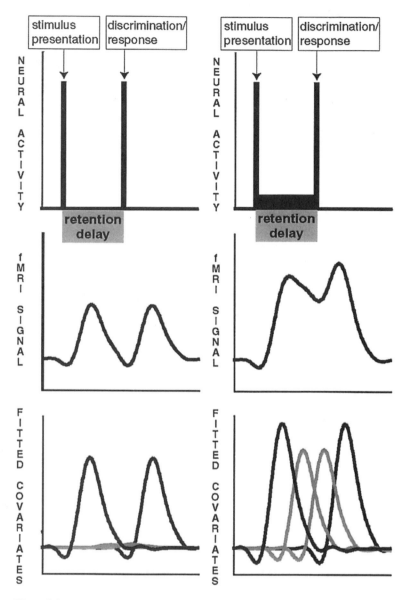

Figure 9.2
Two examples of how the fMRI data analysis model would respond to different neural responses during trials of a delayed-response paradigm. The left panel depicts a scenario in which there is only a brief period of neural activity (first row) associated with both the stimulus presentation and the discrimination/response periods of trials, with no increase above baseline during the bulk of the retention delay. Such neural activity change would lead to a particular profile of fMRI signal change (second row). The model covariates (hemodynamic responses shifted to sequential time points of the trial) scaled by their resulting least-squares coefficients are shown in the third row (gray lines, covariates modeling the retention delay; black lines, covariates modeling the stimulus presentation and the discrimination/response periods). The covariates modeling the retention delay would make only a small contribution to variance explanation. In contrast, the right panel depicts a situation in which there is some neural activity increase relative to baseline during the retention delay. In this case, the covariates modeling the retention delay would tend to explain a larger amount of variance in the fMRI signal than in the scenario in the left panel. In this way, delay-specific brain activity would be detected by the model (from Zarahn et al., 1999).

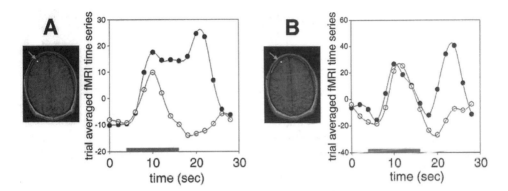

Figure 9.3
(*A*) An example of the time series of the fMRI signal averaged across trials for a PFC region that displayed delay-correlated activity (filled black circles represent activity for delay trials and open circles are trials without a delay). (*B*) An example of a time series where the integrated activity for the presentation of the cue and response during the delay trials (filled black circles) is greater than that observed during the combined presentation of the cue and response in the no-delay trials (open circles). The solid gray bar represents the duration of the delay period of the behavioral task (from Zarahn et al., 1999).

in temporary maintenance of spatial representations in humans. With this event-related fMRI design, we could be confident that activity observed was not due to differences in other components of the task (presentation of the cue or motor response) during the behavioral trials. Most important, these results do not rely on the assumptions of cognitive subtraction. An example of the time series of the fMRI signal averaged across trials for a PFC region that displays delay-correlated activity is shown in figure 9.3A.

In this same study, we also found direct evidence for the failure of cognitive subtraction (see figure 9.3B). We found a region in PFC that did not display sustained activity during the delay (in an event-related analysis) yet showed greater activity in the delay trials as compared to the trials without a delay. In any blocked neuroimaging study, such as those reviewed above, that compares delay versus no-delay trials with subtraction, such a region would be detected and likely be assumed to be a "memory" region. Thus, this result provides empirical grounds for adopting a healthy doubt regarding the inferences drawn from imaging studies that have relied on cognitive subtraction.

Other studies using event-related designs have also investigated the temporal dynamics of neural activity, but during working memory tasks using nonspatial information. For example, Courtney and colleagues (1997) utilized a delayed response task that required the maintenance of faces. Ventral occipitotemporal regions exhibited predominantly transient responses to the stimuli, consistent with a role in perceptual processing, whereas PFC demonstrated sustained activity over the memory delay, consistent with a role in active maintenance of face information. Figure 9.4A illustrates the gradual shift of the relative contribution of perceptual processing to memory processing from posterior to anterior cortical regions.

Cohen and colleagues (1997), in a different fashion than the Zarahn and Courtney studies, utilized a sequential letter n-back task, in which load was manipulated (from 0-back to 3-back) and the rate of stimulus presentation was slowed substantially (10 sec intertrial interval) in order to resolve temporal information. In the n-back task, letters are presented sequentially and the subject is required to respond to any letter that is identical to the one presented one, two, or three trials back. In the 0-back condition, subjects respond to a single prespecified target (such as X). The rationale of the experimental design was that sensory and motor processes would evoke transient increases in activation associated with stimulus presentation and response execution, and would not vary with memory load. Alternatively, areas involved in working memory would vary with memory load. A more refined prediction was made that load-sensitive areas would be dissociated into two types: those involved in active maintenance would exhibit sustained activation throughout the trial, and those involved in other working-memory processes (updating, temporal ordering) would exhibit transient activation but peak higher for increased memory loads. As expected, sensorimotor brain regions exhibited effects of time, but no effects of memory load. The PFC and posterior parietal cortex showed an effect of memory load. Dorsal and ventral regions of PFC (Brodmann's area 9/46 and 44) showed an effect of load but not an interaction with time that was consistent with a role of these regions in active maintenance processes (see figure 9.4B). Ventral PFC (area 44) also showed an effect of the interaction of time and memory load, suggesting a role in transient working-memory processes in addition to more sustained active maintenance processes.

Although PET imaging lacks the resolution to assess the temporal dynamics of neural activity in a manner similar to that in the fMRI studies described above, attempts at isolating maintenance processes with PET have been made. For example, several PET studies have been done with delayed-response tasks during which scanning was performed only during the retention interval (Baker et al., 1996; Fiez et al., 1996; Jonides et al., 1998). Obviously, the delay period must be much longer in these PET studies, in order to allow for adequate data to be obtained (around 30–40 sec), than is typically employed in a single trial (a few seconds) during an fMRI study. Nevertheless, various types of material have been used in these studies, including words and pseudo words (Fiez et al., 1996; Jonides et al., 1998), and objects and spatial information (Baker et al., 1996). These studies provide additional support for a role of PFC in active maintenance processes.

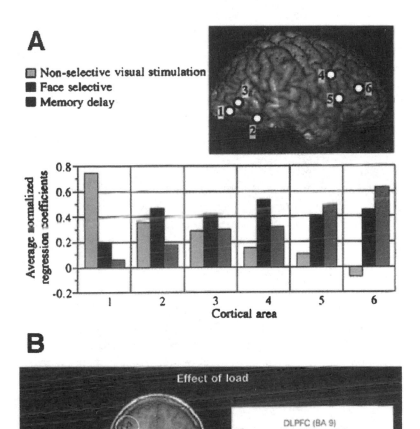

Figure 9.4
(*A*) Data from Courtney et al. (1997) study showing significant regions of activation in a face working-memory task. The graph illustrates the relative contribution of each component of the task (i.e., visual stimulation or memory delay period) to the signal in these regions. (*B*) Data from Cohen et al. (1997) study showing regions of activation that demonstrated a significant effect of load.

The studies described above have all presented stimuli using the visual modality. Two studies have examined activation patterns of working-memory tasks in other sensory modalities. For example, Klingberg et al. (1996) performed a PET study in which subjects were required to actively maintain auditory (pitch of tones), somatosensory (frequencies of a vibrating stimulus), or visual (luminance levels of a monochrome light) information across short delays (2–5 sec). An analysis of the effects of the task (working memory vs. detection) and modality (auditory vs. somatosensory vs. visual) did not reveal a task × modality interaction. The memory task, compared to a baseline detection task, activated a set of overlapping regions within lateral PFC across the different modality types, thus supporting a multimodal role for PFC. A similar conclusion was drawn by Schumacher et al. (1996), based on results of a PET study of subjects performing a verbal working-memory task (the 2-back task) with stimuli presented either visually or aurally. Again, comparison of the memory task to a control detection task revealed almost complete overlap in areas of activation within lateral PFC.

Studies of patients with lesions in PFC have shown impairments on delayed-response tasks (for review, see D'Esposito & Postle, 1999) that suggest the necessity of this cortical region in maintenance processes. However, these studies cannot rule out the possibility that other component processes necessary for successful performance of a delayed-response task, such as retrieval processes, rather than maintenance processes, are dependent on PFC integrity. However, several transcranial magnetic stimulation studies have shown that stimulation over lateral PFC during the delay period of a delayed-response task induces errors (Brandt et al., 1998; Muri et al., 1996; Pascual-Leone & Hallett, 1994). Taken together, imaging and lesion studies provide strong converging evidence for an association between active maintenance and PFC function.

Executive Control Processes

The dual-task paradigm has been used as an effective behavioral tool for probing executive control processes. Sequential performance of two tasks, or parallel performance of two unrelated tasks that engage separate processing mechanisms, is thought to make minimal demands on executive control processes. However, two concurrently performed tasks that require similar processing structures will make greater demands on executive control and will lead to a decrement in performance (Baddeley, 1986). We have tested the idea that PFC is an important neural substrate of executive control by using fMRI to determine whether activation of PFC would be observed while normal human subjects performed a dual-task experiment (D'Esposito et al., 1995). During scanning, subjects concurrently performed a spatial task (mental rotation of visual stimuli) and a verbal task (semantic judgments of auditory stimuli), cognitive challenges that were selected because they have been reported to activate predominantly posterior brain regions (i.e., not PFC regions). We reasoned that any activation in PFC regions would be due to the dual-task nature of the experiment and not to performance of either of the individual tasks per se. Our study did in fact demonstrate lateral PFC activation only during the dual-task condition, and not during either single-task condition.

Another study, utilizing PET, also explored the neural basis of executive control with a dual-task paradigm (Goldberg et al., 1998). Normal subjects were scanned while they performed two cognitive tasks, both individually and simultaneously. One task was the Wisconsin Card Sorting Test (WCST), a complex reasoning task, and the other was a rapidly paced auditory verbal shadowing task. A major difference between this dual-task study, and the one used by D'Esposito et al. (1995), is that one of the cognitive tasks, the WCST, activated PFC when performed individually. When the two tasks were performed simultaneously, there were significant decrements in performance compared with the individual task performance scores, as had been expected. There was less PFC activation under the dual-task condition, however, in contrast to when the WCST was performed separately. These results suggest that under circumstances in which the capacity of executive control is exceeded, cortical activity in PFC may be attenuated. Consideration of these results with those of D'Esposito et al. (1995) leads to a hypothesis that under dual-task conditions, PFC activity may increase to meet the processing demands, up to some level of asymptote, before attenuating. The Goldberg et al. study did not parametrically vary task demands during dual-task performance, however, and thus did not address this hypothesis.

Another PET study has also attempted to assess the neural correlates of deterioration of performance during concurrent performance of two tasks (Klingberg, 1998). In this study, subjects were scanned during performance of an auditory working-memory task, a visual working-memory task, during performance of both tasks, and during a control task. Unlike the D'Esposito et al. (1995) study but similar to the Goldberg et al. (1998) study, each of the single tasks, as compared to the control task, activated PFC. During the dual-task condition, there was no distinct region within PFC (or any other cortical regions) that was activated only in the dual task. Klingberg argued that these results are consistent with the hypothesis that concurrent tasks interfere with each other if they demand activation of the same part of cortex. This conclusion is supported by an earlier study by this group in which it was found that the larger the extent of overlap in the activation of two tasks when performed individually, the greater the decrement in behavioral performance when these two tasks are performed concurrently outside the scanner (Klingberg & Roland, 1997). From the results of the 1998 study, Klingberg also argued that there was not a distinct PFC region which could be associated with any dual-task-specific cognitive process, such as task coordination or divided attention. This evidence does not, of course, rule out the possibility that the PFC supports cognitive operations unique to dual-task performance (e.g., task coordination and shifting attention) as well as working-memory operations, such as active maintenance and rehearsal. In fact, evidence that many different types of distinct operations may engage the PFC will be discussed below.

Studies of patients with frontal injury (McDowell, 1997; Baddeley, 1986) have demonstrated that despite performing comparably to healthy control subjects under single-task conditions, performance of the patients with PFC lesions was significantly inferior to control subject performance under dual-task conditions. Taken together, imaging and behavioral studies with patients provide converging evidence for an association between executive control and PFC function. These data cannot, however, support or refute the notion that a "system" or "controller module" lying within PFC mediates these executive processes. An important issue for future research will be to determine the neural basis of different executive control processes by using paradigms that can more precisely isolate such processes with less complex cognitive paradigms. Such studies will be reviewed in the "Current Issues" section, below.

The Issue of Task Difficulty, Mental Effort, and PFC Function

The issue of task difficulty often arises when interpreting the results of imaging studies of working memory. For example, in the dual-task studies described above, it can be argued that the dual-task condition will always be more difficult than either task condition performed alone. In fact, most tasks that are designed to engage working memory are more difficult and lead to poorer behavioral performance than the corresponding control tasks. Thus, in imaging studies of working memory it seems necessary to eliminate the possibility that PFC activation was simply due to a nonspecific increase in mental effort. We addressed this issue in our dual-task study (D'Esposito, et al., 1995) by having subjects perform the spatial task alone, but at different levels of difficulty. Even during the more difficult condition, when performance was worse than that for the spatial task performed during the dual-task condition, we did not observe any PFC activation. This finding suggested that the PFC activation observed during the dual-task experiment was related specifically to the executive control process required to organize and execute two tasks simultaneously.

Barch and colleagues (1997) have directly addressed this issue and have been able to dissociate working memory from task difficulty in PFC. This study utilized a continuous performance task during which subjects were required to observe a sequence of letters and respond to an X only when it was followed by an A. A factorial design was used with two levels of memory (short versus long delay between cue and the probe) and two levels of difficulty (perceptually degraded versus nondegraded stimuli). This task was ideal to test the issue of task difficulty because behavioral performance was equated between memory conditions (i.e., comparable performance between short delay and long delay conditions) but was significantly worse in the degraded conditions. Thus, task difficulty was increased independently of working-memory demands. The imaging results revealed a region with dorsolateral PFC that showed significantly greater activity in the long, as compared to the short, delay condition, but did not show greater activity as a function of the difficulty manipulation. In contrast, anterior cingulate showed more activity on the more difficult task conditions, but did not show greater activation during the manipulation of the delay period. Thus, a double dissociation between regions responsive to working-memory demands versus task difficulty was demonstrated. Future studies, using event-related designs, can address the issue of task difficulty more directly within each experiment by assessing the differential neural response to correct versus incorrect behavioral responses.

The Specificity of PFC for Working Memory

Single-unit recording studies in monkeys during delayed-response tasks have also observed PFC neurons that are active during periods in addition to the delay period. For example, PFC neurons have been shown to respond during any combination of cue, delay, and response periods (Funahashi et al., 1989; Fuster et al., 1982). Although delay-specific neurons are most common, other types are frequently identified. Thus, the PFC appears to be involved in nonmnemonic processes that may include stimulus encoding, sustained attention to stimuli, preparation for a motor response, and the motor response itself. Most human functional imaging studies of working memory that use cognitive subtraction methodology have not emphasized the role of PFC in nonmnemonic cognitive processes, and sometimes suggest that PFC is specific for working memory. Moreover, the interpretation of some functional imaging studies of other cognitive domains (language, visuoperception) have relied upon posthoc interpretations of observed PFC activation by their task as being due to the engagement of working-memory processes (Cohen et al., 1996; Cuenod et al., 1995). Such an interpretation tacitly assumes that PFC is specific for working memory. The demonstration that the same PFC region activated during tasks which engage working memory is also recruited during nonmnemonic processes would dispute this assumption. In light of the results of the monkey electrophysiological studies cited above, it seems that this pattern of PFC activation would be observed in humans as well. In fact, there are several lines of evidence to support the claim that the PFC is not specific for working memory.

Functional neuroimaging studies of working memory that utilize blocked designs are typically conducted by comparing the signal during a task proposed to engage working memory to a "control" task which does not engage this construct. Since these control tasks are designed not to require working memory, the control task compared to a resting baseline would be a logical candidate for testing the hypothesis that PFC regions which demonstrate activation associated with working memory also display activation in association with nonmnemonic processes. In one such study (D'Esposito, Ballard, et al., 1998), during fMRI scanning, subjects performed a three-condition experiment (working-memory task, non-working-memory task, rest). In the working-memory task, subjects observed serially presented stimuli and determined if each stimulus was the same as that presented two stimuli back (the 2-back task). The non-working-memory task in one experiment required subjects to identify a single predetermined stimulus; in another experiment, subjects were required to make a button press to every stimulus. In all subjects in both experiments, the working-memory task exhibited greater PFC cortical activity compared to the non-working-memory task. In these *same* PFC regions, significantly greater activation was also observed during both non-working-memory tasks compared to rest. This idea is consistent with the idea that human lateral PFC supports processes in addition to working memory. Thus, in this study, the reverse inference of the form "if prefrontal cortex is active, working memory is engaged" was not supported.

McCarthy and colleagues (1994, 1996) have studied similar detection tasks, along with working-memory tasks. Lateral PFC was activated in a spatial working-memory task, as well as during two control tasks (detection of a dot in an object or detection of a red object) relative to a resting baseline. The strength of activation during these detection tasks was noted to be approximately half (and sometimes approaching) the magnitude observed in the working-memory task.

Finally, if we revisit the spatial working-memory experiment performed with an event-related design described above (Zarahn et al., 1999), it can be seen clearly (figure 9.3 left panel, showing fMRI signal) that there is significant activity above baseline in a region of the PFC that displayed activity above baseline even during trials without a delay period. Data from Courtney et al. (1997) demonstrate this point as well. In two of the PFC activated regions (areas labeled 4 and 5) there is some contribution by the nonselective visual stimulation task component (figure 9.4A) in addition to the contribution made by the memory task component. Thus, each of the studies described does not support models that posit neural substrates subserving memory-specific processing, but rather is supportive of models which posit that memory is a property of neural networks which also mediate perceptuomotor processes (Fuster, 1995).

ISSUES

Does Human Prefrontal Cortex Have Functional Subdivisions?

While the evidence presented above suggests that the PFC appears to be critical for the processing of temporarily stored information, it is unclear whether there are functional subdivisions within the PFC which are specialized for particular aspects of working memory. The frontal lobes comprise a large proportion of the cerebral cortex, and PFC represents the largest portion of the frontal lobes. Each of the studies highlighted above has demonstrated activation in lateral PFC. Within lateral PFC, activation has been seen in dorsal portions (Brodmann's areas 9 and 46) as well as ventral portions (Brodmann's areas 44, 45, 47). Medial aspects of the PFC as well as the orbitofrontal cortex have not been consistently activated in working-memory tasks.

There are at least four ways to conceptualize how the operations subserved by the PFC might be organized neuroanatomically (see figure 9.5). First, the PFC as a whole may be involved in all working-memory processes (e.g., simple maintenance operations such as rehearsal, and more complex operations such as retrieval, reordering, performing spatial transformations, etc.) that can be directed at distributed representations in posterior brain regions (model 1). Second, there may be different PFC regions for the temporary maintenance of different types of representations (e.g.,

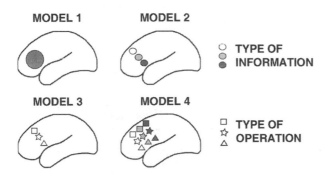

Figure 9.5
Models of prefrontal cortical organization.

spatial, object), regardless of operation (model 2). Third, there may be different PFC regions required for different operations (e.g., maintenance, manipulation), regardless of the type of representation (model 3). Finally, there may be different PFC regions required for either the type of operation or the type of representation (model 4).

Organization by Content?   Goldman-Rakic and colleagues have proposed that the different regions of the PFC are critical for the temporary maintenance of different types of information. Specifically, they have provided evidence that monkey PFC is segregated into one region that retains information about an object's color and shape (ventrolateral PFC) and a second region that retains the object's location in space (dorsolateral PFC) (Wilson et al., 1993). This view is derived from evidence from recording of neurons within a more ventral region, the inferior prefrontal convexity, while monkeys performed spatial-delayed or pattern-delayed response tasks, and from finding that a greater number of neurons in this region responded selectively during the delay period to pattern rather than to location information. Also, lesions comprising the dorsal PFC have been shown to impair spatial working memory (Funahashi et al., 1993; Gross, 1963), whereas other studies reveal impaired non-spatial working memory following more ventral lesions (Mishkin & Manning, 1978; Passingham, 1975).

These findings have led to the hypothesis that lateral PFC is organized in a dorsal/ventral fashion subserving the temporary storage of "what" and "where" information. This hypothesis has the appeal of parsimony, because a similar organization has been identified in the visual system (Ungerleider & Haxby, 1994). Also, anatomical studies in monkeys have demonstrated that parietal cortex (spatial vision regions) projects predominantly to a dorsal region of lateral PFC (Cavada & Goldman-Rakic, 1989; Petrides & Pandya, 1984), whereas temporal cortex (object vision regions) projects more ventrally within lateral PFC (Barbas, 1988).

Functional neuroimaging studies have been able to address this question in humans by determining the pattern of PFC activity during spatial and nonspatial working-memory tasks. Because many such studies have been conducted, we critically examined this literature for evidence for or against the "what" versus "where" model of PFC organization (D'Esposito, Aguirre, et al., 1998). In our review, we plotted the locations of activations from all reported functional neuroimaging studies of spatial and nonspatial working memory on a standardized brain. Based on the animal literature, it is proposed that the human homologue of the principal sulcal region of lateral PFC, the middle frontal gyrus (Brodmann's area 9/46) would subserve spatial working memory, whereas nonspatial working memory would be subserved by a more ventral region, the inferior frontal gyrus (Brodmann's areas 47, 44, 45). In

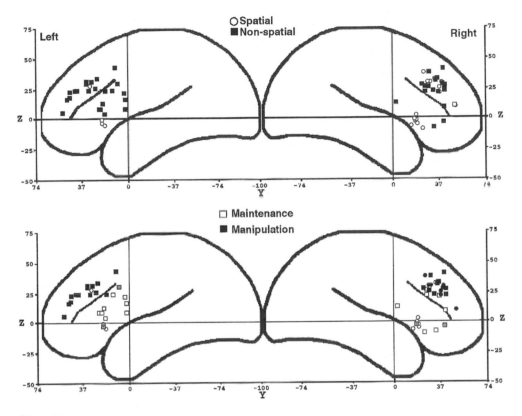

Figure 9.6
Meta-analysis of published functional neuroimaging studies of working memory. Each square represents a significant activation reported in a standardized atlas (Talairach & Tournoux, 1988). Top panel shows activations from either spatial or nonspatial studies; bottom panel reports activations from the same studies reclassified as requiring maintenance or manipulation processes.

this review, we found no evidence for a clear dorsal/ventral dissociation of activation based on the type of information being held in working memory. As illustrated in figure 9.6, there are numerous spatial working-memory studies that have demonstrated activation within ventral PFC and, likewise, nonspatial working-memory studies that have demonstrated activation within dorsal PFC.

In nearly every study reviewed in the above analysis, either spatial or nonspatial working memory was examined within each subject, but not both types of working memory. In an empirical study, we have tested subjects during two different working-memory tasks with different sets of stimuli during fMRI. In the memory condition, subjects attended to serially presented stimuli and determined if a letter or location of a square was the same as that presented two stimuli back. In the control condition, subjects were asked to identify a single predetermined letter or location. Group and individual subject analyses revealed activation in right middle frontal gyrus that did not differ between spatial and nonspatial working memory conditions. Again, these data do not support a dorsal/ventral organization of PFC based on the type of information held in working memory.

Other investigators using virtually identical n-back tasks have found similar results (Owen et al., 1998; Postle et al., 2000). In the Owen study, the spatial 2-back task used required memory for one of three locations that were highlighted by filling in a white box. To equate for difficulty, the nonspatial memory task was performed as a 1-back task and used abstract patterns for stimuli. In the Postle et al. study, the nonspatial 2-back task used Attneave shapes as stimuli that each look distinctive (Attneave & Arnoult, 1956) and were difficult to verbalize (Vanderplas & Garvin, 1959). The spatial 2-back task used identical black circles or Attneave shapes as stimuli in nine different spatial locations on the screen. The results of this study are presented in figure 9.7 (top panel; see also color plate 19). Using a task similar to the 2-back task but with less frequent targets, McCarthy et al. (1996) found that both the spatial (a single square stimulus in 20 different locations) and nonspatial (irregular shapes) conditions activated dorsal PFC, with a ventral extension of the activation in the left hemisphere in the nonspatial task. Since these tasks were not directly compared statistically, it is unclear if an actual difference in the spatial extent of activation between conditions exists.

Four other studies compared spatial and nonspatial working memory tasks; none of these studies found a dorsal/ventral distinction of activation within PFC (Baker et al., 1996; Belger et al., 1998; Smith et al., 1995, 1996). However, in each of these studies there was a suggestion of a hemispheric dissociation between spatial and nonspatial working memory (i.e., greater right PFC activation in spatial paradigms and greater left PFC activation in nonspatial paradigms). These hemispheric differences were found during performance of delayed-response tasks comparing spatial stimuli to nonspatial stimuli—letters (Smith et al., 1996) and objects (Baker et al., 1996; Belger et al., 1998; Smith et al., 1995)—as well as during spatial and nonspatial n-back tasks (Smith et al., 1996). It is important to note that the lateralization of PFC during the n-back task found by Smith and Jonides has not been found in other laboratories (D'Esposito, Aguirre, et al., 1998; Owen et al., 1998; Postle et al., 2000).

Data from one laboratory stand out as an exception to the group of studies presented above in which a dorsal/ventral organization based on the type of information being held in working memory was found (Courtney et al., 1996, 1998). In an initial blocked-design PET study of delayed-response tasks using faces and locations of faces

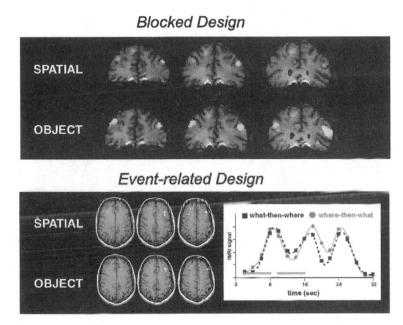

Figure 9.7
(*Top*) Data from a blocked design fMRI experiment by Postle et al. (2000) showing nearly identical bilateral PFC activation associated with spatial and object working memory in an individual subject. (*Bottom*) Data from an event-related fMRI experiment from Postle, D'Esposito et al. (1999) study showing activation maps displaying suprathreshold activity in spatial and object delay periods in dorsolateral PFC in a single subject, illustrating the marked degree of overlap in PFC activity in the two conditions. The graph to the right shows the trial-averaged time series extracted from dorsolateral PFC voxels with object delay-period activity. Again, note the similarity of fMRI signal intensity changes in spatial and object delay periods. (See color plate 19.)

as stimuli (Courtney et al., 1996), it was found that a direct comparison of the two memory conditions revealed that the spatial working-memory task resulted in greater activation within left superior frontal sulcus (Brodmann's areas 8/6), and the face working-memory task resulted in greater activation of right ventral PFC (areas 9/45/46). A confusing finding of this study was that the spatial working-memory task did not produce PFC activation relative to a control task. In a follow-up study using an event-related fMRI design (Courtney et al., 1998), a double dissociation was found between face and spatial working memory. It was observed that within superior frontal sulcus in both hemispheres, there was significantly more sustained activity during spatial than during face working-memory delays. By contrast, left inferior frontal cortex showed significantly more sustained activity during face than during spatial working-memory delays. A particular strength of this study is that a subset of subjects performed a visually guided saccade task, and it was demonstrated that the region which was active during the spatial working-memory delay period was anterior and superior (by approximately 8.5 mm) to the frontal eye fields active during the saccade task. Interestingly, this is the only study of working memory for different types of information in which the nonspatial stimuli used was faces, which may be an important determinant contributing to the dissociation that was found.

We have performed a study using event-related fMRI that examined the neural correlates of the maintenance of spatial versus nonspatial information. Our study differed from Courtney et al. (1998) in that our nonspatial stimuli were objects (Attneave shapes) and we employed a task with a "what-then-where" design, with an object and a spatial delay period incorporated in each trial (see figure 9.7, bottom panel). This task was adapted from a monkey electrophysiology study by Miller and colleagues which provided evidence that there was extensive overlap in "what" and "where" neurons within lateral PFC without a clear segregation (Rao et al., 1997). Similar to this monkey study, even when we modeled only the delay period (similar to Zarahn et al., 1999, discussed above), identical regions of PFC were activated when subjects remembered spatial or object information. Reliable spatial/object differences in the delay period were observed, in contrast, in posterior cortical regions (Postle & D'Esposito, 1999). In fact, these data are consistent with earlier single-unit recording studies of dorsal and ventral regions within lateral PFC during delayed-response tasks that found a mixed population of neurons in both regions which are not clearly segregated by the type of information (i.e., spatial versus nonspatial) being stored (Fuster et al., 1982; Quintana et al., 1988; Rao et al., 1997; Rosenkilde et al., 1981). Other evidence that does not support a dorsal/ventral what/where organization of PFC is that cooling (Bauer & Fuster, 1976; Fuster & Bauer, 1974; Quintana & Fuster, 1993) and lesions of a dorsal region of lateral PFC cause impairments on nonspatial working-memory tasks (Mishkin et al., 1969; Petrides, 1995), and ventral lesions in lateral PFC cause spatial impairments (Butters et al., 1973; Iversen & Mishkin, 1970; Mishkin et al., 1969). Finally, a paper has found that ventral PFC lesions in monkeys did not cause delay-dependent defects on a visual pattern association task and a color-matching task (Rushworth et al., 1997). A critical review of these issues can be found in a paper by Rushworth and Owen (1998). Clearly, further work will be necessary to reconcile the different findings from animal and human studies to determine if the active maintenance of different types of information is subserved by distinct regions of the lateral PFC.

Organization by Process?   Another possible axis along which human lateral PFC may be organized is according to the type of operations performed upon information being stored in working memory rather than the type of information being temporarily stored. Petrides has proposed a two-stage model in which there are two processing systems, one dorsal and the other ventral, within lateral PFC (Petrides, 1994). It is proposed that ventral PFC (Brodmann's areas 45/47) is the site where information is initially received from posterior association areas and where active comparisons of information held in working memory are made. In contrast, dorsal PFC (areas 9/46) is recruited only when active manipulation/monitoring within working memory is required.

To test this alternative hypothesis of PFC organization, we again analyzed the data derived from previously reported working-memory functional neuroimaging studies. We divided all working-memory tasks according to the conditions under which information is being temporarily maintained, rather than according to the type of information being maintained. For example, delayed-response tasks require a subject to maintain information across a *nondistracted* delay period. To achieve accurate performance on this type of task, no additional processing of the stored information is necessary except for its maintenance across a delay period that has no distracting stimuli. Thus, a delayed-response task, engaging "maintenance" processes, should recruit ventral PFC, according to Petrides's model. Alternatively, all other working-memory tasks reported in the literature require either (1) reshuffling of the information being temporarily maintained and/or (2) processing of intervening stimuli during the maintenance of stored information. For example, in self-ordered tasks, subjects must update in working memory each stimulus that they choose, in order to pick a new stimulus correctly (Petrides et al., 1993). The continuous nature of the n-back tasks requires constant reshuffling of the contents held in working memory because different stimuli are simultaneously being stored, inhibited, and dropped from memory (Cohen et al., 1994). Finally, other tasks, such as one in which subjects must compare the first and last notes of an eight-note melody (Zattore et al., 1994), simply require the maintenance of information across a distracted delay. Thus, these types of tasks, engaging "manipulation" processes as well as "maintenance" processes, should additionally recruit dorsal PFC, according to Petrides's model. We thus made an operational distinction between two general types of working-memory tasks used in neuroimaging studies: *maintenance* and *manipulation* tasks.

When all locations of lateral PFC activation reported in the literature are plotted onto a standardized brain according to this classification of tasks as either *maintenance* or *manipulation*, a dorsal/ventral dissociation becomes evident (see bottom panel of figure 9.6), supporting the Petrides model. This model derived initial support from an empirical PET study performed by Owen and colleagues (1996), in which they found dorsal PFC activation during three spatial working memory tasks thought to require greater manipulation/monitoring of remembered information than two other memory tasks, which activated only ventral PFC. Several other functional neuroimaging studies also appear to support Petrides's hypothesis. In a PET study, a running memory task, thought to require updating of the contents in working memory, was compared to a letter span task that did not require such a process (Salmon et al., 1996). When compared directly, greater activation in the running memory task was found in right dorsal PFC (area 9), and to a lesser extent in left dorsal PFC. The letter span task activated only ventral PFC. In another PET study that compared a simple delayed matching task (match a color or pattern) versus a more complex delayed matching task (alternate between matching colors and patterns), only the latter task activated the right dorsal PFC but both tasks activated ventral PFC (Klingberg et al., 1997).

We have tested this process-specific organization of PFC using event-related fMRI (D'Esposito et al., 1999). In our study, subjects were presented two types of trials in random order, in which they were required to either (1) *maintain* a sequence of letters across a delay period or (2) *manipulate* (alphabetize) this sequence during the delay in order to respond correctly to a probe. Similar to the spatial working-memory study described above, we identified brain activity related to the three periods of our task: stimulus presentation, delay, and response. In each subject, activity during the delay period was found in both dorsal and ventral PFC in both types of trials. However, dorsal PFC activity was greater in trials during which information held in working memory was manipulated (figure 9.8). These findings suggest that dorsal PFC may exhibit greater recruitment during conditions where additional processing of information held in working memory is required, and support a process-specific organization of PFC.

A challenge for the further development of the hypothesis that human lateral PFC is organized by processing requirements is determining the psychological constructs

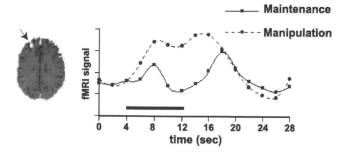

Figure 9.8
Trial averaged time series from voxels within PFC that were significant in the manipulation-maintenance direct contrast. Note the two peaks in the *maintenance* condition corresponding to the stimulus presentation and the probe periods of the trial, whereas in the *manipulation* condition the voxel maintained a high level of activity throughout the delay period. The solid black bar represents the duration of the delay period of the behavioral task.

which differ between tasks that activate dorsal versus ventral PFC. Certainly, there are many possible component processes that may be necessary in tasks which activate dorsal PFC. The component processes that we have labeled "manipulation" will need to be determined. Also, if lateral PFC is functionally subdivided, it will also be important to determine if it is organized hierarchically, with information passing from ventral to dorsal PFC. If a hierarchical organization does exist, it is expected that those tasks which we classified as *manipulation* tasks would activate ventral as well as dorsal PFC.

Two studies have shown that dorsal PFC is recruited during performance of tasks with no overt requirements to manipulate information held in working memory but under increased load conditions (Manoach et al., 1997; Rypma, Prabhakaran, et al., 1999). For example, Rypma et al. observed activation in dorsal PFC in a Sternberg-type item recognition task in which subjects were required to maintain one, three, or six letters in working memory for 5 sec. When subjects were required to maintain three letters in working memory, relative to one letter, activation in frontal regions was limited to left ventral PFC (BA 44). However, when subjects were required to maintain six letters, relative to one letter, additional activation of dorsal PFC was observed, similar to studies in which successful performance required the manipulation of information held in working memory (e.g., D'Esposito et al., 1999; Owen et al., 1996). Two possibilities exist to explain these findings. First, dorsal and ventral PFC may be involved in active maintenance processes, but only dorsal PFC is involved during the manipulation of information. This idea is consistent with the findings by D'Esposito et al.: that the maintenance and manipulation of information during an alphabetization task was directly examined. Alternatively, under conditions during which subjects must actively maintain loads of information that approach or exceed their capacity, dorsal PFC is additionally recruited for the mediation of strategic processes necessary for the maintenance of a high load of information.

Delayed-response tasks like the ones employed by Rypma et al. (1999) and Manoach et al. (1997) involve several component processes for the encoding, retention, and retrieval of information. Since these were blocked designs, it is possible that the recruitment of dorsal PFC observed under conditions of high memory load may have been due to differential recruitment (compared to the low memory load condition) of processes engaged during any or all of these task periods. Thus, we subsequently performed a study using event-related fMRI that allowed us to examine brain activity which correlated with individual components of the task (*encoding*, *delay*, and *response*) in dorsal and ventral PFC while subjects maintained either two or six items in working memory across an unfilled delay period (Rypma & D'Esposito, 1999).

Effects of increased memory load, lateralized to right hemisphere, were observed only in dorsal PFC in the *encoding* period. This result suggests that dorsal PFC plays a greater role in initial encoding of information for subsequent retrieval and not necessarily during the maintenance of such information. It may be that initial encoding of information requires cognitive operations (e.g., monitoring the contents of working memory, updating and coordination of multiple memory buffers) similar to those required in the more complex tasks discussed above.

In summary, the studies reviewed suggest that PFC has functional subdivisions which may be organized by the type of information held in working memory as well as by the type of operation performed on this information. Regarding organization by content, one research group found a dorsal PFC (spatial) vs. ventral PFC (faces) difference in the pattern of activation, whereas other groups have found a hemispheric effect (left PFC, objects; right PFC, spatial). Working-memory tasks that engage "manipulation" processes have consistently found greater activation in dorsal PFC, relative to ventral PFC, regardless of the type of information being maintained and manipulated. Although more work is clearly necessary, these findings represent a significant step toward understanding the functional organization of PFC.

The Role of Non-PFC Regions in Working Memory

This chapter has extensively reviewed the role of the PFC in working memory, and possible ways in which the PFC may be functionally subdivided to support working memory. However, working memory is clearly a complex cognitive system that relies on posterior, as well as anterior, cortical regions. It is likely that subcortical structures such as the basal ganglia and thalamus also play critical roles in this network. Methods have been developed to allow for the study of the interactions among several brain regions within a functional network subserving a cognitive system such as working memory (McIntosh et al., 1996). Such studies, reviewed in another chapter in this volume, will provide a means for extending the knowledge obtained from the activation studies reviewed in this chapter. Finally, in a review of a large number of working-memory studies mentioned above (D'Esposito, Aguirre, et al., 1998), two other cortical regions are consistently activated during tasks that require working memory: lateral and medial premotor areas (Brodmann's area 6 and area 8) and posterior parietal cortex (Brodmann's area 40/7).

Posterior Parietal Cortex   Like PFC, posterior parietal cortex is an area of multimodal association cortex (Mesulam, 1985), that is, it receives from, and projects to, other primary and unimodal association areas all modalities of information (somatosensory, auditory, visual). Smith and Jonides (1998) have emphasized the role of parietal cortex in storage processes in contrast to maintenance/rehearsal processes thought to be subserved by the PFC. In a study of verbal working memory by Awh et al. (1996), an n-back task was designed to separate the brain regions underlying storage and rehearsal. As previously described, the memory condition requires subjects to determine whether or not a letter presented is identical to one presented two letters previously in a sequence. In a "search" control condition, subjects are required to identify a predetermined stimulus (the letter M). In a "rehearsal" control condition, subjects engage in silent rehearsal by repeating each letter silently to themselves until the next letter appears. In this blocked, cognitive subtraction paradigm, it was reasoned that subtraction of the search control condition from the memory condition would reveal activation in brain regions involved in both phonological storage and rehearsal, whereas subtraction of the rehearsal control condition from the memory condition would reveal regions involved only in phonological storage. Finally, by inference, in comparison to the first subtraction, regions involved in rehearsal could be identified as well. These series of subtractions suggested that left ventral PFC (Brodmann's area 44, Broca's area) and premotor areas are involved in subvocal rehearsal (since they did not appear in the [memory–rehearsal] comparison), and posterior parietal cortex participates in phonological storage (since it remained in the [memory–rehearsal] comparison and was also present in the [memory–search] comparison). A similar conclusion was drawn from an earlier PET study of verbal working memory in which subjects performed a delayed response task with letters as stimuli (Paulesu et al., 1993).

A study by Fiez et al. (1996) appeared to contradict the above findings because they failed to find parietal activation when scanning with PET during the retention interval of a task that required the encoding of five words or nonwords and retrieval after scanning of the 40 sec retention interval. These results considered the possibility that parietal activation was actually due to encoding or retrieval processes rather than to storage processes. Jonides and colleagues (1998) subsequently addressed this question directly. These investigators provided behavioral evidence that Fiez et al. (1996) may not have found evidence for parietal activation because their imaging data were heavily influenced by storage of semantic, rather than phonological, representations. Based on empirical PET data using a delayed-response task with only nonwords as stimuli (thus decreasing the likelihood of storing this information in a semantic code), they demonstrated posterior parietal activation during the storage condition, These investigators proposed that left posterior parietal cortex, which is active in most verbal working-memory tasks, is specific to phonological coding and storage. An important finding consistent with this proposal is that patients with verbal working-memory deficits which are abnormal when storing phonological codes are normal when storing semantic and visual codes (Saffran & Marian, 1975; Warrington et al., 1971).

We have recently provided additional evidence that posterior cerebral regions are critical for memory storage by employing an event-related fMRI design (Postle et al., 1999). We used an item-recognition experiment that required memory for the identity and position in the display of either of two letters or five letters (to identify load-sensitive regions), or memory for the identity and position in the alphabet of any of five letters (to identify manipulation-sensitive regions). In each subject, voxels in the left perisylvian cortex showed load, but not manipulation, sensitivity; and regions of PFC in all subjects showed the opposite pattern. This double dissociation provides additional evidence for a role of posterior perisylvian regions in storage processes and also highlights the differential role of this region from PFC. More work is clearly necessary to investigate the functional heterogeneity of posterior parietal cortex, which has evolved as a region as important for working memory function as the PFC.

Premotor Areas   Lateral premotor cortex is consistently activated in working-memory tasks. The location of activation is typically within the precentral sulcus (see D'Esposito, Aguirre, et al., 1998, for review) and likely lies within the frontal eye fields (FEF). Penfield and Boldrey (1937), using electrical stimulation, defined the FEF as the cortex lying around the precentral sulcus at the level of the middle frontal gyrus. Humans with lesions in this region have impaired visually guided (Rivaud et al., 1994) and memory-guided saccades (Pierrot-Deseilligny et al., 1991). Moreover, several PET studies have observed activation in the region around precentral sulcus during voluntary saccades (Anderson et al., 1994; Fox et al., 1985; Sweeney et al., 1996). In the Courtney et al. (1998) study, reviewed earlier, evidence was provided that there are actually two distinct regions within this area surrounding the precentral sulcus: one region that correlates with the retention delay of the memory task and one region that correlates with saccades. Although there may be a distinct region anterior to the FEF involved in temporary maintenance of spatial information, it is possible that the spatial information coded in the FEF is involved in some aspect of memory as well. Some FEF neurons display sustained activity during the delay of memory-guided saccade tasks in nonhuman primates (Bruce & Goldberg, 1985). Also, lesions within the FEF in monkeys (Deng et al., 1986) and humans (Pierrot-Deseilligny et al., 1991) have been shown to impair memory-guided saccades. Finally, increased FEF activity in PET studies of memory-guided saccades occurs even during a comparison with a visually guided saccade control task (Sweeney et al., 1996).

The role of medial premotor areas in working memory has been extensively reviewed by Petit and colleagues (1998). In this study, two regions of interest were examined: dorsomedial PFC that comprises supplementary motor area (SMA) and anterior cingulate cortex (ACC). In an earlier review of the function of these regions, Picard and Strick (1996) proposed that the SMA can be subdivided into the SMA proper, which subserves basic spatial and temporal organization of movement, and a more anterior region, pre-SMA, which subserves additional cognitive demands, such as selection of and preparation for a motor response. Likewise, ACC can be subdivided into a caudal cingulate area that subserves simple motor functions, and a more anterior cingulate area that subserves more complex motor functions. By first identifying the SMA proper and the cingulate motor area by simple motor movements, Petit et al. were able to demonstrate that the location of sustained activity over working memory delays during both spatial and face working-memory tasks was within two distinct areas, pre-SMA and the anterior portion of the ACC. Since these areas were identified by a contrast between sustained activity during working-memory delays as compared with sustained activity during control delays in which subjects were waiting for a cue to make a simple manual motor response, it suggests that the activation of these regions does not reflect simple motor preparation, but rather a state of preparedness for selecting a motor response based on the information held on-line.

Summary

Elucidation of the cognitive and neural architectures underlying human working memory was an important focus of cognitive neuroscience for much of the 1990s. One conclusion that arises from this research is that working memory, a faculty which enables temporary storage and manipulation of information in the service of behavioral goals, can be viewed as neither a unitary nor a dedicated system. Data from numerous imaging studies have been reviewed and have demonstrated that the PFC is critical for several component processes of working memory, such as executive control and active maintenance. Moreover, it appears that the PFC has functional subdivisions which are organized by both the type of information being temporarily maintained and the type of operations performed on this information. In addition to the PFC, other brain regions, such as premotor areas and posterior parietal association cortex, comprise a functional network that may subserve other component processes of working memory function, such as selecting motor responses based on information held-on-line, and on storage processes. Numerous questions remain regarding the neural basis of this complex cognitive system, but imaging studies such as those reviewed in this chapter should continue to provide converging evidence for such questions.

ACKNOWLEDGMENTS

Research was supported by the Charles A. Dana Foundation, the American Federation for Aging Research, and NIH grants NS 01762, AG 09399, and AG 13483.

REFERENCES

Anderson, T. J., Jenkins, I. H., Brooks, D. J., Hawken, M. B., Frackowiak, R. S. J., & Kennard, C. (1994). Cortical control of saccades and fixation in man: A PET study. *Brain* 117, 1073–1084.

Attneave, F., & Arnoult, M. D. (1956). Methodological considerations in the quantitative study of shape and pattern perception. *Psychological Bulletin* 53, 221–227.

Awh, E., Jonides, J., Smith, E. E., Schumacher, E. H., Koeppe, R. A., & Katz, S. (1996). Dissociation of storage and rehearsal in verbal working memory: Evidence from PET. *Psychological Science* 7, 25–31.

Baddeley, A. (1986). *Working Memory*. New York: Oxford University Press.

Baddeley, A. (1998). The central executive: A concept and some misconceptions. *Journal of the International Neuropsychol Society* 4, 523–526.

Baker, S. C., Frith, C. D., Frackowiak, R. S. J., & Dolan, R. J. (1996). Active representation of shape and spatial location in man. *Cerebral Cortex* 6, 612–619.

Barbas, H. (1988). Anatomic organization of basoventral and mediodorsal visual recipient prefrontal regions in the rhesus monkey. *Journal of Comparative Neurology* 276, 313–342.

Barch, D. M., Braver, T. S., Nystrom, L. E., Forman, S. D., Noll, D. C., & Cohen, J. D. (1997). Dissociating working memory from task difficulty in human prefrontal cortex. *Neuropsychologia* 35, 1373–1380.

Bauer, R. H., & Fuster, J. M. (1976). Delayed-matching and delayed-response deficit from cooling dorsolateral prefrontal cortex in monkeys. *Journal of Comparative and Physiological Psychology* 90, 293–302.

Becker, J. T., Mintun, M. A., Diehl, D. J., Dobkin, J., Martidis, A., Madoff, D. C., & DeKosky, S. T. (1994). Functional neuroanatomy of verbal free recall: A replication study. *Human Brain Mapping* 1, 284–292.

Belger, A., Puce, A., Krystal, J. H., Gore, J. C., Goldman-Rakic, P., & McCarthy, G. (1998). Dissociation of mnemonic and perceptual processes during spatial and nonspatial working memory using fMRI. *Human Brain Mapping* 6, 14–32.

Boynton, G. M., Engel, S. A., Glover, G. H., & Heeger, D. J. (1996). Linear systems analysis of functional magnetic resonance imaging in human V1. *Journal of Neuroscience* 16, 4207–4221.

Brandt, S. A., Ploner, C. J., Meyer, B. U., Leistner, S., & Villringer, A. (1998). Effects of repetitive transcranial magnetic stimulation over dorsolateral prefrontal and posterior parietal cortex on memory-guided saccades. *Experimental Brain Research* 118, 197–204.

Bruce, C. J., & Goldberg, M. E. (1985). Primate frontal eye fields. I. Single neurons discharging before saccades. *Journal of Neurophysiology* 53, 603–635.

Butters, N., Butter, C., Rosen, J., & Stein, D. (1973). Behavioral effects of sequential and one-stage ablations of orbital prefrontal cortex in monkey. *Experimental Neurology* 39, 204–214.

Cavada, C., & Goldman-Rakic, P. S. (1989). Posterior parietal cortex in rhesus monkey: II. Evidence for segregated corticocortical networks linking sensory and limbic areas with frontal lobe. *Journal of Comparative Neurology* 287, 422–445.

Cohen, J. D., Forman, S. D., Braver, T. S., Casey, B. J., Servan-Schreiber, D., & Noll, D. C. (1994). Activation of prefrontal cortex in a nonspatial working memory task with functional MRI. *Human Brain Mapping* 1, 293–304.

Cohen, J. D., Perlstein, W. M., Braver, T. S., Nystrom, L. E., Noll, D. C., Jonides, J., & Smith, E. E. (1997). Temporal dynamics of brain activation during a working memory task. *Nature* 386, 604–607.

Cohen, J. D., & Servan-Schreiber, D. (1992). Context, cortex, and dopamine: A connectionist approach to behavior and biology in schizophrenia. *Psychological Review* 99, 45–77.

Cohen, M. S., Kosslyn, S. M., Breiter, H. C., DiGirolamo, G. J., Thompson, W. L., Anderson, A. K., Bookheimer, S. Y., Rosen, B. R., & Belliveau, J. W. (1996). Changes in cortical activity during mental rotation: A mapping study using functional MRI. *Brain* 119, 89–100.

Courtney, S. M., Petit, L., Maisog, J. M., Ungerleider, L. G., & Haxby, J. V. (1998). An area specialized for spatial working memory in human frontal cortex. *Science* 279, 1347–1351.

Courtney, S. M., Ungerleider, L. G., Keil, K., & Haxby, J. V. (1996). Object and spatial visual working memory activate separate neural systems in human cortex. *Cerebral Cortex* 6, 39–49.

Courtney, S. M., Ungerleider, L. G., Keil, K., & Haxby, J. V. (1997). Transient and sustained activity in a distributed neural system for human working memory. *Nature* 386, 608–611.

Cuenod, C. A., Bookheimer, S. Y., Hertz-Pannier, L., Zeffiro, T. A., Theodore, W. H., & Le Bihan, D. (1995). Functional MRI during word generation using conventional equipment: A potential tool for language localization in the clinical environment. *Neurology* 45, 1821–1827.

D'Esposito, M., Aguirre, G. K., Zarahn, E., & Ballard, D. (1998). Functional MRI studies of spatial and non-spatial working memory. *Cognitive Brain Research* 7, 1–13.

D'Esposito, M., Ballard, D., Aguirre, G. K., & Zarahn, E. (1998). Human prefrontal cortex is not specific for working memory: A functional MRI study. *NeuroImage* 8, 274–282.

D'Esposito, M., Detre, J. A., Alsop, D. C., Shin, R. K., Atlas, S., & Grossman, M. (1995). The neural basis of the central executive system of working memory. *Nature* 378, 279–281.

D'Esposito, M., & Postle, B. R. (1999). The dependence of span and delayed-response performance on the prefrontal cortex. *Neuropsychologia* 37, 1303–1315.

D'Esposito, M., Postle, B. R., Ballard, D., & Lease, J. (1999). Maintenance and manipulation of information held in working memory: An event-related fMRI study. *Brain and Cognition* 4, 66–86.

D'Esposito, M., Zarahn, E., & Aguirre, G. K. (1998). Event-related fMRI: Implications for cognitive psychology. *Psychological Bulletin* 125, 155–164.

Deng, S. Y., Goldberg, M. E., Segraves, M. A., Ungerleider, L. G., & Mishkin, M. (1986). The effect of unilateral ablation of the frontal eye fields on saccadic performance in the monkey. In *Advances in Biosciences: Adaptive Processes in Visual and Oculomotor Systems*, E. Keller & D. Zee, eds., 201–208. New York: Pergamon.

Fiez, J. A., Raife, E. A., Balota, D. A., Schwarz, J. P., Raichle, M. E., & Petersen, S. E. (1996). A positron emission tomography study of the short-term maintenance of verbal information. *Journal of Neuroscience* 16, 808–822.

Fox, P. T., Fox, J. M., Raichle, M. E., & Burde, R. M. (1985). The role of cerebral cortex in the generation of voluntary saccades: A positron emission study. *Journal of Neurophysiology* 54, 348–369.

Funahashi, S., Bruce, C. J., & Goldman-Rakic, P. S. (1989). Mnemonic coding of visual space in the monkey's dorsolateral prefrontal cortex. *Journal of Neurophysiology* 61, 331–349.

Funahashi, S., Bruce, C. J., & Goldman-Rakic, P. S. (1993). Dorsolateral prefrontal lesions and oculomotor delayed-response performance: Evidence for mnemonic "scotomas." *Journal of Neuroscience* 13, 1479–1497.

Fuster, J. (1997). *The Prefrontal Cortex: Anatomy, Physiology, and Neuropsychology of the Frontal Lobes*, 3rd ed. New York: Raven Press.

Fuster, J. M. (1995). *Memory in the Cerebral Cortex*. Cambridge, MA: MIT Press.

Fuster, J. M., & Alexander, G. E. (1971). Neuron activity related to short-term memory. *Science* 173, 652–654.

Fuster, J. M., & Bauer, R. H. (1974). Visual short-term memory deficit from hypothermia of frontal cortex. *Brain Research* 81, 393–400.

Fuster, J. M., Bauer, R. H., & Jervey, J. P. (1982). Cellular discharge in the dorsolateral prefrontal cortex of the monkey in cognitive tasks. *Experimental Neurology* 77, 679–694.

Goldberg, T. E., Berman, K. F., Fleming, K., Ostrem, J., Van Horn, J. D., Esposito, G., Mattay, V. S., Gold, J. M., & Weinberger, D. R. (1998). Uncoupling cognitive workload and prefrontal cortical physiology: A PET rCBF study. *NeuroImage* 7, 296–303.

Goldberg, T. E., Berman, K. F., Randolph, C., Gold, J. M., & Weinberger, D. R. (1996). Isolating the mnemonic component in spatial delayed response: A controlled PET 15O-labeled water regional cerebral blood flow study in normal humans. *NeuroImage* 3, 69–78.

Goldman-Rakic, P. S. (1987). Circuitry of the prefrontal cortex and the regulation of behavior by representational memory. In *Handbook of Physiology*, Sec 1, *The Nervous System*, vol 5, F. Plum & V. Mountcastle, eds., 373–417. Bethesda, MD: American Physiological Society.

Goldman-Rakic, P. S. (1996). Regional and cellular fractionation of working memory. *Proceedings of the National Academy of Sciences of the United States of America* 93, 13473–13480.

Gross, C. G. (1963). A comparison of the effects of partial and total lateral frontal lesions on test performance by monkeys. *Journal of Comparative and Physiological Psychology* 56, 41–47.

Iversen, S. D., & Mishkin, M. (1970). Perseverative interference in monkeys following selective lesions of the inferior prefrontal convexity. *Experimental Brain Research* 11, 376–386.

Jonides, J., Schumacher, E. H., Smith, E. E., Koeppe, R. A., Awh, E., Reuter-Lorenz, P. A., Marshuetz, C., & Willis, C. R. (1998). The role of parietal cortex in verbal working memory. *Journal of Neuroscience* 18, 5026–5034.

Jonides, J., Smith, E. E., Koeppe, R. A., Awh, E., Minoshima, S., & Mintum, M. (1993). Spatial working memory in humans as revealed by PET. *Nature* 363, 623–625.

Kimberg, D., & Farah, M. (1993). A unified account of cognitive impairments following frontal damage: The role of working memory in complex, organized behavior. *Journal of Experimental Psychology: Learning, Memory, and Cognition* 122, 411–428.

Klingberg, T. (1998). Concurrent performance of two working memory tasks: Potential mechanisms of interference. *Cerebral Cortex* 8, 593–601.

Klingberg, T., Kawashima, R., & Roland, P. E. (1996). Activation of multi-modal cortical areas underlies short-term memory. *European Journal of Neuroscience* 8, 1965–1971.

Klingberg, T., O'Sullivan, B. T., & Roland, P. E. (1997). Bilateral activation of fronto-parietal networks by incremental demand in a working memory task. *Cerebral Cortex* 7, 465–471.

Klingberg, T., & Roland, P. E. (1997). Interference between two concurrent tasks is associated with activation of overlapping fields in the cortex. *Cognitive Brain Research* 6, 1–8.

Manoach, D. S., Schlaug, G., Siewert, B., Darby, D. G., Bly, B. M., Benfield, A., Edelman, R. R., & Warach, S. (1997). Prefrontal cortex fMRI signal changes are correlated with working memory load. *NeuroReport* 8, 545–549.

McCarthy, G., Blamire, A. M., Puce, A., Nobre, A. C., Bloch, G., Hyder, F., Goldman-Rakic, P., & Shulman, R. G. (1994). Functional magnetic resonance imaging of human prefrontal cortex activation during a spatial working memory task. *Proceedings of the National Academy of Sciences USA* 91, 8690–8694.

McCarthy, G., Puce, A., Constable, R. T., Krystal, J. H., Gore, J. C., & Goldman-Rakic, P. (1996). Activation of human prefrontal cortex during spatial and nonspatial working tasks measured by functional MRI. *Cerebral Cortex* 6, 600–611.

McDowell, S., Whyte, J., & D'Esposito, M. (1997). Working memory impairments in traumatic brain injury: Evidence from a dual-task paradigm. *Neuropsychologia* 35, 1341–1353.

McIntosh, A. R., Grady, C. L., Haxby, J. V., Ungerleider, L. G., & Horwitz, B. (1996). Changes in limbic and prefrontal functional interactions in a working memory task for faces. *Cerebral Cortex* 6, 571–584.

Mesulam, M. M. (1985). *Principles of Behavioral Neurology*. Philadelphia: F. A. Davis.

Mishkin, M., & Manning, F. J. (1978). Non-spatial memory after selective prefrontal lesions in monkeys. *Brain Research* 143, 313–323.

Mishkin, M., Vest, B., Waxler, M., & Rosvold, H. E. (1969). A re-examination of the effects of frontal lesions on object alternation. *Neuropsychologia* 7, 357–363.

Muri, R. M., Vermersch, A. I., Rivaud, S., Gaymard, B., & Pierrot-Deseilligny, C. (1996). Effects of single-pulse transcranial magnetic stimulation over the pretrontal and posterior parietal cortices during memory guided saccades in humans. *Journal of Neurophysiology* 76, 2102–2106.

Norman, D. A., & Shallice, T. (1986). Attention to action: Willed and automatic control of behavior. In *Consciousness and Self-Regulation: Advances in Research and Theory*, R. J. Davidson, G. E. Schawartz, & D. Shapiro, eds., 1–18. New York: Plenum.

O'Sullivan, E. P., Jenkins, I. H., Henderson, L., Kennard, C., & Brooks, D. J. (1995). The functional anatomy of remembered saccades: A PET study. *NeuroReport* 6, 2141–2144.

Owen, A. M., Evans, A. C., & Petrides, M. (1996). Evidence for a two-stage model of spatial working memory processing within the lateral frontal cortex: A positron emission tomography study. *Cerebral Cortex* 6, 31–38.

Owen, A. M., Stern, C. E., Look, R. B., Tracey, I., Rosen, B. R., & Petrides, M. (1998). Functional organization of spatial and nonspatial working memory processing within the human lateral frontal cortex. *Proceedings of the National Academy of Sciences USA* 95, 7721–7726.

Pascual-Leone, A., & Hallett, M. (1994). Induction of errors in a delayed response task by repetitive transcranial magnetic stimulation of the dorsolateral prefrontal cortex. *NeuroReport* 5, 2517–2520.

Passingham, R. (1975). Delayed matching after selective prefrontal lesions in monkeys. *Brain Research* 92, 89–102.

Paulesu, E., Frith, C. D., & Frackowiak, R. S. J. (1993). The neural correlates of the verbal component of working memory. *Nature* 362, 342–345.

Penfield, W., & Boldrey, E. (1937). Somatic motor and sensory representation in the cerebral cortex of man as studied by electrical stimulation. *Brain* 60, 389–443.

Petersen, S. E., Fox, P. T., Posner, M. I., Mintun, M., & Raichle, M. E. (1988). Positron emission tomographic studies of the cortical anatomy of single-word processing. *Nature* 331, 585–589.

Petit, L., Courtney, S. M., Ungerleider, L. G., & Haxby, J. V. (1998). Sustained activity in the medial wall during working memory delays. *Journal of Neuroscience* 18, 9429–9437.

Petrides, M. (1994). Frontal lobes and working memory: Evidence from investigations of the effects of cortical excisions in nonhuman primates. In *Handbook of Neuropsychology*, F. Boller & J. Grafman, eds., vol. 9, 59–82. Amsterdam: Elsevier Science.

Petrides, M. (1995). Impairments on nonspatial self-ordered and externally ordered working memory tasks after lesions of the mid-dorsal lateral part of the lateral frontal cortex of monkey. *Journal of Neuroscience* 15, 359–375.

Petrides, M., Alivisatos, B., Evans, A. C., & Meyer, E. (1993). Dissociation of human mid-dorsolateral from posterior dorsolateral frontal cortex in memory processing. *Proceedings of the National Academy of Sciences USA* 90, 873–877.

Petrides, M., Alivisatos, B., Meyer, E., & Evans, A. C. (1993). Functional activation of the human frontal cortex during the performance of verbal working memory tasks. *Proceedings of the National Academy of Sciences USA* 90, 878–882.

Petrides, M., & Pandya, D. N. (1984). Projections to the frontal cortex from the posterior parietal region in the rhesus monkey. *Journal of Comparative Neurology* 228, 105–116.

Picard, N., & Strick, P. L. (1996). Motor areas of the medial wall: A review of their location and functional activation. *Cerebral Cortex* 6, 342–353.

Pierrot-Deseilligny, C., Rivaud, S., Gaymard, B., & Agid, Y. (1991). Cortical control of memory-guided saccades in man. *Experimental Brain Research* 83, 607–617.

Posner, M. I., Petersen, S. E., Fox, P. T., & Raichle, M. E. (1988). Localization of cognitive operations in the human brain. *Science* 240, 1627–1631.

Postle, B. R., Berger, J. S., & D'Esposito, M. (1999). Functional neuroanatomical double dissociation of mnemonic and nonmnemonic processes contributing to working memory. *Proceedings of the National Academy of Sciences USA* 96, 12959–12964.

Postle, B. R., & D'Esposito, M. (1999). "What"-then-"Where" in visual working memory: An event-related fMRI study. *Journal of Cognitive Neuroscience* 11, 585–597.

Postle, B. R., Stern, C. E., Rosen, B. R., & Corkin, S. (2000). An fMRI investigation of cortical contributions to spatial and nonspatial visual working memory. *NeuroImage*, 11, 409–423.

Ptito, A., Crane, J., Leonard, G., Amsel, R., & Caramanos, Z. (1995). Visual-spatial localization by patients with frontal-lobe lesions invading or sparing area 46. *NeuroReport* 6, 1781–1784.

Quintana, J., & Fuster, J. M. (1993). Spatial and temporal factors in the role of prefrontal and parietal cortex in visuomotor integration. *Cerebral Cortex* 3, 122–132.

Quintana, J., Yajeya, J., & Fuster, J. (1988). Prefrontal representation of stimulus attributes during delay tasks. I. Unit activity in cross-temporal integration of motor and sensory-motor information. *Brain Research* 474, 211–221.

Rao, S. C., Rainer, G., & Miller, E. K. (1997). Integration of what and where in the primate prefrontal cortex. *Science* 276, 821–824.

Rivaud, S., Muri, R. M., Gaymard, B., Vermersch, A. I., & Pierrot-Deseilligny, C. (1994). Eye movement disorders after frontal eye field lesions in humans. *Experimental Brain Research* 102, 110–120.

Rosen, B. R., Buckner, R. L., & Dale, A. M. (1998). Event-related fMRI: Past, present, and future. *Proceedings of the National Academy of Sciences USA* 95, 773–780.

Rosenkilde, C. E., Bauer, R. H., & Fuster, J. M. (1981). Single cell activity in ventral prefrontal cortex of behaving monkeys. *Brain Research* 209, 375–394.

Rushworth, M. F. S., Nixon, P. D., Eacott, M. J., & Passingham, R. E. (1997). Ventral prefrontal cortex is not essential for working memory. *Journal of Neuroscience* 17, 4829–4838.

Rushworth, M. F. S., & Owen, A. M. (1998). The functional organization of lateral frontal cortex: Conjecture or conjuncture in the electrophysiology literature. *Trends in Cognitive Sciences* 2, 46–43.

Rypma, B., & D'Esposito, M. (1999). The roles of prefrontal brain regions in components of working memory: Effects of memory load and individual differences. *Proceedings of the National Academy of Sciences USA* 96, 6558–6563.

Rypma, B., Prabhakaran, V., Desmond, J. E., Glover, G. H., & Gabrieli, J. D. E. (1999). Load-dependent roles of frontal brain regions in maintenance of working memory. *NeuroImage* 9, 216–226.

Saffran, E. M., & Marian, S. M. (1975). Immediate memory for word lists and sentences in a patient with deficient auditory short-term memory. *Brain and Language* 2, 420–433.

Salmon, E., Van der Linden, M., Collette, F., Delfiore, G., Maquet, P., Degueldre, C., Luxen, A., & Franck, G. (1996). Regional brain activity during working memory tasks. *Brain* 119, 1617–1625.

Sarter, M., Bernston, G., & Cacioppo, J. (1996). Brain imaging and cognitive neuroscience: Toward strong inference in attributing function to structure. *American Psychologist* 51, 13–21.

Schumacher, E. H., Lauber, E., Awh, E., Jonides, J., Smith, E. E., & Koeppe, R. A. (1996). PET evidence for an amodal verbal working memory system. *NeuroImage* 3, 79–88.

Shallice, T. (1988). *From Neuropsychology to Mental Structure.* Cambridge: Cambridge University Press.

Smith, E. E., & Jonides, J. (1998). Neuroimaging analyses of human working memory. *Proceedings of the National Academy of Sciences USA* 95, 12061–12068.

Smith, E. E., Jonides, J., & Koeppe, R. A. (1996). Dissociating verbal and spatial working memory using PET. *Cerebral Cortex* 6, 11–20.

Smith, E. E., Jonides, J., Koeppe, R. A., Awh, E., Schumacher, E. H., & Minoshima, S. (1995). Spatial versus object working memory: PET investigations. *Journal of Cognitive Neuroscience* 7, 337–356.

Sternberg, S. (1969). The discovery of processing stages: Extensions of Donders' method. *Acta Psychologica* 30, 276–315.

Swartz, B. E., Halgren, E., Fuster, J. M., Simpkins, E., Gee, M., & Mandelkern, M. (1995). Cortical metabolic activation in humans during a visual memory task. *Cerebral Cortex* 5, 205–214.

Sweeney, J. A., Mintun, M. A., Kwee, S., Wiseman, M. B., Brown, D. L., Rosenburg, D. R., & Carl, J. R. (1996). Positron emission tomography study of voluntary saccadic eye movements and spatial working memory. *Journal of Neurophysiology* 75, 454–468.

Talairach, J., & Tournoux, P. (1988). *Co-planar Stereotaxic Atlas of the Human Brain.* New York: Thieme Medical Publishers.

Ungerleider, L. G., & Haxby, J. V. (1994). "What" and "where" in the human brain. *Current Opinion in Neurobiology* 4, 157–165.

Vanderplas, J. M., & Garvin, E. A. (1959). The association of random shapes. *Journal of Experimental Psychology* 57, 147–163.

Vazquez, A. L., & Noll, D. C. (1998). Nonlinear aspects of the BOLD response in functional MRI. *NeuroImage* 7, 108–118.

Verin, M., Partiot, A., Pillon, B., Malapani, C., Agid, Y., & Dubois, B. (1993). Delayed response tasks and prefrontal lesions in man—Evidence for self generated patterns of behavior with poor environmental modulation. *Neuropsychologia* 31, 1379–1396.

Warrington, E. K., Logue, V., & Pratt, R. T. C. (1971). The anatomical localisation of selective impairment of auditory-verbal short-term memory. *Neuropsychologia* 9, 377–387.

Wilson, F. A., Scalaidhe, S. P., & Goldman-Rakic, P. S. (1993). Dissociation of object and spatial processing domains in prefrontal cortex. *Science* 260, 1955–1958.

Zarahn, E., Aguirre, G. K., & D'Esposito, M. (1996). Delay-specific activity within prefrontal cortex demonstrated during a working memory task: A functional MRI study. *Society of Neuroscience Abstracts* 22, 968.

Zarahn, E., Aguirre, G. K., & D'Esposito, M. (1997). A trial-based experimental design for fMRI. *NeuroImage* 6, 122–138.

Zarahn, E., Aguirre, G. K., & D'Esposito, M. (1999). Temporal isolation of the neural correlates of spatial mnemonic processing with fMRI. *Cognitive Brain Research* 7, 255–268.

Zattore, R. J., Evans, A. C., & Meyer, E. (1994). Neural mechanisms underlying melodic perception and memory for pitch. *Journal of Neuroscience* 14, 1908–1919.

III SPECIAL POPULATIONS

10 Functional Neuroimaging of Cognitive Aging

Roberto Cabeza

INTRODUCTION

One type of brain dysfunction that will affect all of us if we live long enough is normal aging. During aging, the brain undergoes a series of deleterious changes, including gray and white matter atrophy, synaptic degeneration, blood flow reductions, and neurochemical alterations. As in the case of brain dysfunction due to accidents or stroke, normal aging is accompanied by a variety of cognitive deficits. As we age, we are more likely to be distracted by internal and external stimuli, we forget more easily what we did and what we have to do, and it becomes increasingly difficult for us to manage several pieces of information at the same time or to perform simultaneous tasks. It seems indisputable that these age-related cognitive deficits are in great part a consequence of the age-related decline endured by the brain. Yet, although cognitive aging and neural aging have been thoroughly studied in isolation, the relations between the two phenomena are still largely unexplored. Whereas the *neuroscience of aging* and the *cognitive psychology of aging* are well developed, the *cognitive neuroscience of aging* is still in its infancy.

One way of relating neural and cognitive aspects of aging is to correlate measures of brain integrity, such as brain volume, to measures of cognitive ability, such as memory performance. Recently, functional neuroimaging techniques, such as positron emission tomography (PET) and functional magnetic resonance imaging (fMRI), have provided a more direct link between cerebral aging and cognitive aging. PET and fMRI studies can now reveal which brain regions are activated during a certain cognitive task, and how this activity is affected by aging.

The chapter consists of three main parts. The first part, Introduction, briefly summarizes findings provided by neural and cognitive measures of aging, as well as the attempts to correlate the two types of measures. The second part, Functional Neuroimaging of Cognitive Aging, reviews PET and fMRI studies comparing brain activity in young and older adults during the performance of cognitive tasks. The third part, Issues, discusses some current issues in the field of functional neuroimaging of cognitive aging.

A Model of Neurocognitive Aging

At present, our knowledge concerning neural and cognitive aging phenomena and their relations is too limited to allow the construction of a comprehensive and realistic model of neurocognitive aging. Nevertheless, a rudimentary model can help iden-

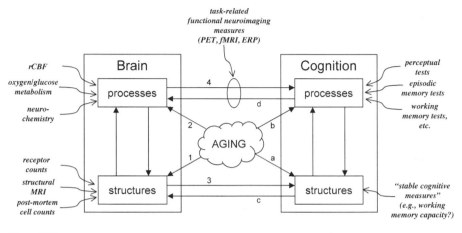

Figure 10.1
A simple model of neurocognitive aging.

tify the different aspects of the problem, and this is the goal of the simple model in figure 10.1. This model has two main components: brain and cognition. Both brain and behavior are partitioned into structures and processes. This distinction is artificial but useful in conceptual terms. Structures and processes interact with each other and differ only in degree: structures are more stable (e.g., neurons, memory stores), whereas processes are more dynamic (e.g., blood flow, cognitive operations).

Aging is assumed to have direct effects on both the brain and cognition. Although any change in cognition implies a change in the brain, it is useful to differentiate between *neurogenic effects* (arrows 1–4) and *psychogenic effects* (arrows a–d). To illustrate a neurogenic causal chain, aging could lead to atrophy of gray matter in the prefrontal cortex (PFC) and to deficits in dopaminergic function, which in turn cause alterations in working memory structures and processes. As an example of a psychogenic chain, aging could be associated with an increase in the use of semantic strategies during episodic retrieval, and this change could result in age-related increase in left PFC activity. Neurogenic and psychogenic effects interact and it is impossible to place a clear boundary between them. For example, a decline in neural function may lead to a compensatory change in cognitive strategies, which in turn leads to a change in brain function. The text around the model corresponds to some of the empirical measures available for elements of the model: neural measures (left), cognitive measures (right), and task-related functional neuroimaging measures (top).

The next section reviews evidence provided by neural measures, the following section reviews findings contributed by cognitive measures, and the last section of the Introduction discusses the relation between these two types of measures.

Neuroscience of Aging

This section briefly reviews structural and functional changes in the aging brain. Several comprehensive reviews on age-related neural changes are available (e.g., DeKosky & Palmer, 1994; Kemper, 1994; Madden & Hoffman, 1997; Raz, 2000); to avoid redundancy, only their conclusions are reviewed here.

Structural Changes The most obvious aspect of brain structure is brain volume. Postmortem studies indicate that with aging the weight and volume of the brain shrink at a slow but persistent rate of about 2% per decade (Kemper, 1994). This atrophy may reflect neuronal death and/or neuronal atrophy (e.g., Esiri, 1994) due to dendritic "debranching" and synaptic loss (Kemper, 1994). Consistent with postmortem studies, in vivo MRI studies show significant negative correlations between overall brain volume and age (e.g., r = −.41 in Raz et al., 1997). Postmortem and in vivo studies also converge on the idea that age-related atrophy affects some brain regions more than others. If the median of age-volume correlations across studies is used as a comparative measure, then the regions most affected are PFC (−.47) and neostriatum (caudate: −.47; putamen: −.44). In contrast, temporal (−.27) and parietal (−.29) cortices, the hippocampus (−.31), and the cerebellum (−.29) show only moderate shrinkage with age (Raz, 2000). Finally, some regions, such as primary sensory areas and the pons, show little or no volume reductions with age. It is important to note that the relation between atrophy and function could vary across the brain; and hence, the same amount of atrophy (e.g., 10%) could have very different effects depending on the region affected. Figure 10.2 illustrates the finding that age-related decline in PFC is more pronounced than in hippocampal regions. The moderate shrinkage of the hippocampus in normal aging is interesting because it contrasts with the severe damage suffered by this structure in Alzheimer's disease (AD). It has been proposed that whereas PFC atrophy is a characteristic of healthy aging, hippocampal atrophy may be a sign of pathologic aging (Raz, 2000).

Age-related atrophy in white matter can be as pronounced as in gray matter, and is probably due to a loss of myelin (Kemper, 1984). Volumetric MRI analyses show white matter atrophy primarily in PFC regions (Raz et al., 1997). This atrophy is not as pronounced as grey matter atrophy in PFC, but it is larger than white matter atrophy in other brain areas (e.g., parietal cortex). However, the most conspicuous age-related white matter change in MRI images is not atrophy, but the appearance of

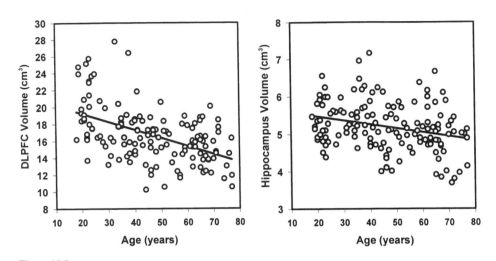

Figure 10.2
Scatter plots and simple linear regression of volume on age for dorsolateral PFC and hippocampus (from Raz et al., 1997).

the bright patches and spots known *white matter hyperintensities* (WMHs). WMHs are assumed to reflect a reduction in white matter density (Raz, 2000) and to have a variety of vascular and nonvascular causes.

Aging is also associated with an accumulation of certain chemicals and pathological structures inside or outside brain neurons. The lipid lipofuscin accrues inside cerebral and cerebellar neurons as a function of age, but its effects on neural function and behavior are still unknown (Kemper, 1994). In contrast, age-related aggregation of iron is more likely to have a deleterious effect by catalyzing the cytotoxic effects of free radicals (Marti et al., 1998). Iron accumulation is pronounced in the basal ganglia, and in accordance with the atrophy pattern in which (phylogenetically and ontogenetically) late structures are more affected, it alters primarily the caudate and the putamen but has a smaller effect on the globus pallidus (Raz, 2000). Although gross accumulation of amyloid plaques and neurofibrillary tangles is a diagnostic feature of AD, these histologic features are present to a lesser extent in the normal aging brain (Schochet, 1998).

Functional Changes   Age-related changes in brain function include alterations in neurochemistry, blood flow, and in the metabolism of oxygen and glucose. Changes in number of receptors and/or concentration of enzymes and neurotransmitters have been reliably observed for serotonin, acetylcholine, and dopamine (Strong, 1998). As in the case of atrophy, receptor losses are conspicuous in the PFC, where significant reductions in serotonergic (e.g., Wang et al., 1995), cholinergic (Lee et al., 1996), and dopaminergic (e.g., de Keyser et al., 1990) receptors have been demonstrated. Serotonin function is associated with mood regulation, and depressive mood in older adults could contribute to their cognitive deficits (Strong, 1998). The cholinergic system is critical for learning and memory, and its decline is one of the causes of memory decay in AD patients (Weinstock, 1995). Significant age-related decreases in cholinergic receptors of the muscarinic type have been demonstrated not only in PFC, but also in the basal ganglia and hippocampus (DeKosky & Palmer, 1994). Although age-related decreases in dopamine content are modest (DeKosky & Palmer, 1994), considerable reductions in the number of striatal D$_2$ receptors have been demonstrated, both postmortem and in vivo (Strong, 1998). Dopamine is primarily associated with motor function, but its modulatory effect on frontal function is also critical for cognitive function (Volkow et al., 1998). Alterations in dopaminergic fronto-striatal loops contribute to cognitive deficits in Parkinson's disease (PD) and may also be an important component of cognitive decline in normal aging (Bashore, 1993; Prull et al., 2000).

In living humans, regional cerebral blood flow (rCBF) has been investigated mainly with the xenon[133] nontomographic imaging technique, which measures rCBF only in the cortex, or with the ^{15}O-PET technique, which measures rCBF throughout the brain (Madden & Hoffman, 1997). The results of most of these studies indicate that aging is associated with a decline in rCBF over the entire cortex. The distribution of blood flow between frontal and posterior regions also changes with age: whereas middle-aged adults show more rCBF in anterior than in posterior regions (hyperfrontality), older adults display more rCBF in posterior than in anterior regions (hypofrontality; West, 1996). Fluorodeoxyglucose PET provides a measure of glucose metabolism in living humans. In contrast with blood flow data, findings regarding age-related changes in glucose metabolism have been inconsistent, with some studies finding significant age-related decreases in some regions (e.g., PFC; Kuhl et al., 1984) and others showing no differences whatsoever (for a review, see Madden & Hoffman, 1997).

In sum, normal aging is associated with a series of changes in brain anatomy and physiology. Gray matter atrophy is maximal in frontal and neostriatal regions; moderate in temporal, parietal, hippocampal, and cerebellar regions; and minimal in primary sensory areas. Frontal regions are also affected by white matter atrophy, and striatal regions by iron deposits. Functional changes include alterations in neurotransmitter systems, blood flow, and metabolism. Age-related reductions in acetylcholine receptors are prominent in frontal, striatal, and hippocampal regions, and for dopamine receptors in the neostriatum. Changes in cholinergic and dopaminergic function could underlie age-related deficits in memory and frontal functions. Age-related reductions in blood flow have been observed over the entire cortex, whereas results for glucose metabolism have been inconclusive. Thus, the regions most affected by age-related neural changes are frontal and neostriatal regions, followed by hippocampal, temporal, parietal, and cerebellar regions. This pattern is consistent with the idea that those structures which appeared late during phylogenesis and develop late during ontogenesis are more vulnerable ("last in, first out"; for a review see Raz, 2000).

Cognitive Psychology of Aging

While neuroscientists were busy gathering information about the effects of aging on brain structures and functions, cognitive psychologists were independently engaged in measuring and explaining age-related decline in cognitive functions. This section summarizes basic cognitive aging findings and theories.

Data   This section reviews cognitive aging data in areas where functional neuro-imaging studies have been conducted: (1) visual perception and attention; (2) episodic memory and priming; and (3) working memory and executive functions. Because excellent reviews on cognitive aging data are available (e.g., Balota et al., 2000; McDowd & Shaw, 2000; Schneider & Pichora-Fuller, 2000; Spencer & Raz, 1995; Verhaeghen et al., 1993; Zacks et al., 2000), repetition is reduced by relying on these reviews whenever possible.

VISUAL PERCEPTION AND ATTENTION   Traditionally, psychologists have focused on the effects of aging on higher-order cognitive processes and paid little attention to age-related changes in sensory and perceptual processes. This situation has changed in recent years, partly due to new evidence of strong correlations between age-related sensory/perceptual decline and cognitive decline (e.g., Lindenberger & Baltes, 1994). There are three main explanations for the close link between age-related deficits in perception and in cognition (Baltes & Lindenberger, 1997; Schneider & Pichora-Fuller, 2000): (1) perceptual decline causes cognitive decline; (2) cognitive decline causes perceptual decline; and (3) perceptual and cognitive decline have a common cause. These three alternatives have different implications concerning the neural basis of age-related information-processing deficits. In the second case, for example, age-related perceptual deficits could reflect changes in regions associated with higher-order processes (e.g., PFC) rather than in regions associated with perceptual processes (e.g., occipital cortex).

   In the case of vision, sensory deficits are primarily due to the decline of eye structures, including cornea, iris, lens, and humors (for a review, see Schneider & Pichora-

Fuller, 2000). These changes lead to decreases in sharpness, contrast, and brightness of retinal images, even after optical correction. Although visual pathways and the striate cortex are not markedly altered by aging, age-related deficits are also found in higher-order visual processes, such as peripheral vision and motion perception (Schneider & Pichora-Fuller, 2000). Age-related peripheral vision deficits are more pronounced under divided attention conditions. In general, older adults show deficits in attentionally demanding tasks, such as visual search, divided attention, and task switching (McDowd & Shaw, 2000). Perception involves a spectrum of cognitive operations from low-level analyses of the sensory input to semantic processing and identification of objects and words. Evidence suggests that in visual word identification tasks, sensory processing is more sensitive to age-related slowing than is access to word meaning (see Madden et al., 1996).

EPISODIC MEMORY AND PRIMING A considerable amount of evidence suggests the existence of at least five different memory systems: episodic memory, priming, working memory, semantic memory, and procedural memory (Tulving, 1995). Episodic memory refers to encoding and retrieval of information about personally experienced past events (Tulving, 1983). Priming occurs when a past experience (e.g., reading the word *assassin*) facilitates cognitive performance (e.g., completing _SS_SS___) in the absence of a conscious intention to retrieve the experience (for a review, see Roediger & McDermott, 1993). Working memory is discussed below, but semantic and procedural memory are not considered here because they have not yet been the focus of functional neuroimaging studies of cognitive aging (see, however, PET of a lexical decision task in Madden et al., 1996). The effects of aging on episodic memory and priming can be summarized in a simple statement: aging effects are considerable on episodic memory but negligible on priming. This statement is generally correct, even if some forms of episodic memory are more affected than others (for reviews, see Balota et al., 2000; Spencer & Raz, 1995; Zacks et al., 2000) and priming tests occasionally show significant age effects (for a review, see La Voie & Light, 1994).

Age-related episodic memory deficits may reflect difficulties during encoding, during retrieval, or both. Behavioral measures cannot easily distinguish between these alternatives, because they can only assess encoding success on the basis of retrieval performance. In contrast, functional neuroimaging methods can provide separate measures of encoding and retrieval, and hence provide very useful information regarding this issue. In addition to the encoding/retrieval distinction, two other distinctions are critical concerning the effects of aging on episodic memory: recall vs. recognition and context vs. content memory. In general, age effects are larger on recall tests than on recognition tests, and on context memory tests (e.g., source tests, temporal order tests) than on content memory tests (e.g., recognition) (Spencer & Raz,

1995). More generally, older adults tend to be more impaired on tests that require strategic retrieval, such as recall and context memory tests, than on those which require only associative retrieval, such as simple recognition tests (Moscovitch, 1992).

WORKING MEMORY AND EXECUTIVE FUNCTIONS According to Baddeley's model (Baddeley, 1986, 1998), working memory consists of two slave systems—the phonological loop and the visuospatial sketchpad—and a central executive. The slave systems are assumed to maintain verbal or visuospatial information for a brief period of time, and are roughly equivalent to the concept of short-term memory. The central executive, on the other hand, is assumed to have a supervisory role and to distribute attentional resources among different operations performed on information in working memory. In general, simple short-term memory tasks show modest age effects, whereas tasks involving executive processes show large age effects. For example, the meta-analysis of Verhaeghen et al. (1993) indicated that the effects size of aging is -0.31 for an auditory digit span task but -0.81 for tasks involving executive operations, such as the working-memory span task (Daneman & Carpenter, 1980). Older adults are also impaired on problem solving tasks that involve shifting strategies and inhibiting responses, such as the Wisconsin Card Sorting Test (WCST) (e.g., Haaland et al., 1987; Parkin & Lawrence, 1994).

Theories Older adults' cognitive decline has been attributed to deficits in (1) attentional resources, (2) processing speed, and (3) inhibition. Several other hypotheses have been proposes, but they are usually variations of these three main views.

ATTENTIONAL RESOURCES According to Kahneman's (1973) economic metaphor, cognitive processes are fueled by a limited supply of attentional resources. Craik and collaborators (Craik, 1983, 1986; Craik & Byrd, 1982) suggested that aging is associated with a reduction in the amount of attentional resources, which results in deficits in demanding cognitive tasks. This view is supported by evidence that older adults' memory performance resembles that of young adults under divided attention conditions (e.g., Anderson et al., 1998; Jennings & Jacoby, 1993). A corollary of the reduced attentional resources view, the *environmental support hypothesis* (Craik, 1983, 1986), predicts that age-related differences should be smaller when the task provides a supportive environment which reduces attentional demands. Consistent with this hypothesis, age-related deficits in episodic retrieval tend to be smaller on recognition tests (more environmental support) than on recall tests (less environmental support) (Spencer & Raz, 1995)

PROCESSING SPEED According to Salthouse and collaborators, older adults' cognitive deficits are primarily a consequence of a general age-related reduction in processing speed (for a review, see Salthouse, 1996). Slow processing is assumed to impair cognitive performance because of two mechanisms: (1) the time required by early operations reduces the time available for later operations (*limited time mechanism*); and (2) the products of early operations are lost or irrelevant by the time later operations are completed (*simultaneity mechanism*). This view emphasizes general aging mechanisms rather than task-specific mechanisms. For example, age-related memory deficits are not considered memory deficits per se, but rather consequence of a general slowing phenomenon. This view is supported by evidence that processing speed declines steadily with age, that this slowing shares considerable variance with age-related deficits in cognitive measures, and that processing speed is a strong mediator of cognitive decline in structural equation models (for a review, see Salthouse, 1996).

INHIBITION   The inhibition view of Hasher and Zacks (e.g., Hasher & Zacks, 1988; Zacks et al., 2000) attributes age-related cognitive deficits to a decline in the inhibitory control of working-memory contents. Such control involves three functions (Hasher et al., 1999): (1) to stop partially activated goal-irrelevant information from entering working memory (*access* function); (2) to dampen the activation of information that is no longer relevant to the current task (*suppression* function); and (3) to block strong inappropriate responses, thereby allowing weak appropriate responses (*restraint* function). When inhibitory control fails, goal-irrelevant information gains access to working memory, and the resulting "mental clutter" impairs working-memory operations, including the encoding and retrieval of episodic information (Zacks et al., 2000). Evidence supporting the inhibition view include results showing that, compared to young adults, older adults make more indirect semantic associations and better remember disconfirmed solutions and to-be-forgotten information (for a review, see Zacks et al., 2000).

In summary, this section has mentioned a few examples of the effects of aging on visual perception and attention, episodic memory and priming, and working memory and executive functions. In general, age-related perceptual deficits are highly correlated with age-related cognitive deficits, increase as a function of attentional demands, and are less pronounced in semantic aspects of object identification. The effects of aging on episodic memory are quite large, whereas those on priming tend to be small. Age-related deficits on episodic memory may be due to problems in encoding, retrieval or both, and tend to be larger on recall and context memory than on recognition. Age effects on working memory are more pronounced on tests involving executive functions than on simple short-term memory tasks. Age-related cognitive deficits have usually been interpreted in terms of reduced attentional resources, processing speed, or inhibitory control.

Cognitive Neuroscience of Aging

Linking Age-Related Cognitive Deficits to the Brain   The previous two sections briefly reviewed the progress made in neuroscience of aging and cognitive psychology of aging. Unfortunately, the relation between these two domains—the cognitive neuroscience of aging—has received very little attention. The main goal of this new discipline is to link neural and cognitive aspects of aging (for reviews, see Moscovitch & Winocur, 1992, 1995; Prull et al., 2000). There are several different ways to address this problem, but this section will mention only three: (1) making inferences from psychological theories of aging; (2) using patients with focal brain damage and degenerative disease as models of cognitive aging; and (3) interpreting age-related cognitive deficits in terms of general cognitive neuroscience models. These three strategies are briefly discussed below.

Although the psychological theories of cognitive aging discussed in the previous section do not make explicit predictions concerning the neural basis of aging, some expectations may be inferred. If age-related cognitive deficits reflect reduced attentional resources, then it is reasonable to assume that they involve brain areas associated with attention, such as PFC and anterior cingulate, thalamic, and parietal regions (Posner & Petersen, 1990). Also, this view suggests that brain function in older adults should resemble brain function in young adults under divided attention, and that age-related differences in brain function should decrease as environmental support increases (Anderson & Craik, 2000). In contrast, if age-related cognitive deficits reflect a general slowing phenomenon, then the neural correlates of these deficits can be assumed to be similar across tasks, and possibly to involve changes in neural transmission speed due to white matter alterations. Likewise, they could involve alterations in regions that play a role in the coordination of cognitive operations and motor responses, such as the cerebellum and the striatum. Finally, if age-related cognitive deficits reflect a deficiency in inhibitory mechanisms, then they are likely to involve regions associated with such mechanisms, such as PFC and anterior cingulate regions. Also, the inhibition view would predict that some brain regions should be more activated in older adults than in young adults, and that these activations should be negatively correlated with performance. It is important to emphasize that these inferences are mediated by assumptions concerning the roles of different brain regions in attention, processing speed, and inhibition, which require their own corroboration.

An alternative strategy is to reason by analogy from brain-damaged patients (Prull et al., 2000): if patients with damage in specific brain regions display cognitive deficits that are *qualitatively* similar to the ones displayed by elderly adults, then age-related cognitive deficits may be related to alterations in these specific regions. Conversely, if damage of a certain brain area yields a kind of cognitive deficit that is uncommon in healthy aging, then it is unlikely that such area is a major contributor to cognitive aging. Let us consider three neuropsychological syndromes: frontal damage, Parkinson disease (PD), and medial-temporal amnesia. Frontal patients show in augmented fashion many of the cognitive deficits displayed by healthy elderly, including difficulties with recall, context memory, working memory, and executive functions. Also, both frontal patients and elderly adults show deficits on tests that require task switching and inhibition, such as the WCST (Moscovitch & Winocur, 1995). This and other evidence have provided strong support for the view that frontal dysfunction is one of the main causes of age-related cognitive decline (West, 1996).

The pattern of cognitive deficits in PD patients is also quite similar to that of healthy aging, probably because dopamine deficits that characterize PD compromise the operation striatal-frontal circuits (Alexander et al., 1986), thereby leading to features of frontal dysfunction (Prull et al., 2000). PD could be a better model of cognitive aging than frontal damage, because frontal dysfunction in healthy aging is likely to be global rather than focal, and functional rather than structural. Actually, as mentioned previously, aging is associated with alterations in the dopaminergic system (see above), and hence it is possible that frontal-like deficits in old age reflect the dysfunction of this system (Prull et al., 2000).

Finally, older adults show deficits in episodic memory, which is a function severely impaired in medial-temporal amnesics. Although this would suggest that medial-temporal dysfunction is a main contributor to cognitive decline, episodic memory deficits are different in medial-temporal amnesics and healthy elderly. For example, whereas healthy elderly tend to be more impaired in recall than in recognition (Spencer & Raz, 1995), there is evidence that medial-temporal amnesics are equally impaired in recall and recognition (Haist et al., 1992; see, however, Hirst et al., 1988). Medial-temporal deficits do not seem to be a general component of cognitive aging, but rather they might be a precursor of AD (Prull et al., 2000).

A third strategy to link age-related cognitive deficits to the brain is to account for these deficits within a general cognitive neuroscience model. For example, one model that has been explicitly applied to explain patterns of preserved and impaired functions in healthy aging is Moscovitch's memory model (Moscovitch, 1992; Moscovitch & Umiltà, 1991). This model has four main components: (1) a posterior cortical component that mediates perceptual priming; (2) a medial temporal/hippocampal component that mediates associative episodic memory; (3) a frontal system that mediates strategic episodic memory and rule-based procedural memory; and (4) a basal ganglia component that mediates sensorimotor procedural memory. This model can account for minimal age effects on perceptual priming on the assumption that the posterior cortical component is relatively resistant to aging. It can also account for larger age

effects on recall and context memory than on recognition on the assumption that episodic memory is mediated by two systems: an associative medial-temporal system and
a strategic frontal system. The associative system automatically encodes information
that has been consciously apprehended, and it automatically retrieves it whenever an
appropriate cue is presented. This system cannot distinguish veridical from false
memories, organize the retrieval output, or guide a retrieval search. These "intelli-
gent" functions are provided by the strategic frontal system, which controls the operation of the associative medial-temporal system. This view predicts that age effects
should be more pronounced on episodic memory tests that more dependent on the
strategic system, such as recall and context memory, than on tasks that rely primarily
on the associative system, such as recognition. The controlled strategic system consumes more attentional resources than the automatic strategic system, and hence, it is
more sensitive to an age-related reduction of these resources (Moscovitch & Winocur,
1995). Also, as mentioned above, there is evidence that the integrity of the PFC is
more sensitive to aging than that of medial-temporal regions.

Empirical Evidence in Cognitive Neuroscience of Aging   Whether inspired by psychological theories, neuropsychological findings, or cognitive neuroscience models,
hypotheses concerning the neural basis of cognitive aging must be corroborated by
empirical evidence. There are two basic approaches to gathering this evidence: correlational and task-related functional neuroimaging. The difference between these two
approaches is depicted in figure 10.1.

   The correlational approach involves associating a neural measure, typically volumetric MRI or rCBF (left side of figure 10.1) and a cognitive measure (right side of
figure 10.1). Consider three examples of the correlational approach (for a review,
see Raz, 2000). First, a group of studies correlated the volume of medial temporal
regions, such as the hippocampus or the hippocampal formation with measures of
episodic memory performance. The results of these studies have been contradictory,
with some studies showing a moderate positive correlation (e.g., Golomb et al., 1994),
other studies showing a lack of correlation (e.g., Raz, Gunning-Dixon et al., 1998),
and still other studies showing negative correlations (e.g., Kohler et al., 1998).
Second, in some studies the volume of the PFC was correlated with measures of working memory. For example, Raz, Dupuis, et al. (1998) found weak positive correlations
between the volume of the dorsolateral PFC and working memory, both verbal and
nonverbal. However, these associations were nonsignificant after adjustment for age.
Finally, a few studies correlated functional measures, such as rCBF or glucose or oxygen metabolism, with cognitive performance data collected outside the scanner.
Eustache et al. (1995), for example, found significant correlations between word-pair
cued recall (from Wechsler Memory Scale) and oxygen consumption in bilateral hip-

pocampal and left thalamic regions. These correlations remained significant after adjustment for age.

In general, the results of correlational studies using structural neural measures have not provided consistent associations between age-related cognitive deficits and specific brain regions. As illustrated in figure 10.1, one possible reason for this outcome is that the relation between brain structures and cognitive functions is quite indirect. Age-related changes in brain structures can affect cognitive functions only if they are associated with changes in brain function. The relation between brain function and cognitive performance is more direct, and this could be one of the reasons why functional-correlational studies, such as the one by Eustache et al. (1995), are more likely to find significant correlations. Yet, the relation between brain activity and cognitive performance in these studies is still oblique; age-related difference in resting brain activity is not directly associated with cognitive performance. For example, older adults may show reduced resting rCBF in a certain region but recruit this region as much as young adults during a cognitive challenge. Conversely, a region may not show age-related rCBF differences during rest, but these differences may become apparent under the demands of cognitive tasks (Anderson & Craik, 2000).

In contrast, task-related functional neuroimaging measures (see top of figure 10.1) do not assess brain activity and cognitive performance independently, but in direct relation to each other. In contrast to correlational studies, if a brain region shows an age-related difference in brain activity during a particular cognitive task, then it is quite likely that this region is involved in the age-related differences found in the performance of the task. Despite a series of problems discussed at the end of the chapter, these measures are probably our best chance of identifying the particular brain regions underlying specific age-related cognitive deficits. Task-related functional neuroimaging measures are reviewed below.

FUNCTIONAL NEUROIMAGING OF COGNITIVE AGING

This section reviews functional neuroimaging studies that compared brain activity in young and old healthy subjects. This field is quite new, and only about a dozen studies have been published. Except for one fMRI study (Rypma & D'Esposito, 2000), all these studies measured rCBF with ^{15}O-PET. The studies are classified in three groups: (1) visual perception and attention (see table 10.1); (2) episodic memory and priming (see table 10.2); and (3) working memory and executive processes (see table 10.3). With only a few studies in each group, it is impossible to abstract general patterns of results or arrive at definite conclusions. Nevertheless, a few results in each

Table 10.1
Effects of Aging on Brain Activity Associated with Perception and Attention

Study/Contrast	Behavior	Y = O[a]	Y > O, Y not O[b]	O > Y, O not Y[c]
Grady et al. (1994)				
Face matching minus sensorimotor	Accur: Y = O RTs: Y < O	B18, B19 (ventral), B37	R18 (lingual)	B37, B47, B46, LIns
Location matching minus sensorimotor	Accur: Y = O RTs: Y < O	B19 (dorsal), B7	B18 (lingual and Cu)	B37, L19, M7(pCu), L10, L8, R47, LIns
Madden et al. (1996)				
Lexical decision minus passive encoding	Accur: ceiling RTs: Y = O	B18 (lingual and fusiform)	L18 (lingual and fusiform)	
Passive encoding minus sensorimotor	Accur: ceiling RTs: Y = O		L32/10, L20	
Madden, Turkington et al. (1997)				
Central attention minus passive	Accur: Y = O RTs: Y = O		L32, L10	
Divided attention minus central	Accur: Y > O RTs: Y < O		B18 (lingual and inf occipital)	L32, L6, R9

Note: The numbers correspond to Brodmann areas activated in each contrast.
Y, young; O, old; B, bilateral; L, left; R, right.
[a] Regions that were significantly activated in both groups when taken separately.
[b] Regions that were more activated in the young group than in the old group, or that were activated in the young but not in the old group.
[c] Regions that were more activated in the old group than in the young group, or that were activated in the old group but not in the young group.

cognitive domain have been replicated by two or more studies, and these results are summarized and related to theories of aging at the end of this section.

Visual Perception and Attention

One of the first activation studies of cognitive aging, Grady et al. (1994), focused on visual cognition. This study investigated the effects of aging on object and spatial visual processing by comparing rCBF in young and older adults on a face-matching task and location-matching task. In both tasks, older adults performed as accurately as young adults but their responses were significantly slower. Both groups showed the expected dissociation between ventral and dorsal visual processing pathways (Ungerleider & Mishkin, 1982): compared to a sensorimotor task, the face-matching task yielded occipitotemporal activations, whereas the location-matching task yielded occipitoparietal activations (see table 10.1). As illustrated by figure 10.3, during both the face-matching and the location-matching tasks, older adults showed less activity than young adults in occipital regions (lingual gyrus and cuneus) but more activity outside the occipital cortex (temporal, medial parietal, PFC, and insular regions). According to the authors, this pattern suggests that young adults engaged visual areas

Face Matching   Location Matching

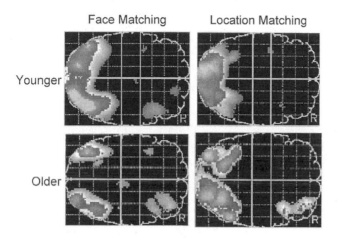

Figure 10.3
Areas of significant rCBF increase during face matching and location matching in young and older adults (from Grady et al., 1994).

before the ventral-dorsal bifurcation more efficiently, whereas older adults had to rely also on areas either farther along in the ventral and dorsal pathways, including PFC, or outside these pathways. They also proposed that the extra processing performed by these additional regions could account for slower reaction times in older adults.

Words are also assumed to be processed along the ventral visual pathway. Accordingly, Madden et al. (1996) predicted that a lexical decision task (word/nonword decision) would yield an activation pattern similar to that of the face-matching task in Grady et al.'s (1994) study. Madden et al. compared the lexical decision task to a task in which subjects made the same response to words and nonwords (passive encoding of letter features), which was in turn compared to a simple sensorimotor task. Consistent with Grady et al., ventral pathway activity during the lexical decision task was weaker in older adults than in young adults (see table 10.1). Unlike Grady et al., however, these age-related rCBF differences were not associated with differences in reaction times (RTs). Age-related decreases in ventral pathway activity were also found in the passive encoding condition, although more anteriorly, in Brodmann area (BA) 20. Additionally, the passive encoding task yielded an age-related rCBF decrease in medial PFC (left BA 32/10), which contrasts with the age-related PFC increase found by Grady et al., although that difference was dorsolateral rather than medial. In short, Madden et al. replicated Grady et al.'s finding of age-related decrease in the ventral pathway but not their finding of an age-related increase in PFC.

A subsequent study by Madden et al. (1997) replicated both findings. This study investigated the neural correlates of selective and spatial attention in young and older adults. Subjects had to indicate which of two target letters was included in the matrix. In the Central condition, the target always occurred in the center of the matrix, whereas in the Divided condition, it could appear in any of the nine matrix locations. Young adults were more accurate and faster than older adults in the Divided condition, but not in the Central and Passive conditions. Replicating Grady et al. (1994), in the Divided-Central contrast, older adults showed weaker activity than young adults in occipital regions but stronger activity than young adults in PFC (see table 10.1). The authors suggested that older adults were not able to perform the search task on the basis of letter identification processes mediated by the ventral pathway, and had to rely on higher-order control processes (e.g., rehearsal, monitoring) mediated by the frontal lobes.

In summary, the studies in this section converged on a very interesting finding: age-related rCBF decreases in occipital cortex coupled with an age-related rCBF increases in PFC (Grady et al., 1994; Madden et al., 1997). This finding was interpreted as reflecting altered perceptual mechanisms in older adults that are compensated for by increased PFC involvement (Grady et al., 1994; Madden et al., 1997). According to Grady et al. (1994), the engagement of PFC could account for older adults' slower responses.

Episodic Memory and Priming

In a seminal study in this area, Grady al. (1995) investigated age effects on the neural correlates of episodic memory for faces. Subjects tried to remember unfamiliar faces and then performed a forced-choice recognition test. During encoding, young adults showed stronger activations than older adults in left temporal, left PFC, and anterior cingulate regions (table 10.2). There was also a nonsignificant age-related decrease in the right hippocampus. During recognition, there were age-related decreases in activation in right parietal and occipital regions, but right PFC activity was similar in both groups. Thus, age effects occurred during both encoding and recognition, but they were more prominent during encoding. The authors suggested that older adults failed to engage the appropriate encoding network, encoded faces insufficiently, and, as a consequence, showed poorer recognition performance. They contrasted these results with those of Grady et al.'s (1994) face-matching task, in which compensatory activations could have allowed older adults to maintain accuracy at the expense of speed.

A second study in the memory domain was conducted by Schacter and collaborators (1996). In this study, young and older adults were scanned while recalling words (stem cued-recall) in conditions of high and low recall performance. Regions associated with the low recall condition were assumed to reflect retrieval effort, and those

Table 10.2
Effects of Aging on Brain Activity Associated with Episodic Memory and Priming

Study/Contrast	Behavior	Y = O	Y > O, Y not O	O > Y, O not Y
Grady et al. (1995)				
Face encoding minus two control tasks			L37, L45/47, M32, RHipp†	
Face recognition minus two control tasks	Accur: Y > O RTs: Y = O	R10/46, R47	R7, R19	
Schacter et al. (1996)				
High recall minus stem completion	Accur: Y > O	BHipp		
Low recall—stem completion	Accur: Y > O		B10	R46†, L45†, R4/6†
Cabeza, Grady et al. (1997)				
PLS: encoding	Accur: Y = O	R22/42, R40	L46, L8, L6, L1/2/3, L19	BIns, R18, M24
PLS: retrieval (both Rn and Rc)	Accur: Y = O	R10	R9m, R47, R9, R39, R20/21, midbrain	M31(Cun/pCun), L47, M32/6, L22
Madden, Turkington et al. (1999)				
Encoding minus Baseline	Accur: ceiling RTs: Y < O			L thalamus Red nuclcus
Recognition minus Baseline	Accur: Y > O RTs: Y < O	R10, L8	B Th	R10, L8, R8/9, L10, L47, L6/8
Backman et al. (1997)				
Baseline minus Priming	Priming: Y = O	R19		
Recall minus Baseline	Accur: Y > O	B10/46, B32	L Cb, L22 (Wernicke)	B36
Cabeza et al. (2000)				
Item memory minus order memory	Accur: Y = O	L28, B38, Caud	LSyl	L10, Cb
Order memory minus item memory	Accur: Y > O	B39, L9	R10, M19/18 (Cun/pCun), R39/19	
Anderson et al. (2000)				
Full-attention: encoding minus recall		L9/10/46, L20, B21, B37, B40, L22, L18	L45–47, B44, M6, R4, L37–38, R21–22, R18	R9/10/46, L20, L37, R22, L19, R41, B40
Full-attention: recall minus encoding	Accur: Y > O	L11, R47, R10, M32, BIns, precun, Cb, ptm, bs	B10, R9, M23, cun, th	L45/46, L47, R4, M32, L19, cun, bs

Note: See note of table 10.1.

associated with the high recall condition to reflect recollection of target words. In the high recall condition, young and older adults showed similar hippocampal activations (see table 10.2). In the low recall condition, anterior PFC regions were more activated in young and than in older adults, whereas posterior PFC regions showed a non-significant trend in the opposite direction. According to the authors, the similar hippocampal activations may reflect a commonality in the way young and older adults remember past events, whereas differences in PFC activity may reflect a change in retrieval strategies. The age-related reduction in anterior PFC activity suggests a problem engaging the mental set of episodic retrieval (Nyberg et al., 1995), whereas the age-related increase in posterior PFC activity suggests the adoption of inefficient retrieval strategies (e.g., a phonetic strategy involving Broca's area, left BA 45).

The combined results of Grady et al. (1995) and Schacter et al. (1996) suggested two conclusions: (1) age-related reductions in hippocampal activity occur during encoding (Grady et al.) but not during retrieval (Schacter et al.); and (2) age-related reductions in PFC activity occur for recall (Schacter et al.) but not for recognition (Grady et al.). However, these differences might reflect discrepancies in the materials employed in the two studies (novel nonverbal information in Grady et al. vs. well-learned verbal information in Schacter et al.). To investigate this issue, Cabeza, Grady et al. (1997) compared the effect of aging on encoding, recognition, and recall, using the same kind of materials (word pairs). Older adults showed lower activity than young adults in left PFC and occipitotemporal regions during encoding, and in right PFC and parietal regions during recognition and recall (see table 10.2). According to the authors, these age-related reductions reflected altered memory networks during both encoding and retrieval. Regions showing age-related increases included the right insula during encoding, the cuneus/precuneus area during recognition, and the left PFC during recall (see table 10.2). Because the left PFC is associated with word generation and its augmented activity in older adults could have aided their cued recall performance, the authors interpreted the age-related increase in left PFC activity as compensatory. Consistent with the hemispheric encoding/retrieval asymmetry (HERA) model (Nyberg, Cabeza, & Tulving, 1996; Tulving et al., 1994), PFC activity in young subjects was left-lateralized during encoding and right-lateralized during recall. In contrast, older adults showed little PFC activity during encoding and a more bilateral pattern of PFC activation during retrieval (see figure 10.7A). This bilateral pattern was also interpreted as compensatory: to counteract neurocognitive deficits, older adults would engage both prefrontal cortices in a task for which young adults recruit only one prefrontal cortex. The age-related reduction in hemispheric asymmetry is further discussed at the end of the functional neuroimaging review.

Madden, Turkington, et al. (1999) also investigated both encoding and retrieval (see table 10.2). Subjects made living/nonliving decisions about words while trying

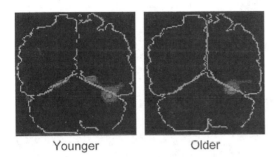
Younger   Older

Figure 10.4
Deactivations associated to priming in young and older adults (from Bäckman et al., 1997).

to memorize them, and then performed a recognition test. During encoding, young adults did not show any significant activation, but there were two regions showing significant age-related increases: the left thalamus and the red nucleus. According to the authors, the living/nonliving task was not difficult enough to elicit activations in young adults, and the thalamic activation in older adults could reflect increased attention during encoding. The recognition condition replicated the finding of Cabeza, Grady et al. (1997): PFC activity was right-lateralized in young subjects but bilateral in old subjects (see figure 10.7B). According to the authors, their results extended Cabeza et al.'s finding to conditions in which older adults perform more poorly than young adults. The activation data of Madden, Turkington et al. (1999b) was subsequently investigated by conducting a stepwise regression analysis of RT data that distinguished between exponential (*tau*) and Gaussian (*mu*) components of RT distributions (Madden, Gottlob, et al., 1999). During recognition, young adults' right frontal activity was related only to *mu* (right BA 10), whereas older adults showed activations related to both *mu* and *tau* (right BA 10, left BA 41). Since *tau* is associated with task-specific decision processes and *mu* is associated with residual sensory coding and response processes, the authors concluded that attentional demands were greater for older adults, possibly leading to the recruitment of additional regions.

As discussed earlier, older adults tend to be impaired in explicit but not in implicit memory. Bäckman and collaborators (1997) investigated the neural basis of this dissociation. Young and old subjects were presented word stems and tried to complete them, either with the first word that came to mind (Priming condition) or with studied words (Recall condition). As expected, age-related rCBF differences were considerable in the recall condition but minimal in the priming condition. In both groups, priming was associated with a similar right occipital deactivation (see table 10.2 and figure 10.4). This deactivation did not reach significance in the young group, possibly due to a lack of statistical power. During recall, older adults showed activations similar to those of young adults in bilateral PFC and cingulate regions. As in Cabeza, Grady et al. (1997), left PFC activations during recall were significant in older adults but not in young adults (see figure 10.7C). Compared to young adults, older adults showed weaker activations in the cerebellum and Wernicke's area, and stronger activations in bilateral medial temporal regions. According to Bäckman et al., the age-related decrease in the cerebellum could reflect impaired self-initiated retrieval and processing speed, whereas the one in Wernicke's area suggested a deficit in visual-auditory recoding. The most surprising finding of this study was the age-related increase in medial temporal regions. The authors related this finding to the aforementioned distinction between a frontal strategic system and a medial temporal associative system (e.g., Moscovitch, 1992). Bäckman et al. suggested that older adults might rely on nonstrategic processes to a greater extent than young adults.

Age effects are usually larger on context memory than on item memory (Spencer & Raz, 1995). To investigate the neural basis of this differential effect, Cabeza et al. (2000) compared rCBF in young and older adults during item retrieval (recognition) and temporal-order memory (recency). There were three main results (see table 10.2). First, younger adults engaged right PFC more during temporal-order retrieval than during item retrieval, whereas older adults did not. This result is consistent with the hypothesis that context memory deficits in older adults are due to PFC dysfunction. Second, ventromedial temporal activity during item memory was relatively unaffected by aging. This finding concurs with evidence that item memory is relatively preserved in older adults (e.g., Spencer & Raz, 1995) and with the aforementioned idea that medial temporal regions are involved in automatic retrieval operations (e.g., Moscovitch, 1992). Finally, replicating the results of Cabeza, Grady et al. (1997), older adults showed weaker activations than young adults in the right PFC but stronger activations than young adults in the left PFC. The age-related increase in left PFC activity was again interpreted as compensatory.

As mentioned in the Introduction, one piece of evidence supporting the reduced attentional resources view is evidence that when attention is divided during encoding, young adults' memory performance resembles that of older adults (e.g., Anderson et al., 1998). To investigate this phenomenon, Anderson et al. (2000) scanned young and old subjects while encoding or recalling word pairs under full attention (FA) or divided attention (DA). Under FA conditions, there were age-related reductions in left PFC activity during encoding and age-related increases in left PFC activity during retrieval (see table 10.2). These results are consistent with Cabeza, Grady et al. (1997). One of the most interesting findings of Anderson et al. was that some left PFC activations during encoding (BAs 45/46 and 44/9) were similarly affected by divided attention and by aging. This finding is consistent with the reduced attentional resources view, and suggests that poor memory performance in older adults is partly due to impaired encoding operations mediated by the left PFC (Cabeza, Grady et al., 1997; Grady et al., 1995).

In summary, age-related differences in brain activity were observed for episodic encoding and retrieval but not for priming. During encoding, age-related decreases in activation were observed primarily in left PFC (Anderson et al., 2000; Cabeza, Grady et al., 1997; Grady et al., 1995) and the medial temporal lobes (Grady et al., 1995). During retrieval, they were typically observed in the right PFC (Anderson et al., 2000; Cabeza et al., 2000; Cabeza, Grady et al., 1997; Schacter et al., 1996) but not in medial temporal regions (Bäckman et al., 1997; Cabeza et al., 2000; Schacter et al., 1996). Cabeza, Grady et al. (1997) found an age-related increase in the left PFC during retrieval, and interpreted it as compensatory. This finding was replicated in several studies (Anderson et al., 2000; Bäckman et al., 1997; Cabeza et al., 2000; Madden, Turkington et al., 1999b). Finally, paralleling behavioral data, young and older adults showed a similar occipital deactivation during primed word stem completion (Bäckman et al., 1997).

Working Memory and Executive Functions

Grady and collaborators (1998) investigated the effects of aging on the neural correlates of working memory for faces (see table 10.3). In each trial, subjects saw an unfamiliar face and after a varying delay (1–21 sec), they selected a face from two alternatives. Older adults were slower and less accurate than young adults, but these differences were relatively small. According to the authors, similar levels of performance and a considerable overlap on activation patterns suggest that basic working memory mechanisms are relatively preserved in older adults. At the same time, there were three interesting age-related differences. First, young adults showed greater activity in right frontal BA 45, and activation in this area increased with longer delays in the young but not in the old. The authors suggested that young subjects were better able to engage this region as task difficulty increased. Second, older adults showed greater activity in left frontal BA 9/45, possibly reflecting a compensatory mechanism or increased task demands. Thus, as in Cabeza, Grady et al. (1997), an age-related decrease in right PFC activity was accompanied by an age-related increase in left PFC activity. Finally, as delay extended from 1 to 6 sec, activation of the left medial temporal cortex increased in young adults but decreased in older adults. This result was interpreted as suggesting that older adults have difficulties initiating memory strategies which recruit medial temporal regions (see Grady et al., 1995), or sustaining medial temporal activity beyond very short retention intervals.

Reuter-Lorenz et al. (2000) investigated the effects of aging on the lateralization of the neural correlates of verbal and spatial working memory. Subjects maintained let-

Table 10.3
Effects of Aging on Brain Activity Associated with Working Memory and Executive Functions

Study/Contrast	Behavior	Y = O	Y > O, Y not O	O > Y, O not Y
Grady et al. (1998)				
Face working memory minus sensorimotor control	accur: Y > O speed: Y > O	L44/45, R11, L19, R19/37	L45/ins, R45	L9/45, R19
Increase with longer delays		L11/10/46, R9/8/1–2, B21, L39, Cb, R41/42, M18/31,	R45/46, Cb, LHC	L19, mBr
Decrease with longer delays		R6,11/47,45, M32, B19, R19, mBr/Th	R6, M23/31, Lins	Rins, LTh, LHC
Reuter-Lorenz et al. (2000)				
Letter working memory minus control	accur: Y > O speed: Y > O	left parietal	left PFC	right PFC
Location working memory minus control	speed: Y > O	bilateral parietal	right PFC	left PFC
Rypma & D'Esposito (2000)				
Letter WM: encoding, maintenance, retrieval	accur: Y = O speed: Y > O		B9/46 during retrieval	
Nagahama et al. (1997)				
Card sorting—matching	accur: Y > O speed: Y > O	L9/46, B10, L18 (Cun)	L46/44, L10, L40, B39, L19, R18, Cun/pCun, Cb	R10/11/47†
Jonides et al. (2000)				
High-recency DMS– low-recency DMS	accur/speed: Y > O		L45	
Esposito et al. (1999)				
WCST (correlations with age)	accur: Y > O		(−cor) L9, R32, L39/40, LCb	(+cor) B9, L18, R17, R30/19
RPM (correlations with age)	accur: Y > O		(−cor) L40, B37, L21, L36, BCb	(+cor) L9, B10, L23, B22

Note: See note of table 10.1. DMS = delayed matched to sample; WCST = Wisconsin Card Sorting Test; RPM = Raven's Progressive Matrices.

ters or spatial locations in short-term memory for 3 sec and then responded whether or not any of the letters or locations matched a probe. The main finding of the study was that in young adults, PFC activity was left-lateralized for verbal task and right lateralized for spatial task, whereas in older adults, it was bilateral for both tasks (see figure 10.7D). Thus, consistent with Cabeza, Grady et al. (1997), hemispheric asymmetry was reduced in older adults. Like Cabeza, Grady et al. (1997), Reuter-Lorenz and collaborators interpreted the age-related reduction in lateralization as compensatory. Since there were no age-related differences in activation in posterior brain regions, the authors concluded that frontal components of the working memory network are more vulnerable to aging than posterior components (e.g., parietal cortex). Finally, in some dorsolateral frontal regions older adults showed greater left activation for spatial working memory and greater right activation for verbal working memory. This "paradoxical laterality" does not seem to be efficient, because it was associated with slower RTs in the verbal task; faster older adults showed a bilateral activation pattern.

An fMRI study conducted by Rypma and D'Esposito (2000) employed an event-related paradigm to disentangle the effects of aging on three successive working-memory stages: stimulus encoding, memory maintenance, and memory retrieval. On each trial, subjects encoded two or six letters, maintained them for an unfilled 12-sec interval, and responded to a probe letter. fMRI signal changes during encoding, maintenance, and retrieval were modeled with covariates consisting of shifted impulse response functions. fMRI analyses focused on two regions of interest within the PFC: dorsolateral (BAs 9 and 46) and ventrolateral (BAs 44, 45, and 47). Ventrolateral regions did not show significant age-related differences during any stage. Dorsolateral regions showed an age-related decrease during the retrieval stage, but not during the encoding and maintenance stages. Thus, Rypma and D'Esposito's study suggested that age-related working-memory deficits are related to a dysfunction in dorsolateral PFC regions during the retrieval stage of the working-memory process. The differential effect of aging on ventrolateral and dorsolateral PFC regions (see also Rypma et al., 2000) is important because these two areas are assumed to reflect different working memory operations. Functional neuroimaging data (for reviews, see Cabeza & Nyberg, 2000; D'Esposito, this volume) generally support the hypothesis that ventrolateral regions are involved in simple short-term operations, whereas dorsolateral regions are involved in higher-level executive operations, such as monitoring (Owen, 1997; Petrides, 1994, 1995). Thus, Rypma and D'Esposito's finding is consistent with behavioral evidence that old adults are more impaired in executive functions than in short-term memory processes (e.g., Verhaeghen et al., 1993).

The effect of aging on executive functions was investigated by Nagahama et al. (1997), using a modified version of the Wisconsin Card Sorting Test. Compared to a number-matching task, card sorting was associated with left dorsolateral PFC, bilateral frontopolar, and cuneus regions in both groups. Age-related reductions in activation were found in several regions, including left PFC, bilateral parietal, and cerebellar gyrus, possibly reflecting wider strategy use in younger adults. The right ventrolateral PFC was activated in older adults but not in young adults, although the age effect was nonsignificant. Nagahama et al. suggested that this activation could reflect greater effort to maintain selective attention. The left dorsolateral prefrontal as well as lingual, precuneus, and right parahippocampal regions showed significant negative correlations between number of perseverative errors and rCBF during card sorting. Since the number of perseverative errors was also negatively correlated with age, the authors interpreted these regions as reflecting age-related deficits in set-shifting ability.

Esposito et al. (1999) investigated two tests assumed to reflect executive functions, the Wisconsin Card Sorting Test (WCST) and Raven's Progressive Matrices (RPM). Instead of comparing a group of young adults and a group of older adults, Esposito et al. investigated a relatively large group of subjects (N = 41) ranging from 18 to 80 years of age. During RPM, regions activated by the young were less activated by the old (e.g., parahippocampal, fusiform, and parietal regions), whereas regions deactivated by the young were less deactivated by the old (e.g., frontopolar and superior temporal regions). The authors suggested this attenuation of activation/deactivation patterns could reflect an age-related reduction in mental flexibility. During WCST, however, old adults also showed activations (e.g., frontopolar cortex, cuneus, parahippocampal gyrus) and deactivations (e.g., left prefrontal, anterior cingulate, and cerebellar regions) not shown by the young. According to Esposito et al., these age-related differences may reflect a failure to engage appropriate and suppress inappropriate networks, or a compensatory use of alternative networks.

One of the main conclusions of this study is that age-related changes in brain activity are task-specific. For example, in young adults, the left PFC (BAs 9/45/46) was activated during both WCST and RPM, whereas in older adults, it was activated during RPM but deactivated during WCST. The authors suggested that age-related changes are more pronounced in regions associated with processes critical for a particular task, such as PFC associated with working memory in the case of WCST and occipito-temporal regions associated with visual processing in the case of RPM. Using a method reported by Cabeza, McIntosh et al. (1997), Esposito et al. also investigated the effect of aging on the interactions between the regions involved in WCST and RPM. The results of these covariance analyses indicated that PFC-parietal interactions within the working-memory system and temporal-parietal-hippocampal interactions within posterior visuospatial processing systems are altered in older adults. The authors interpreted this finding in terms of disconnectivity and systems failure.

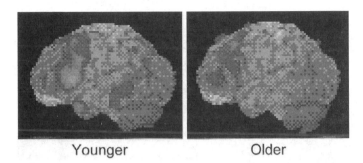

Younger   Older

Figure 10.5
Left PFC activation associated with inhibition in young and older adults (from Jonides et al., 2000). (See color plate 21.)

An important executive function is to resolve conflict between competing processes or responses, and this function is assumed to involve inhibition. Jonides et al. (2000) investigated the effects of aging on the neural correlates of inhibition. In each trial of the task, subjects maintained four target letters for 3 sec and then decided whether a probe matched any of the four target letters. In a high-recency condition, half of the probes did not match any target letter in the current trial but matched a target letter in the immediately preceding trial. In the low-recency condition, in contrast, the probe did not match any target letter in the two preceding trials. Thus, inhibitory control was critical in the high-recency but not in the low-recency condition. The high-recency minus the low-recency condition yielded an activation in the left PFC (Jonides et al., 1998). An ROI analysis indicated that in older adults this activation was significantly weaker than in young adults and was not reliable (see figure 10.5 and color plate 21). A combined measure of accuracy and reaction times yielded an interference effect for negative trials in which the probe matched a target letter in the preceding trial. Since this interference effect was larger for older than for young adults, the authors concluded that aging diminishes the efficacy of the left PFC in inhibiting the interfering effects of prepotent processes.

Conclusions

Main Findings and Their Interpretations To summarize, studies using task-related functional neuroimaging measures have provided five main sets of findings:

1. During perception and attention, age-related decreases in occipital activity were coupled with age-related increases in PFC activity (Grady et al., 1994; Madden et al., 1997).

2. During encoding, older adults showed weaker activations in left PFC (Anderson et al., 2000; Cabeza, Grady, et al., 1997; Grady et al., 1995) and medial temporal regions (Grady et al., 1995). Left PFC activity was found to be similarly affected by aging and divided attention (Anderson et al., 2000).

3. During episodic retrieval, age-related decreases in right PFC activity (Anderson et al., 2000; Cabeza et al., 2000; Cabeza et al., 1997a; Schacter et al., 1996) were often accompanied by age-related increases in left PFC activity (Anderson et al., 2000; Bäckman et al., 1997; Cabeza et al., 2000; Cabeza, Grady et al., 1997; Madden, Turkington, et al., 1999). In general, medial temporal activations were not reduced by aging (Bäckman et al., 1997; Cabeza et al., 2000; Schacter et al., 1996).

4. During priming, young and older adults showed a similar right occipital deactivation (Bäckman et al., 1997). Even if this deactivation did not reach significance in the old, the similar location in both groups suggests likeness rather than unlikeness. It is worth noting that in contrast with healthy elderly, AD patients have recently been found to be impaired in priming and to show priming-related occipital activations instead of deactivations (Bäckman et al., 2000).

5. During working memory, older adults often showed weaker PFC activations in the hemisphere primarily engaged by the young but stronger PFC activations in the contralateral hemisphere (Grady et al., 1998; Nagahama et al., 1997). Age-related changes in PFC activity were localized to dorsolateral areas during retrieval (Rypma & D'Esposito, 2000) and could involve inhibition-related activations in left PFC (Jonides et al., 2000). Medial temporal activity may be also altered by aging, particularly at longer delays (Grady et al., 1998).

In general, age-related decreases in activation were interpreted as reflecting inefficient neurocognitive processing in older adults, whereas age-related increases in activation were interpreted as compensatory. Unlike cognitive psychologists, who normally try to attribute age-related changes to one main factor, such as reduced attentional resources (e.g., Craik & Byrd, 1982) or inhibitory control (Hasher & Zacks, 1988), functional neuroimaging researchers attributed these changes to a complex interplay between different age effects on a variety of brain regions. It is worth noting that these multi-factorial accounts could also shed light on old problems in the cognitive aging literature. For instance, the close association between perceptual and cognitive age-related deficits has been attributed to an effect of perception on cognition, to an effect of cognition on perception, or to a common cause (Baltes & Lindenberger, 1997; Schneider & Pichora-Fuller, 2000). The idea that age-related changes in perceptual mechanisms could be compensated by increased frontal activity at the expense of processing speed (Grady et al., 1994) suggests a more complex mechanism in which perception and cognition affect each other and contribute to different aspects of age-related differences in performance (e.g., accuracy vs. reaction times).

Even if functional neuroimaging researchers have favored multifactorial explanations, it is interesting to consider a few examples of functional neuroimaging findings that are consistent with cognitive aging theories. For example, the reduced attentional resources view is consistent with evidence that age-related differences in activation decrease as a function of environmental support (for a discussion, see Anderson & Craik, 2000). For example, a recent study by Grady et al. (1999) found that age-related differences in activation during episodic encoding were attenuated by conditions providing more environmental support, such as pictorial stimuli and semantic processing. Also, age-related decreases in right PFC activity during retrieval were repeatedly observed for associative cued-recall tests (Anderson et al., 2000; Cabeza, Grady, et al., 1997; Schacter et al., 1996), whereas several studies did not find them for recognition (Grady et al., 1995; Madden, Turkington et al., 1999). Cabeza, Grady et al. (1997a) observed them for both recognition and recall, but this study employed an associative recognition test, which may tap episodic recollection (Donaldson & Rugg, 1998; Yonelinas, 1997). Another example of results consistent with the reduced attentional resources view is Anderson et al. (2000) finding of regions that are affected similarly by aging and by divided attention.

The reduced inhibitory control view predicts not only weaker activations in regions that control inhibitory effects but also stronger activations in regions that were not properly suppressed. An example of the first type of evidence is Jonides et al.'s (2000) finding that a left prefrontal activation associated with interference control was abated by aging. An instance of the second type of result is Cabeza, Grady et al.'s (1997) finding of an age-related increase in insular activity during encoding. When this activation was correlated with subsequent recall performance a significant negative correlation emerged (see figure 10.6), suggesting that engaging insular regions during encoding is detrimental and could reflect a lack of inhibition in older adults (Cabeza, Grady et al., 1997a).

Finally, the effects of aging on PFC and medial temporal activations during episodic retrieval are generally consistent with the Moscovitch's (1992) memory model. While PFC activations during retrieval often showed age-related decreases (Anderson et al., 2000; Cabeza et al., 2000; Cabeza, Grady et al., 1997; Schacter et al., 1996), medial temporal activations were found to be as strong as (Cabeza et al., 2000; Schacter et al., 1996), or even stronger than (Bäckman et al., 1997) in older adults than in young adults. This pattern is consistent with Moscovitch's distinction between a frontal strategic retrieval system and a medial-temporal associative retrieval system, and with his assumption that the frontal system is more sensitive to aging than the

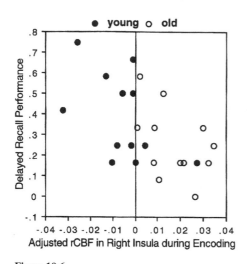

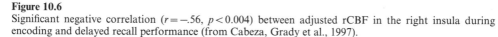

Figure 10.6
Significant negative correlation ($r = -.56$, $p < 0.004$) between adjusted rCBF in the right insula during encoding and delayed recall performance (from Cabeza, Grady et al., 1997).

medial temporal system (Moscovitch & Winocur, 1995). This pattern could also explain why older adults tend to be more impaired on context memory, which is more dependent on the frontal lobes, than on item memory, which is more dependent on the medial temporal lobes (Cabeza et al., 2000). In contrast with episodic retrieval, episodic encoding has been associated with age-related decreases in medial temporal regions (Grady et al., 1994). Medial temporal dysfunction could underlie age-related deficits in feature binding (Mitchell et al., in press).

Hemispheric Asymmetry Reduction in Older Adults   Despite the small number of task-related PET and fMRI studies of cognitive aging, there is one aging finding that has been replicated by several studies: an age-related attenuation in hemispheric asymmetry. This effect has been observed during episodic memory retrieval and working memory.

In functional neuroimaging studies of long-term memory, PFC activity tends to be left-lateralized during semantic retrieval and episodic encoding but right-lateralized during episodic retrieval (HERA model, e.g., Nyberg, Cabeza, & Tulving, 1996; Tulving et al., 1994). However, several studies have found that while young adults showed right-lateralized PFC activations during episodic retrieval, older adults showed a bilateral activation pattern. The first study to identify this effect was Cabeza, Grady et al. (1997a). In this study, frontal activity during associative cued-recall was clearly right-lateralized in young adults and clearly bilateral in the older adults (see figure 10.7A and color plate 20). This finding was also observed by Madden, Turkington et al. (1999b) during a word recognition test (see figure 10.7B), and by Bäckman et al. (1997C) during a word-stem cued-recall test (figure 10.7C).

Functional neuroimaging studies of working memory have identified a different kind of hemispheric asymmetry: PFC activations tend to be left-lateralized for verbal stimuli and right-lateralized for spatial stimuli (for review, see D'Esposito, 2000; Smith & Jonides, 1997). Consistent with this pattern, in Reuter-Lorenz et al.'s (2000) study young adults' PFC activity was left-lateralized in a verbal working-memory task and right lateralized in a spatial working-memory task. In contrast, PFC activity in older adults bilateral in both tasks (see figure 10.7D).

Although the age-related attenuation of hemispheric asymmetry is easier to identify when young adults' activations are distinctly lateralized, it may also occur in conditions where lateralization in young adults is less obvious. In those cases, the effect may be observed only as a "hemispheric shift," that is, an age-related decrease in one hemisphere accompanied by an age-related increase in the other hemisphere (Anderson et al., 2000; Grady et al., 1998; Nagahama et al., 1997). Anderson et al. (2000), for example, found during recall an age-related decrease in right PFC activity coupled with an age-related increase in left PFC. Likewise, in the Grady et al. (1998) face working memory study, older adults showed weaker activations in the right PFC but stronger activations in the left PFC. It is still unclear whether these activation "shifts" reflect a reduction in lateralization or an entirely different phenomenon.

As for explanations of the age-related attenuation in lateralization, two hypotheses have been suggested. Cabeza et al. (1997a) proposed that greater bilaterality in older adults could serve a compensatory function: older adults might counteract neurocognitive deficits by recruiting both hemispheres in tasks for which young adults normally engage only one hemisphere. In the case of episodic retrieval, the additional recruitment of the left PFC would compensate for episodic deficits. Consistent with this idea, Bäckman and colleagues (1999) found that during retrieval the left PFC was more activated in early AD patients than in healthy elderly adults (see also Becker et al., 1996). Thus, young adults, normal older adults, and early AD patients could be viewed as three points on a continuum of decreasing episodic memory ability and increasing compensatory processes (Bäckman et al., 1999). The compensatory hypothesis is also consistent with evidence that brain damage may lead to a shift in lateralized activation patterns. For example, Buckner et al. (1996) reported that a unilateral localization of cognitive tasks in the left PFC is shifted to right PFC when left PFC is damaged. Also, it has been reported that bilateral activation, with involvement of regions homologous to the ones responsible for normal function, may facilitate recovery after brain injury (Engelien et al., 1995).

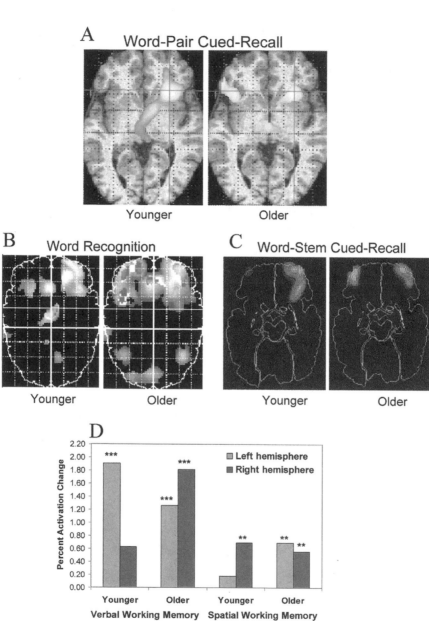

Figure 10.7
Examples of an age-related attenuation in hemispheric asymmetry: unilateral activations in young adults coupled with bilateral activations in older adults. (*A*) Brain activity during recall (data from Cabeza, Grady, et al., 1997 re-analyzed with SPM). (*B*) Brain activity during recognition (from Madden, Turkington et al., 1999). (*C*) Brain activity during word-stem cued recall (from Bäckman et al., 1997). (*D*) Brain activity during verbal and spatial working memory (from Reuter-Lorenz, 2000; **p < .03; ***p < .001). (See color plate 20.)

In contrast to Cabeza, Grady et al.'s (1997) *optimistic* interpretation, a *pessimistic* account is also possible: the attenuation in hemispheric asymmetry could reflect a difficulty in engaging specialized neural mechanisms. The idea that aging is associated with a dedifferentiation of brain systems is supported by studies showing that correlations between different cognitive measures (e.g., knowledge vs. perceptual tasks) increase with age (Baltes & Lindenberger, 1997).

Although it is not an easy task, compensatory and dedifferentiation hypotheses can be tested. One method would be to correlate rCBF in regions showing age-related increases in activation with measures of cognitive performance: a positive correlation would favor the compensatory account, whereas a negative or a null correlation would support the dedifferentiation account. Unfortunately, reliable rCBF-performance correlations are difficult to find, given the small number of subjects used in functional neuroimaging experiments (see, however, Cabeza, Grady, et al., 1997; Madden et al., 1997; Madden, Gottlob et al., 1999; Madden, Turkington, et al., 1999). Another alternative is to compare groups of elderly who differ in degree of cognitive impairment. These different ways of clarifying the meaning of age-related changes in activation are discussed in the next part of the chapter.

ISSUES

This section discusses some of the main problems faced by researchers conducting task-related functional neuroimaging studies of cognitive aging, and considers some possible solutions. The issues are organized according to the four main components of a functional neuroimaging experiment: subjects, tasks and design, behavioral performance, and activations. Since these four elements are intimately related, several of the issues discussed below could be classified under a different heading.

Subjects

When selecting healthy elderly subjects, one is faced with a dilemma. On one hand, one would like to select elderly adults who are perfectly healthy and who are matched to young adults in all possible variables except age. One the other hand, one would also like to investigate a sample of older adults that is representative of the general elderly population. This is a general problem of cognitive aging research, but some aspects of it are particularly thorny in functional neuroimaging studies. In this section, I briefly discuss three issues concerning the selection of elderly subjects in these studies: health screening, cognitive performance, and subgroups of elderly.

In most functional neuroimaging studies of cognitive aging, subjects fill out a simple health questionnaire and are excluded if they respond positively to items concerning past neurological or psychiatric episodes, hypertension, and medication use. Although subjects with brain damage must be excluded, dismissal based on past psychiatric events is not so obvious. For example, simply by having lived longer, older adults are more likely to have experienced a depressive episode. Hypertension excludes about 20% of elderly candidates and rightly so: it may not only affect blood flow measures, and it is associated with covert cerebrovascular damage (Skoog, 1998). Subjects are also excluded if they are taking any medication that could affect blood flow. However, clear guidelines about which drugs actually do so are not available. Several studies have included objective measures, such as structural MRI or a complete medical exam as part of the health screening (e.g., Grady et al., 1994, 1998; Madden et al., 1996, 1997, Madden, Turkington, et al., 1999). Structural MRI allows the exclusion of subjects showing signs of brain atrophy or white matter hyperintensities indicative of cerebrovascular disease, and its use will probably become more common in the future, because structural MRI is usually included in fMRI studies. A study by D'Esposito et al. (1999) showed age-related changes in the coupling between neural activity and blood oxygenation level dependent (BOLD) fMRI signal, which could reflect differences in the properties of the vascular bed or vascular pathology. Future fMRI studies may have to include special screening procedures to address this issue. This trend toward more accurate and stricter screening procedures will eventually require an examination of the impact of exclusion criteria on the generalizability of functional neuroimaging results.

A second issue concerning subject selection is the level of cognitive impairment of the elderly sample. Differences in this dimension could help explain some of inconsistencies in the data. For example, Cabeza, Grady et al. (1997) found regions that were more activated in old than in young adults during memory retrieval, suggesting functional compensation, whereas Grady et al. (1995) did not. This inconsistency could be related to the fact that during the scans the elderly group in Cabeza, Grady et al.'s study performed as well as the young group, whereas the elderly group in Grady et al.'s study performed significantly worse than the young group. In other words, the results of functional neuroimaging studies of cognitive aging may depend on the level of cognitive performance displayed by the elderly sample investigated. One way of addressing this problem is to have two groups of elderly subjects, one that shows significant deficits in the task investigated and one that does not. Comparing high-performing and low-performing elderly subjects could help identify the kinds of age-related changes in neural function that are actually associated with deficits in cognitive performance.

Finally, a third issue is the existence of different subgroups within the elderly population. Most research on aging has focused on general effects of aging on the brain and cognition. This work has identified brain regions and cognitive tasks that are particularly affected by aging. However, there is evidence that the brain regions and tasks most affected by aging may vary across the elderly population. In the memory domain, for example, age-related deficits in context memory (source, temporal order, etc.) are usually attributed to PFC dysfunction, and age-related deficits in content memory (e.g., recognition), to medial temporal lobe dysfunction. Although age effects are generally more pronounced in context memory (e.g., Spencer & Raz, 1995) and the frontal lobes (e.g., Raz et al., 1997), some elderly adults could be more impaired in item memory and medial temporal function. In Glisky et al.'s (1995) study, neuropsychological tests were used to classify elderly subjects as either high or low in frontal lobe function, and as either high or low in medial temporal lobe function. Subjects low in frontal function were impaired in context memory but not in content memory, whereas those subjects low in medial temporal lobe function showed the converse pattern. If there are different aging patterns, as this study suggests, then it is critical for functional neuroimaging studies to take this into account when selecting subjects.

Tasks and Design

Cognitive tasks are never "pure"; they always involve a complex blend of different cognitive operations. In functional neuroimaging studies, this means that the set of brain regions associated with a particular task may reflect any of the cognitive operations engaged by the task. Thus, when age-related differences in activation are found in a certain region, it is very difficult to determine what component of the task is actually responsible for the age effect. This could explain some inconsistent findings. For example, Cabeza, Grady et al. (1997a) found a significant age-related reduction in PFC activity during verbal recognition, whereas Madden, Turkington et al. (1999b) did not. Recognition memory is assumed to involve two different processes, recollection and familiarity (e.g., Mandler, 1980), and there is evidence that the former is more sensitive to aging than the latter (e.g., Jennings & Jacoby, 1997). The associative recognition test used by Cabeza et al. involves a larger recollection component than the recognition test employed by Madden et al. (Donaldson & Rugg, 1998; Yonelinas, 1997); hence it is more likely to show aging effects. Similarly, many of the inconsistent findings in studies using nominally the same tasks could reflect variations in the specific processing components tapped by the particular tasks employed.

The traditional approach to the problem of task complexity is the subtraction method, which attempts to isolate a process A by comparing a target task, involving processes A and B, to a reference task involving only process B. There are two main problems with this method, and they are both magnified by between-subject comparisons. The first problem is that neural activity identified by the subtraction method reflects the target task as much as the reference task. Thus, an age-related decrease in the difference between a target task and a reference task may reflect an age-related decrease in activation in the target task or an age-related increase in the reference task. For example, if a PFC activation in a recognition-minus-reading subtraction is weaker in older adults, this could indicate that older adults did not activate this region as much as young adults during recognition, or that older adults activated the region more than young adults during reading. This problem is not solved by the inclusion of low-level sensory-motor baselines, because these tasks are also associated with age-related differences in brain activity (Grady et al., 1994). The search for an "absolute baseline" has been as successful as the pursuit of the Holy Grail. One way of ameliorating this problem is to have more than one baseline condition (e.g., Grady et al., 1995) or to use a multivariate technique, such as PLS (e.g., Cabeza, Grady, et al., 1997a).

The second problem is the assumption of "pure insertion" (Friston et al., 1996; Jennings, et al., 1997), that is, the idea that the addition of process A does not alter process B, and hence process B is exactly the same in the target task and in the reference task. When different groups of subjects are being compared the problem is augmented: it is not only possible that process A affects process B, but also that the effect differs across groups. One possibility is that the "insertion effect" is more pronounced in older adults because they have fewer processing resources (Craik & Byrd, 1982) and, hence, are more sensitive to the addition of cognitive components. Another possibility is that this effect is stronger in young adults, because their cognitive operations are assumed to be more flexible or fluid (e.g., Salthouse, 1996), and, consequently, more likely to change when combined with other operations.

The problems of the subtraction method can be partially circumvented by using parametric or event-related designs. In a parametric design, the process of interest varies across conditions while other aspects of the task remain relatively constant. For example, the number of letters held in a working memory task could be 2, 4, or 6, thereby varying working memory load within the same task. Parametric designs attenuate the problem of age-related differences in the baseline task, but they are not free of difficulties. For example, if the activation of a certain region increases as a function of the manipulation in one group but not the other, it is important to confirm that there were no ceiling or floor effects in one of the groups. When the component processes of a task have different time courses, event-related fMRI provides another way of disentangling them. For example, Rypma and D'Esposito (2000) differentiated encoding, maintenance, and retrieval stages of working memory, and found significant age effects only in the latter.

Performance

Brain activity can vary as a function of performance measures, such as accuracy (e.g., Nyberg, McIntosh et al., 1996) and reaction times (e.g., McIntosh et al., 1998; Rypma & D'Esposito, 2000). Therefore, it is an issue whether differences in brain activity between young and old subjects reflect the effects of aging or differences in performance levels. If the elderly group performs more poorly than young adults, then differences in brain activity between the young and older adults could reflect differences in task performance rather than differences in age. This is a typical "chicken and egg problem": do older adults perform poorly because their brain activity is different, or is their brain activity different because they perform poorly?

One approach to this problem is to equate cognitive performance in young and old groups, for example, by scanning high-functioning elderly subjects who perform as well as young adults (e.g., Cabeza, Grady et al., 1997). When cognitive performance is similar in the young and old groups, then differences in brain activity between the two groups can be safely attributed to aging. Unfortunately, this situation entails a different problem: if older adults can perform as well as the young despite a different pattern of activation, then there is a chance that these activation differences are inconsequential for cognitive performance. Thus, researchers are faced with a dilemma: if the relation of brain activity to performance is clear, then its relation to aging is uncertain; if the relation of brain activity to aging is clear, then its relation to performance is uncertain.

A possible solution to this dilemma is to compare brain activity in young and older adults both when performance is poorer in older adults and when performance is similar in both groups. One way of doing this is to introduce test performance as a factor within a factorial design. In the aforementioned study by Cabeza et al. (2000) comparing item and temporal-order memory, encoding conditions were manipulated so that each test had "high" and "low" performance conditions. Because the effects of this factor did not interact with group differences in brain activity, the authors assumed that the group differences could be attributed to aging rather than to performance differences.

Another method to address the confounding between age and performance differences is to analyze brain activity in direct relation to performance. For example, partial least squares (PLS) analyses may used to identify patterns of correlation between brain activity and behavior, and to determine whether these patterns are common or differ across young and older adults (Grady et al., 2000; McIntosh et al., 1999).

Finally, event-related fMRI paradigms have provided a new solution to the problem of performance differences: by analyzing only those trials in which performance was successful, group differences in performance can be controlled. The solution,

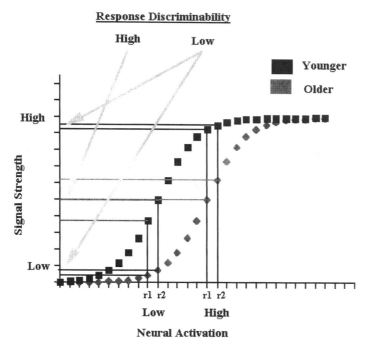

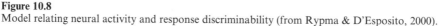

Figure 10.8
Model relating neural activity and response discriminability (from Rypma & D'Esposito, 2000).

however, is not perfect; brain activity during correct trials is probably different when overall performance is high (i.e., successful performance without much effort) than when it is low (i.e., successful performance with considerable effort). In conditions in which reaction times provide a good estimate of trial difficulty, RTs could be also used for selecting trials and matching performance across groups.

In this context, it is worth noting that the relation between RTs and brain activity may be different in young and older adults. Rypma and D'Esposito (2000), for example, found that higher PFC activity predicted slower responses in young adults but faster responses in older adults (see however, Grady et al., 1998). The authors accounted for this finding by assuming that, due to a sigmoid relationship between neuronal input and firing probability, there is an optimal level of activation for maximal response discriminability, and that this optimal activation level is higher for older adults than for young adults (see figure 10.8). Thus, within a certain range, increases in activation may be beneficial for older adults and detrimental for young adults. This brings us to issues concerning the interpretation of age-related differences in activation.

Activations

After subjects have been appropriately selected, task components suitably analyzed, and performance differences properly controlled, researchers are still faced with the fundamental problem of interpreting the age-related differences in activation they have found. The issues in this area can be divided into three groups: (1) determining what kinds of age-related differences in activation have occurred; (2) interpreting aging effects on the activation of a circumscribed region; and (3) evaluating global network changes. These three groups of issues are considered in turn below.

Determining the kinds of age-related differences found is not a trivial problem. First, an important issue is whether the two groups engaged different brain regions or the same region with different strengths. The first kind of difference may be called "qualitative" and the second, "quantitative." The distinction between qualitative and quantitative differences is not always easy. For example, quantitative differences may appear as qualitative due to threshold effects. Also, when two groups show activations in neighboring areas (e.g., BAs 45 and 46), these could be interpreted as "different" activations or as the "same" activation in different locations. Second, another knotty problem is whether age-related differences in activation reflect changes in neural architecture or in cognitive architecture (see Price & Friston, this volume). In other words, did young and older adults engage different regions to perform the same cognitive operations, or did they recruit different regions to perform different cognitive operations? If one wants to know if the neural correlates of process A change with age, it is critical that both groups engage process A to the same extent. At the same time, if aging is associated with a shift from process A to process B, then the neural correlates of *both* processes should be investigated in *both* groups. The main problem, of course, is how to determine exactly the processes engaged by human subjects, since cognitive tasks can be performed in many different ways and introspective reports provide very limited information about the actual operations performed by the subjects.

A second set of issues arises at the time of interpreting age-related differences in activation. At this early stage of the game, researchers have usually interpreted these differences in terms of one main dimension: whether these differences are "detrimental" or "beneficial" for cognition. In general, age-related decreases in activation have been interpreted as detrimental and age-related increases as beneficial. For example, if older adults did not activate a region activated by young adults, or activated it to a lesser extent, this might be interpreted as indicating that older adults did not recruit the region as much as young adults, and hence their cognitive performance suffered. In contrast, when older adults activated a region more than young adults, this could suggest that the additional activity served a compensatory function (e.g., Cabeza,

Grady et al., 1997; Grady et al., 1994). Unfortunately, the relation between neural activity and cognitive performance is not so simple; a decrease in activation may reflect more efficient processing (Karni et al., 1995) and an increase in activation may reflect unnecessary or even obstructive operations (Cabeza, Grady et al., 1997). Thus, age-related decreases in activation can be beneficial or detrimental, as can age-related increases in activation.

One method to distinguish between these alternative interpretations is to correlate brain activity with cognitive performance: if the correlation is positive, increases are probably beneficial and decreases are probably detrimental, whereas if the correlation is negative, then the converse interpretations could be made (see figure 10.6). The problem with correlations, however, is that they may reflect differences between subjects, rather than differences in performance per se. The interpretations in these two cases can be diametrically different. For example, if correlations are due to subject differences, a negative correlation may suggest that the activation was actually beneficial for performance but that the region was recruited only by subjects who had difficulty with the task. This issue may be explained with a simple analogy: although breathing is beneficial for running (it increases oxygenation), the correlation between breathing rate and running performance may be negative because poor runners need to breathe faster than good runners. Event-related fMRI can provide a solution for this problem. Event-related paradigms allow separate measures for successful and unsuccessful trials. Brain activity associated with successful trials can be safely interpreted as beneficial, providing stronger grounds for attributing age-related decreases to inefficient processing and age-related increases to functional compensation. Conversely, brain activity associated with unsuccessful trials can be interpreted as ineffectual or detrimental, with age-related changes interpreted accordingly.

Finally, although most studies have interpreted age-related differences in terms of local changes (e.g., PFC dysfunction), these differences may also reflect more global changes. In the aforementioned study by Cabeza, Grady et al. (1997), for example, the left PFC (BA 47) was more active during encoding than during recall in young adults, but it was more active during recall than during encoding in older adults (figure 10.9). It is difficult to interpret this result in terms of a local neural phenomenon, because the same region was less activated or more activated in older adults, depending on the task. In contrast, this kind of finding suggests a global change in which the same region can have different roles in the two age groups, depending on its interactions with other regions within the network subserving the task.

To investigate this issue, a follow-up study applied structural equation modeling to the encoding and recall PET data of both groups (Cabeza, McIntosh et al., 1997). Figure 10.10 (and color plate 22) shows the main results of this network analysis. In the young group, there was a shift from positive interactions involving the left PFC

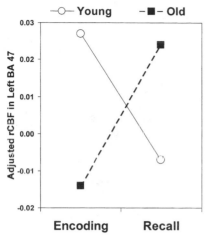

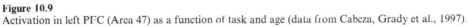

Figure 10.9
Activation in left PFC (Area 47) as a function of task and age (data from Cabeza, Grady et al., 1997).

during encoding to positive interactions involving the right PFC during recall (HERA pattern), whereas in the older group, PFC interactions were mixed during encoding and bilaterally positive during recall. Thus, these results suggest that the age-related decrease in left PFC activation during encoding does not reflect a local change in the left PFC but a global change in memory networks. More generally, these results support the idea that age-related changes in brain activation during a cognitive task are partly due to age-related changes in effective connectivity in the neural network underlying the task. If this idea is correct, then functional neuroimaging researchers will have to be cautious when interpreting age-related changes in activation without any information about global network changes. They will also have to cautions when interpreting similar patterns of brain activity in young and old adults. Actually, McIntosh et al. (1999) have shown that even if young and old adults recruit a similar set of brain regions, the functional interconnections between these regions can be quite different in the two groups. These differences in connectivity can occur even if old adults perform as well as young adults, suggesting that similar performance levels do not imply similar neural systems.

Concluding Remarks

In summary, task-related functional neuroimaging studies have investigated the effects of aging on neural activity during cognitive performance. During perception and attention, age-related decreases in occipital activity were coupled with age-related increases in prefrontal activity. During encoding, older adults showed weaker activa-

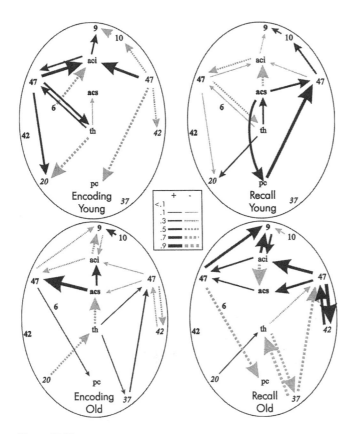

Figure 10.10
Results of a path analysis of activations during encoding and recall in young and older adults. Only path coefficients with a difference of >0.50 between encoding and recall conditions are displayed. Positive coefficients appear in solid red arrows and negative coefficients in segmented blue arrows, with the thickness of the arrow representing the strength of the effect (from Cabeza, McIntosh et al., 1997). (See color plate 22.)

tions in left prefrontal and medial temporal regions. During episodic retrieval, age-related decreases in right prefrontal activity were often accompanied by age-related increases in left prefrontal activity, whereas medial temporal activations were not reduced by aging. Priming was associated with right occipital activations in both young and older adults. During working memory, older adults often showed weaker prefrontal activations in the hemisphere primarily engaged by the young, but stronger prefrontal activations in the contralateral hemisphere. Age-related reductions during working memory affected dorsolateral prefrontal regions as well as regions associated with inhibition. The most consistent finding has been an age-related reduction in hemispheric asymmetry, found during both episodic retrieval and working memory.

In general, age-related decreases in activation have been attributed to inefficient cognitive processing and age-related increases in activation, to compensatory mechanisms. However, several issues must be addressed before definite conclusions can be reached. First, the selection of elderly participants must be examined. Screening procedures should provide enough confidence that age-related differences in activation are not artifacts generated by brain atrophy or cerebrovascular pathology. Given the large variability of cognitive decline in the aging population, cognitive performance must be controlled, or, even better, manipulated. The assumption that aging affects are similar across the aging populations may be incorrect, and it may be necessary to differentiate various patterns of aging. Second, the problems associated with tasks and designs in functional neuroimaging experiments are augmented by the inclusion of aging as a factor. Aging may affect task components differently, and this may appear as inconsistencies in the data if those components are not identified. The problems of the subtraction method, its relativity and "pure insertion" assumption, are even more serious when between-subject comparisons are added to the equation. Parametric methods and event-related fMRI can provide partial relief to these troubles Third, the close coupling between brain activity and cognitive performance has a downside: group differences in activity may just reflect performance differences. Manipulating and statistically controlling performance may ameliorate this problem. Finally, the most serious issue of all is the interpretation of age-related differences in activation: Are they detrimental, beneficial, or irrelevant? Do they reflect a local change or a global transformation of neurocognitive networks?

This long list of issues may seem overwhelming, but the progress in this area has been so fast that it is reasonable to expect they will be addressed before long. In just half decade, functional neuroimaging of cognitive aging has dramatically improved our chances of understanding the neural basis of age-related cognitive deficits. Even if several problems await resolution, the future of the cognitive neuroscience of aging has never been so bright.

ACKNOWLEDGMENTS

I thank Nicole Anderson, Cheryl Grady, David Madden, Lars Nyberg, Naftali Raz, and Endel Tulving for helpful comments, and NSERC and AHFMR (Canada) for financial support.

REFERENCES

Alexander, G. E., Delong, M. R., & Strick, P. L. (1986). Parallel organization of functionally segregated circuits linking basal ganglia and cortex. *Annual Review of Neuroscience* 9, 357–381.

Anderson, N. D., & Craik, F. I. M. (2000). Memory in the aging brain. In *Handbook of Memory*, E. Tulving & F. I. M. Craik, eds., Oxford: Oxford University Press.

Anderson, N. D., Craik, F. I. M., & Naveh-Benjamin, M. (1998). The attentional demands of encoding and retrieval in younger and older adults: I. Evidence from divided attention costs. *Psychology and Aging* 13, 405–423.

Anderson, N. D., Iidaka, T., McIntosh, A. R., Kapur, S., Cabeza, R., & Craik, F. I. M. (2000). The effects of divided attention on encoding- and retrieval related brain activity: A PET study of younger and older adults. *Journal of Cognitive Neuroscience*.

Bäckman, L., Almkvist, O., Andersson, J., Nordberg, A., Winblad, B., Rineck, R., & Lågström, B. (1997). Brain activation in young and older adults during implicit and explicit retrieval. *Journal of Cognitive Neuroscience* 9, 378–391.

Bäckman, L., Almkvist, O., Nyberg, L., & Andersson, J. (2000). Functional changes in brain activity during priming in Alzheimer's disease. *Journal of Cognitive Neuroscience* 12, 134–141.

Bäckman, L., Andersson, J., Nyberg, L., Winblad, B., Nordberg, A., & Almkvist, O. (1999). Brain regions associated with episodic retrieval in normal aging and Alzheimer's disease. *Neurology* 52, 1861–1870.

Baddeley, A. (1986). *Working Memory*. New York: Oxford University Press.

Baddeley, A. (1998). The central executive: A concept and some misconceptions. *Journal of the International Neuropsychological Society* 4, 523–526.

Balota, D. A., Dolan, P. O., & Duchek, J. M. (2000). Memory changes in healthy young and older adults. In *Handbook of Memory*, E. Tulving & F. I. M. Craik, eds., Oxford: Oxford University Press.

Baltes, P. B., & Lindenberger, U. (1997). Emergence of a powerful connection between sensory and cognitive functions across the adult life span: A new window to the study of cognitive aging? *Psychology and Aging* 12, 12–21.

Bashore, T. R. (1993). Differential effects of aging on the neurocognitive functions subserving speeded mental processing. In *Adult Information Processing: Limits on Loss*, J. Cerella, J. Rybash, W. Hoyer, & M. L. Commons, eds., 37–76. San Diego: Academic Press.

Becker, J. T., Mintun, M. A., Aleva, K., Wiseman, M. B., Nichols, T., & DeKosky, S. T. (1996). Compensatory reallocation of brain resources supporting verbal episodic memory in Alzheimers's disease. *Neurology* 46, 692–700.

Buckner, R. L., Corbetta, M., Schatz, J., Raichle, M. E., & Petersen, S. E. (1996). Preserved speech abilities and compensation following prefrontal damage. *Proceedings of the National Academy of Sciences USA* 93, 1249–53.

Cabeza, R., Anderson, A. D., Mangels, J., Nyberg, L., & Houle, S. (2000). Age-related differences in neural activity during item and temporal-order memory retrieval: A positron emission tomography study. *Journal of Cognitive Neuroscience* 12, 197–206.

Cabeza, R., Grady, C. L., Nyberg, L., McIntosh, A. R., Tulving, E., Kapur, S., Jennings, J. M., Houle, S., & Craik, F. I. M. (1997a). Age-related differences in neural activity during memory encoding and retrieval: A positron emission tomography study. *Journal of Neuroscience* 17, 391–400.

Cabeza, R., McIntosh, A. R., Tulving, E., Nyberg, L., & Grady, C. L. (1997). Age-related differences in effective neural connectivity during encoding and recall. *Neuroreport* 8, 3479–3483.

Cabeza, R., & Nyberg, L. (2000). Imaging Cognition II: An empirical review of 275 PET and fMRI studies. *Journal of Cognitive Neuroscience* 12, 1–47

Craik, F. I. M. (1983). On the transfer of information from temporary to permanent memory. *Philosophical Transactions of the Royal Society of London* B302, 341–359.

Craik, F. I. M. (1986). A functional account of age differences in memory. In *Human Memory and Cognitive Capabilities, Mechanisms, and Performances*, F. Lix & H. Hagendorf, eds., (499–522), Amsterdam: Elsevier Science Publishers B. V.

Craik, F. I. M., & Byrd, M. (1982). Aging and cognitive deficits: The role of attentional resources. In *Aging and cognitive processes*, F. I. M. Craik & S. Trehub, eds., 191–211, New York: Plenum.

Daneman, M., & Carpenter, P. A. (1980). Individual differences in working memory and reading. *Journal of Verbal Learning and Verbal Behavior* 19, 450–466.

de Keyser, J., De Backer, J.-P., Vauquelin, G., & Ebinger, G. (1990). The effect of aging on the D_1 dopamine receptors in human frontal cortex. *Brain Research* 528, 308–310.

DeKosky, S. T., & Palmer, A. M. (1994). Neurochemistry of aging. In *Clinical neurology of aging*, 2nd ed., M. L. Albert & J. E. Knoefel, eds., 79–101. New York: Oxford University Press.

D'Esposito, M., Zarahn, E., Aguirre, G. K., & Rypma, B. (2000). The effect of normal aging on the coupling of neural activity to the BOLD hemodynamic response. *Neuroimage* 10, 6–14.

Donaldson, D. I., & Rugg, M. D. (1998). Recognition memory for new associations: Electrophysiological evidence for the role of recollection. *Neuropsychologia* 36, 337–395.

Engelien, A., Silbersweig, D., Stern, E., Huber, W., Doring, W., Frith, C., & Frackowiak, R. S. (1995). The functional anatomy of recovery from auditory agnosia: A PET study of sound categorization in a neurological patient and normal controls. *Brain* 118, 1395–1409.

Esiri, M. (1994). Dementia and normal aging: neuropathology. In *Dementia and Normal Aging*, F. A. Huppert, C. Brayne, & D. W. O'Connor, eds. Cambridge, UK: Cambridge University Press.

Esposito, G., Kirby, G. S., Van Horn, J. D., Ellmore, T. M., & Faith Berman, K. (1999). Context-dependent, neural system-specific neurophysiological concomitants of ageing: Mapping PET correlates during cognitive activation. *Brain* 122, 963–979.

Eustache, F., Rioux, P., Desgranges, B., Marchal, G., Petit-Taboue, M. C., Dary, M., Lechevalier, B., & Baron, J. C. (1995). Healthy aging, memory subsystems and regional cerebral oxygen consumption. *Neuropsychologia* 33, 867–87.

Friston, K. J., Price, C. J., Fletcher, P., Moore, C., Frackowiak, R. S., & Dolan, R. J. (1996). The trouble with cognitive subtraction. *Neuroimage* 4, 97–104.

Glisky, E. L., Polster, M. R., & Routhieaux, B. C. (1995). Double dissociation between item and source memory. *Neuropsychology* 9, 229–235.

Golomb, J., Kluger, A., de Leon, M. J., Ferris, S. H., Convit, A., Mittelman, M., Cohen, J., Rusinek, H., De Santi, S., & George, A. E. (1994). Hippocampal formation size in normal human aging: A correlate of delayed secondary memory performance. *Learning and Memory* 1, 45–54.

Grady, C. L., Maisog, J. M., Horwitz, B., Ungerleider, L. G., Mentis, M. J., Salerno, J. A., Pietrini, P., Wagner, E., & Haxby, J. V. (1994). Age-related changes in cortical blood flow activation during visual processing of faces and location. *Journal of Neuroscience* 14(3, Pt 2), 1450–1462.

Grady, C. L., McIntosh, A. R., Bookstein, F., Horwitz, B., Rapoport, S. I., & Haxby, J. V. (1998). Age-related changes in regional cerebral blood flow during working memory for faces. *Neuroimage* 8, 409–425.

Grady, C. L., McIntosh, A. R., Horwitz, B., Maisog, J. M., Ungerleider, L. G., Mentis, M. J., Pietrini, P., Schapiro, M. B., & Haxby, J. V. (1995). Age-related reductions in human recognition memory due to impaired encoding. *Science* 269, 218–221.

Grady, C. L., McIntosh, A. R., Horwitz, B., & Rapoport, S. I. (2000). Age-related changes in the neural correlates of degraded and nondegraded face processing. *Cognitive Neuropsychology* 217, 165–186.

Grady, C. L., McIntosh, A. R., Raja, M. N., Beig, S., & Craik, F. I. M. (1999). The effects of age on the neural correlates of episodic encoding. *Cerebral Cortex* 9, 805–814.

Haaland, K. Y., Vranes, L. F., Goodwin, J. S., & Garry, P. J. (1987). Wisconsin Card Sorting Test performance in a healthy elderly population. *Journal of Gerontology* 42, 345–346.

Haist, F., Shimamura, A. P., & Squire, L. R. (1992). On the relationship between recall and recognition memory. *Journal of Experimental Psychology: Learning, Memory, and Cognition* 18, 691–702.

Hasher, L., & Zacks, R. T. (1988). Working memory, comprehension and aging: A review and a new view. *Psychology of Learning and Motivation* 22, 193–225.

Hasher, L., Zacks, R. T., & Macy, C. P. (1999). Inhibitory control, circadian arousal, and age. In *Attention and Performance, XVII: Cognitive Regulation of Performance: Interaction of Theory and Application*, D. Gopher & A. Koriat, eds. Cambridge, MA: MIT Press.

Hirst, W., Johnson, M. K., Phelps, E. A., & Volpe, B. T. (1988). More on recognition and recall in amnesics. *Journal of Experimental Psychology: Learning, Memory, & Cognition* 14, 758–762.

Jennings, J. M., & Jacoby, L. L. (1993). Automatic versus intentional uses of memory: Aging, attention, and control. *Psychology & Aging* 8, 283–293.

Jennings, J. M., & Jacoby, L. L. (1997). An opposition procedure for detecting age-related deficits in recollection: Telling effects of repetition. *Psychology & Aging* 12, 352–361.

Jennings, J. M., McIntosh, A. R., Kapur, S., Tulving, E., & Houle, S. (1997). Cognitive subtractions may not add up: the interaction between semantic processing and response mode. *Neuroimage* 5, 229–39.

Jonides, Marshuetz, C., Smith, E. E., Reuter-Lorenz, P. A., Koeppe, R. A., & Hartley, A. (2000). Brain activation reveals changes with age in resolving interference in verbal working memory. *Journal of Cognitive Neuroscience* 12, 188–196.

Jonides, J., Smith, E. E., Marshuetz, C., Koeppe, R. A., & Reuter-Lorenz, P. A. (1998). Inhibition in verbal working memory revealed by brain activation. *Proceedings of the National Academy of Sciences USA* 95, 8410–8413.

Kahneman, D. (1973). *Attention and Effort.* Englewood Cliffs, NJ: Prentice-Hall.

Karni, A., Meyer, G., Jezzard, P., Adams, M. M., & et al. (1995). Functional MRI evidence for adult motor cortex plasticity during motor skill learning. *Nature* 377, 155–158.

Kemper, T. (1984). Neuroanatomical and neuropathological changes in normal aging and in dementia. In *Clinical Neurology of Aging*, M. Albert, ed., 9–52. New York: Oxford University Press.

Kemper, T. (1994). Neuroanatomical and neuropathological changes during aging and in dementia. In *Clinical Neurology of Aging*, 2nd ed., M. L. Albert & E. J. E. Knoepfel, eds., 3–67. New York: Oxford University Press.

Kohler, S., Black, S. E., Sinden, M., Szekely, C., Kidron, D., Parker, J. L., Foster, J. K., Moscovitch, M., Winocur, G., Szalai, J. P., & Bronskill, M. J. (1998). Hippocampal and parahippocampal gyrus atrophy in relation to distinct anterograde memory impairment in Alzheimer's disease: An MR volumetric study. *Neuropsychologia* 26, 129–142.

Kuhl, D. E., Metter, E. J., Riege, W. H., & Hawkins, R. A. (1984). The effect of aging on patterns of local cerebral glucose utilization. *Annals of Neurology* 15, S133–S137.

La Voie, D., & Light, L. L. (1994). Adult age differences in repetition priming: A meta-analysis. *Psychology and Aging* 9, 539–553.

Lee, K. S., Frey, K. A., Koeppe, R. A., Buck, A., Mulholland, G. K., & Kuhl, D. E. (1996). In vivo quantification of cerebral muscarinic receptors in normal human aging using positron emission tomography and [^{11}C]tropanyl benzilate. *Journal of Cerebral Blood Flow & Metabolism* 16, 303–10.

Lindenberger, U., & Baltes, P. B. (1994). Sensory functioning and intelligence in old age: A strong connection. *Psychology and Aging* 9, 339–355.

Madden, D. J., Gottlob, L. R., Denny, L. L., Turkington, T. G., Provenzale, J. M., Hawk, T. C., & Coleman, R. E. (1999). Aging and recognition memory: Changes in regional cerebral blood flow associated with components of reaction time distributions. *Journal of Cognitive Neuroscience* 11, 511–520.

Madden, D. J., & Hoffman, J. M. (1997). Application of positron emission tomogrphy to age-related cognitive changes. In *Brain Imaging in Clinical Psychiatry*, K. R. R. Krishman & P. M. Doraiswamy, eds. New York: M. Dekker.

Madden, D. J., Turkington, T. G., Coleman, R. E., Provenzale, J. M., DeGrado, T., R., & Hoffman, J. M. (1996). Adult age differences in regional cerebral blood flow during visual word identification: Evidence from H215O PET. *Neuroimage* 3, 127–142.

Madden, D. J., Turkington, T. G., Provenzale, J. M., Denny, L. L., Hawk, T. C., Gottlob, L. R., & Coleman, R. E. (1999). Adult age differences in functional neuroanatomy of verbal recognition memory. *Human Brain Mapping* 7, 115–135.

Madden, D. J., Turkington, T. G., Provenzale, J. M., Hawk, T. C., Hoffman, J. M., & Coleman, R. E. (1997). Selective and divided visual attention: Age-related changes in regional cerebral blood flow measured by H2150 PET. *Human Brain Mapping* 5, 389–409.

Mandler, G. (1980). Recognizing: The judgement of previous occurrence. *Psychological Review* 87, 252–271.

Martin, W. R., Ye, F. Q., & Allen, P. S. (1998). Increasing striatal iron content associated with normal aging. *Movement Disorders* 13, 281–286.

McDowd, J. M., & Shaw, R. J. (2000). Attention and aging: A Functional perspective. In *Handbook of Aging and Cognition II*, F. I. M. Craik & T. A. Salthouse, eds. Mahwah, NJ: Erlbaum.

McIntosh, A. R., Lobaugh, N. J., Cabeza, R., Bookstein, F., & Houle, S. (1998). Convergence of neural systems processing stimulus associations and coordinating motor responses. *Cerebral Cortex* 8, 648–659.

McIntosh, A. R., Sekuler, A. B., Penpeci, C., Rajah, M. N., Grady, C. L., Sekuler, R., & Bennett, P. J. (1999). Recruitment of unique neural systems to support visual memory in normal aging. *Current Biology* 9, 1275–1278.

Mitchell, K. J., Johnson, M. K., Raye, C. L., & D'Esposito, M. (in press). fMRI evidence of age-related hippocampal dysfunction in feature binding in working memory. *Cognitive Brain Research*.

Moscovitch, M. (1992). Memory and working-with-memory: A component process model based on modules and central systems. *Journal of Cognitive Neuroscience* 4, 257–267. (Special Issue: Memory Systems).

Moscovitch, M., & Umiltà, C. (1991). Conscious and nonconscious aspects of memory: A neuropsychological framework of modules and central systems. In *Perspectives in Cognitive Neuroscience*, R. G. Lister & H. J. Weingartner, eds. Oxford: Oxford University Press.

Moscovitch, M., & Winocur, G. (1992). The neuropsychology of memory and aging. In *The Handbook of Aging and Cognition*, F. I. M. Craik & T. A. Salthouse, eds., 315–372. Hillsdale, NJ: Erlbaum.

Moscovitch, M., & Winocur, G. (1995). Frontal lobes, memory, and aging. *Annals of the New York Academy of Sciences* 769, 119–150.

Nagahama, Y., Fukuyama, H., Yamaguchi, H., Katsumi, Y., Magata, Y., Shibasaki, H., & Kimura, J. (1997). Age-related changes in cerebral blood flow activation during a card sorting test. *Experimental Brain Research* 114, 571–577.

Nyberg, L., Cabeza, R., & Tulving, E. (1996a). PET studies of encoding and retrieval: The HERA model. *Psychonomic Bulletin & Review* 3, 135–148.

Nyberg, L., McIntosh, A. R., Houle, S., Nilson, L.-G., & Tulving, E. (1996b). Activation of medial temporal structures during episodic memory retrieval. *Nature* 380, 715–717.

Nyberg, L., Tulving, E., Habib, R., Nilsson, L.-G., Kapur, S., Houle, S., Cabeza, R., & McIntosh, A. R. (1995). Functional brain maps of retrieval mode and recovery of episodic information. *Neuroreport* 7, 249–252.

Owen, A. M. (1997). The functional organization of working memory processes within human lateral frontal cortex: the contribution of functional neuroimaging. *European Journal of Neuroscience* 9, 1329–39.

Parkin, A. J., & Lawrence, A. (1994). A dissociation in the relation between memory tasks and frontal lobe tests in the normal elderly. *Neuropsychologia* 32, 1523–1532.

Petrides, M. (1994). Frontal lobes and working memory: evidence from investigations of the effects of cortical excisions in nonhumans primates. In *Handbook of Neuropsychology*, F. Boller & J. Grafman, eds., vol. 9, 59–82. Amsterdam: Elsevier.

Petrides, M. (1995). Functional organization of the human frontal cortex for mnemonic processing: Evidence from neuroimaging studies. *Annals of the New York Academy of Sciences* 769, 85–96.

Posner, M. I., & Petersen, S. E. (1990). The attention system of the human brain. *Annual Review of Neurosciences* 13, 25–42.

Prull, M. W., Gabrieli, J. D. E., & Bunge, S. A. (2000). Memory and aging: A cognitive neuroscience perspective. In *Handbook of Aging and Cognition II*, F. I. M. Craik & T. A. Salthouse, eds. Mahwah, NJ: Erlbaum.

Raz, N. (2000). Aging of the brain and its impact on cognitive performance: Integration of structural and functional findings. In *Handbook of Aging and Cognition II*, F. I. M. Craik & T. A. Salthouse, eds. Mahwah, NJ: Erlbaum.

Raz, N., Dupuis, J. H., Briggs, S. D., McGavran, C., & Acker, J. D. (1998a). Differential effects of age and sex on the cerebellar hemispheres and the vermis: A prospective MR study. *American Journal of Neuroradiology* 19, 65–71.

Raz, N., Gunning, F. M., Head, D., Dupuis, J. H., McQuain, J., Briggs, S. D., Loken, W. J., Thornton, A. E., & Acker, J. D. (1997). Selective aging of the human cerebral cortex observed in vivo: Differential vulnerability of the prefrontal gray matter. *Cerebral Cortex* 7, 268–82.

Raz, N., Gunning-Dixon, F. M., Head, D., Dupuis, J. H., & Acker, J. D. (1998b). Neuroanatomical correlates of cognitive aging: evidence from structural magnetic resonance imaging. *Neuropsychology* 12, 95–114.

Reuter-Lorenz, P., Jonides, J., Smith, E. S., Hartley, A., Miller, A., Marshuetz, C., & Koeppe, R. A. (2000). Age differences in the frontal lateralization of verbal and spatial working memory revealed by PET. *Journal of Cognitive Neuroscience* 12, 174–187.

Roediger, H. L., & McDermott, K. B. (1993). Implicit memory in normal human subjects. In *Handbook of Neuropsychology*, F. Boller & J. Grafman, eds., vol. 8. Amsterdam: Elsevier.

Rypma, B., & D'Esposito, M. (2000). Isolating the neural mechanisms of age-relate changes in human working memory. *Nature Neuroscience*, 3, 509–515.

Rypma, B., Prabhakaran, V., Desmond, J. D., & Gabrieli, J. D. E. (2000). Age differences in prefrontal cortical activity in working memory. Manuscript submitted for publication.

Salthouse, T. A. (1996). The processing speed theory of adult age differences in cognition. *Psychological Review* 103, 403–428.

Schacter, D. L., Savage, C. R., Alpert, N. M., Rauch, S. L., & Albert, M. S. (1996). The role of hippocampus and frontal cortex in age-related memory changes: A PET study. *Neuroreport* 7, 1165–1169.

Schneider, B. A., & Pichora-Fuller, M. K. (2000). Implications of perceptual deterioration for cognitive aging research. In *Handbook of Aging and Cognition II*, F. I. M. Craik & T. A. Salthouse, eds. Mahwah, NJ: Erlbaum.

Schochet, S. S., Jr. (1998). Neuropathology of aging. *Neurologic Clinics* 16, 569–80.

Skoog, I. (1998). Status of risk factors for vascular dementia. *Neuroepidemiology* 17, 2–9.

Smith, E. E., & Jonides, J. (1997). Working memory: A view from neuroimaging. *Cognitive Psychology* 33, 5–42.

Spencer, W. D., & Raz, N. (1995). Differential effects of aging on memory for content and context: A meta-analysis. *Psychology & Aging* 10, 527–539.

Strong, R. (1998). Neurochemical changes in the aging human brain: Implications for behavioral impairment and neurodegenerative disease. *Geriatrics* 53 (Suppl. 1), S9–12.

Tulving, E. (1983). *Elements of Episodic Memory*. Oxford: Oxford University Press.

Tulving, E. (1995). Organization of memory: Quo vadis? In *The Cognitive Neurosciences*, M. S. Gazzaniga, ed. Cambridge, MA: MIT Press.

Tulving, E., Kapur, S., Craik, F. I. M., Moscovitch, M., & Houle, S. (1994). Hemispheric encoding/retrieval asymmetry in episodic memory: Positron emission tomography findings. *Proceedings of the National Academy of Sciences USA* 91, 2016–2020.

Ungerleider, L. G., & Mishkin, M. (1982). Two cortical visual systems. In *Analysis of Visual Behavior*, D. J. Ingle, M. A. Goodale, & R. J. W. Mansfield, eds., 549–589. Cambridge, MA: MIT Press.

Verhaeghen, P., Marcoen, A., & Goossens, L. (1993). Facts and fiction about memory aging: A quantitative integration of research findings. *Journal of Gerontology* 48, 157–171.

Volkow, N. D., Gur, R. C., Wang, G. J., Fowler, J. S., Moberg, P. J., Ding, Y. S., Hitzemann, R., Smith, G., & Logan, J. (1998). Association between decline in brain dopamine activity with age and cognitive and motor impairment in healthy individuals. *American Journal of Psychiatry* 155, 344–349.

Wang, G. J., Volkow, N. D., Logan, J., Fowler, J. S., Schlyer, D., MacGregor, R. R., Hitzemann, R. J., Gur, R. C., & Wolf, A. P. (1995). Evaluation of age-related changes in serotoning 5-HT$_2$ and dopamine D$_2$ receptor availability in healthy human subjects. *Life Sciences* 56, 249–253.

Weinstock, M. (1995). The pharmacotherapy of Alzheimer's disease based on the cholinergic hypothesis: An update. *Neurodegeneration* 4, 249–256.

West, R. L. (1996). An application of prefrontal cortex function theory to cognitive aging. *Psychological Bulletin* 120, 272–292.

Yonelinas, A. P. (1997). Recognition memory ROCs for item and associative information: The contribution of recollection and familiarity. *Memory & Cognition* 25, 747–763.

Zacks, R. T., Hasher, L., & Li, K. Z. H. (2000). Human memory. In *Handbook of Aging and Cognition II*, F. I. M. Craik & T. A. Salthouse, eds. Mahwah, NJ: Erlbaum.

11 Functional Neuroimaging of Neuropsychologically Impaired Patients

Cathy J. Price and Karl J. Friston

INTRODUCTION

This chapter addresses some critical issues that arise when performing brain imaging experiments on patients with neurological insult and psychological impairment. In the 1990s, neuropsychology per se has been fundamentally augmented by the ability to measure the neurophysiological correlates of cognitive processing. This has led to a revision of some cognitive models and a shift in emphasis from cognitive science to cognitive neuroscience. Despite the abundant literature from imaging studies and neuropsychology, there are many issues of interpretation that remain unresolved. In this chapter, we consider some basic questions about how neuroimaging can be used to inform the neuropsychological characterization of patients and some of the logical limitations or restrictions on the inferences that can be made. In particular, we focus on the conditions that are necessary to draw tenable conclusions when a patient's brain activates in an abnormal way relative to normal subjects. The chapter is divided into three sections. In this introductory section, we review the expectations of neuropsychology and neuroimaging. The second section provides some examples of how neuroimaging experiments have been used to inform normal and abnormal models of brain function, and the third section addresses some of the implicit assumptions and limitations that are encountered.

Neuropsychological Studies of Cognitively Impaired Patients

Neuropsychology is the study of patients with functional deficits in which the neuronal pathophysiology is known to a lesser or greater extent. Neuropsychological investigations have contributed to our understanding of normal brain function by informing models of cognition and functional anatomy. Typically, models of cognition are engendered or modified by neuropsychological studies when patients demonstrate a double dissociation in the impairment of selective functions. For instance, different types of dyslexia point to a double dissociation in reading processes: some patients retain the ability to read words with regular spelling-to-sound correspondence but fail to read words that do not follow spelling rules. In contrast, other patients suffer the reverse dissociation. This particular double dissociation has been used to infer the independence of two routes to reading (see Coltheart, 1981).

With respect to normal functional anatomy, the inferences that can be drawn from brain-damaged patients are based on the lesion deficit model. To be informative, the lesion deficit model requires a patient with a selective brain lesion and a selective cognitive deficit. The function of the damaged brain region is simply equated with the lost cognitive skill. Some classic examples of the lesion deficit model, as applied to neuropsychological patients, were documented by the 19th-century neurologists. For instance, postmortem studies demonstrated that a patient who had been impaired at articulating language had damage encompassing the third frontal convolution (Broca, 1861) and a patient with a deficit in speech comprehension had damage to the left posterior temporal cortex (Wernicke, 1874). By deduction, Broca's area was associated with speech production and Wernicke's area was associated with speech comprehension. Wernicke developed the model further to predict that patients could have intact speech comprehension and production but a deficit in integrating these regions in order to repeat what was heard. This type of disconnection syndrome, referred to as conduction aphasia, was demonstrated by Lichtheim (1885) in a patient who had damage to the white matter tract that connects Broca's area with Wernicke's area (the arcuate fasciculus). By clinical descriptions and localization of lesions, Wernicke and Lichtheim were able to demonstrate that disorders of language arose either from damage to the "centers of memory images" or from disconnections between the so-called centers.

Limitations of the Lesion Deficit Model

The shortcomings of the lesion deficit model are becoming increasingly appreciated. For a number of reasons, it is very difficult to ascribe a function to a particular region that has been damaged. Perhaps the most obvious is that pathological (as opposed to experimental) lesions seldom conform to functionally homogeneous neuroanatomical systems. Furthermore, the neuropsychological profile is usually complicated, involving more than one functional deficit, and these deficits can be obscured by the compensatory measures adopted by the patient to overcome them. Any reasonable relationship between the functional deficit and the brain systems involved is therefore usually impossible to establish. Another problem with the lesion deficit model, which has a history dating from the 19th century (Goltz, 1881) is that the results of lesion studies are properly interpreted only by referring to the connections between cortical areas: damage to a selected area may impair nearby connections, and therefore the responsiveness of undamaged areas. Indeed, it is impossible to distinguish between the impact of a lesion due to the loss of neuronal infrastructure per se and the more pervasive dysfunction of distributed systems of which the lesioned area is a component. These considerations mean that all that can be concluded from a lesion deficit study is that the neuronal systems intrinsic to the lesioned area, or the connections passing through this area, were necessary for the cognitive function. One cannot say that this region was either sufficient for, or uniquely identifiable with, the function in question.

Expectations of Neuroimaging with Brain-Damaged Patients

With the advent of functional neuroimaging, it is hoped that some of the incompleteness of the lesion deficit model can be remedied by studying brain activity in normal and brain-damaged subjects. Functional imaging offers several fundamental advantages over the lesion deficit model. The most obvious is that brain activity can be observed, noninvasively, in subjects who have normal psychological and physiological responses. The other major advantage is that, unlike the lesion deficit model, functional imaging is not limited to a particular region of the brain that has been damaged; rather, the system of distributed cortical areas that sustain sensory, motor, or cognitive tasks can be identified. This systems-level approach has several important implications. First, unlike the lesion deficit model, it does not assume that cognitive processes or operations are localized in discrete anatomical modules, but allows for functional specialization that is embodied in the interactions among two or more areas. In relation to patient studies, the systems-level approach enables one to identify where there is abnormal function in the absence of structural damage and where the responsiveness of an undamaged region is context dependent (responds normally) in some tasks and abnormally in others.

Most neuroimaging studies assume that different tasks will be associated with a different set of cortical areas, and experiments aim to identify the areas where there are changes in regional cerebral activity in response to changes in task or to pathology. Irrespective of whether a cognitive function is localized in one or more than one brain region, the existence of a distinct set of regions for one task relative to another is embodied in the concept of functional segregation. A different perspective on functional brain systems is functional integration. Whereas functional segregation refers to the specialization evident when different cognitive processes are associated with activity in different brain regions, functional integration refers to the integration of these regions where the interactions among regions may be profoundly task dependent (see chapter 3 in this volume). This distinction between studies of functional segregation and functional integration is crucial for imaging patients because some patients suffer from abnormal functional segregation (the function of a discrete cortical area is abnormal) and some patients suffer from abnormal functional integration (abnormal interactions among different brain regions). More specifically, as described by Wernicke and Lichtheim (see above), patients may behave abnormally following (1) damage to an area of gray matter with a particular specialization (e.g., Broca's area or Wernicke's area), (2) damage to white matter that connects gray matter regions (e.g., the arcuate fasciculus), or (3) no detectable pathological damage but a failure to integrate activity during particular tasks. The latter two cases correspond to anatomical and functional disconnection syndromes, respectively, and in these cases a functional deficit will be revealed only by looking at how different regions interact.

Functional imaging can assess these functional interactions in terms of correlations between the responses of two regions. These correlations may be expressed during some tasks but not during others. Functional neuroimaging therefore provides a potential means to test directly the disconnection syndromes described by the 19th-century neurologists. Current advances in diffusion weighted magnetic resonance imaging may allow one to measure lesions in anatomical connections directly. This will, it is hoped, confer a more integrative perspective on the lesion deficit model.

Functional neuroimaging experiments aim to characterize the basic relationship between the cognitive processes elicited by a task and the neuronal responses that underpin them. In this chapter, the discussion of this relationship will be in terms of the task analysis, cognitive architectures, and neuronal architectures. A task consists of the cognitive and sensorimotor processes that it comprises. Task analysis is the decomposition of a task into these component processes, whose existence is inferred on the basis of neuropsychological, psychophysiological, and psychophysical studies. The cognitive architecture is any particular set of processes and the serial or parallel interactions among them. The neuronal architecture relates to how a particular cognitive architecture is implemented in the brain by neuronal dynamics in distributed cortical areas, subareas, and neuronal populations. It is the relationship between the neuronal and cognitive architecture that underlies the interpretation of brain imaging data in the context of neuropsychological impairment. This requires a comprehensive and valid task analysis that specifies the cognitive architecture and enables mapping from the cognitive to the neural domain. The problems of specifying a complete task analysis are addressed below in the section "Issues."

With respect to neuroimaging studies of cognitively impaired patients, the most seemingly straightforward application is the investigation of how a neuropsychological deficit is characterized in terms of abnormal brain function. The idea is that brain activity observed when patients perform a task can be compared with that when normal subjects perform the same task. Differences between patients and normals can then be ascribed to the neuropsychological syndrome. In other words, it might be expected that the alteration of neuronal responses in the damaged brain will shed some light on the physiological underpinnings of a cognitive deficit. There are fundamental limitations when using neuroimaging in this way. We will discuss these limitations in the section "Issues." The most critical point relates to task performance. By definition, patients will have reduced performance relative to normals on tasks that reveal a cognitive impairment. In severe cases, the patients may not be able to perform a task at all. In this case it is meaningless to perform neuroimaging experiments that attempt to compare normal and abnormal brain activity because failure to activate could be due either to a loss of neuronal responsiveness or to a failure to perform the task. Neuroimaging studies of patients are therefore interpretable relative to normal subjects only if (1) the patients retain the ability to perform the task normally or (2) the patients activate normally (i.e., one variable is kept constant).

Of course, these restrictions severely limit the range of experiments that can be performed in an ideal fashion with patients. They also have a critical impact on the types of questions that can be addressed. Nevertheless, it may still be possible to equate cognitive symptoms to abnormal neuronal responses when patients perform significantly above chance but significantly below normal controls. For example, in the case of reduced accuracy, analysis of functional imaging data can model correct responses separately from incorrect responses. Patients can then be compared to normals on trials (or blocks of trials) where performance is matched. This is most effectively achieved by analyzing single events (trials) using an event-related design (in fMRI or ERP studies), but if performance is only mildly impaired, it is also possible to analyze blocks of trials (in PET or blocked fMRI designs) where the mean normal and patient performances are the same. Another approach to discounting performance differences is to enter normal and patient response measures (e.g., reaction times) into the analysis as confounds.

Once performance is matched, abnormal neuronal responses can be attributed to changes in either the cognitive architecture (cognitive reorganization) or changes in the neuronal architecture (neuronal reorganization). Cognitive reorganization occurs when a patient uses a different set of cognitive processes to perform the same task either because a new cognitive procedure has been learned or because of increased demands on normal cognitive processes, particularly attention. Neuronal reorganization is mediated by changes in the strength of preexisting connections. It does not indicate a rewiring of the neuronal system because in the mature brain, neuronal systems and extrinsic connections are fully established. Changes in the strength of preexisting connections may result from learning-dependent plasticity or may simply be a direct consequence of brain damage that can disrupt neuronal responses at, or distant from, the lesion site.

Evidence for either cognitive or neuronal reorganization (in the context of normal task performance) has implications for both abnormal and normal models of processing. In either case, abnormal activations fall into three categories: (1) activation is

Table 11.1
Informing Models of Abnormal Cognitive Processing from Abnormal Brain Activation

Underactivation	1. Damage to local tissue
	2. Damage to distant tissue (e.g., a diaschisis)
	3. Cognitive reorganization
Overactivation	1. Learning-related plasticity
	2. Disinhibition of duplicated neuronal system
	3. Cognitive reorganization

Table 11.2
Informing Models of Normal Cognitive Processing from Abnormal Brain Activation

Underactivation	1. Redundant area (area not necessary for task performance)
	2. Connections between damaged and underactive area
Overactivation	1. Duplicated neuronal system
	2. Alternative cognitive strategies

greater for normals than for patients (underactivity); (2) activation is greater for patients than normals (overactivity); and (3) the same regions activate but there are alterations in the effective connectivity between regions. Table 11.1 summarizes how abnormal activation in the context of normal performance can inform abnormal models of cognitive processing.

Table 11.1 indicates that areas of underactivity in the patients could indicate damage to the tissue itself, damage to the inputs into the underresponsive region (a diaschisis), or changes in cognitive strategy (cognitive reorganization). In contrast, areas of overactivity in patients can reflect a disinhibition of a duplicate neuronal system that can implement the same task, learning-related plasticity, or cognitive reorganization. Table 11.2 summarizes how abnormal activation in the context of normal performance can inform normal models of cognitive processing.

Table 11.2 indicates that areas of underactivity (in the context of normal task performance) can be used to infer that normal activation was not necessary to perform the task (activation was redundant). If there is a known site of brain damage that is distant from a region of underactivity, we can also infer that the damaged region encompassed inputs to the underactive region (i.e., make implications about the normal connections between regions). Areas of overactivity in the patient (in the context of normal task performance) can be used to infer which regions of the brain are able to take over the function of damaged regions. The more difficult issue is to distinguish whether the functional reorganization is cognitive or neuronal in nature (see the section "Issues"). The ideas summarized in tables 11.1 and 11.2 are reprised in the next section, which provides examples of the types of neuroimaging studies that can be performed with neurologically damaged patients.

FUNCTIONAL NEUROIMAGING OF NEUROPSYCHOLOGICALLY IMPAIRED PATIENTS

This section is divided into two parts. The first, "Informing Models of Abnormal Functional Anatomy," provides examples of how functional imaging can inform models of abnormal processing; the second, "Informing Models of Normal Functional Anatomy," provides examples of how functional imaging can inform models of normal processing.

Informing Models of Abnormal Functional Anatomy

The advantage of functional neuroimaging, as discussed above, is that it can identify distributed brain systems responding to a particular task. This means that, unlike the lesion deficit model, functional neuroimaging can detect (1) normal functionality at a site of brain damage, (2) abnormal functionality distant from the site of known brain damage, and (3) abnormal functionality in the absence of brain damage. Critically, some of these effects may be task specific, depending on which inputs are being used. In patients, for example, a nondamaged region can perform normally in some tasks and abnormally in other tasks, depending on whether input from a disconnected region is required.

Below we report functional imaging studies of (1) semantic dementia and (2) Broca's aphasia, where dysfunctional integration can be attributed directly to structural damage; (3) studies of schizophrenia where there is no obvious anatomical damage to account for the functional disintegration; and (4) studies of language recovery following aphasia, where functionality is preserved by activation of peridamage tissue, duplicated neuronal systems, or cognitive reorganization.

"Semantic dementia" is the term used to describe patients suffering from a progressive deterioration in semantic knowledge and name retrieval while other cognitive and language functions remain relatively intact (Warrington, 1975; Sasanuma and Monoi, 1975; Hodges et al., 1992). The anatomical correlates, according to the lesion deficit model, lie in bilateral temporal lobes; cortical atrophy commences in the anterior temporal poles and then spreads posteriorly as the disease progresses. Application of the lesion deficit model leads to the inference that the damaged anterior temporal lobes are the site of the impaired semantic and naming processes. Functional neuroimaging allows us to evaluate whether patients show response changes in the damaged anterior temporal lobe or whether damage to the anterior temporal lobe results in abnormal activation in other (intact) regions of the language system.

This approach was used by Mummery et al. (1999) with four semantic patients and six age-matched control subjects. Semantic similarity judgments were used to activate the semantic system, and perceptual (visual size) judgments were used as a control condition. In order to exclude the possibility that the abnormal responses detected in the patients were a direct consequence of impaired performance (see above), scans in which patients had impaired performance relative to the normals were removed from the analysis. The results revealed that both patients and normals activated the left inferior frontal, left temporoparietal cortex, left middle temporal cortex, anterior cingulate, and right cerebellum. Unlike the normals, the patients did not activate the left posterior inferior temporal cortex or the right temporoparietal junction. Neither of these regions evidenced any structural damage on structural MRI scans, but damage to the left posterior inferior temporal region in other patients has been associated with naming deficits (Foundas et al., 1998) and may account for the impairment all the patients had in naming.

Remarkably, the regions where there was structural damage (the anterior temporal cortices) were more active in the patients than in the normals. These results demonstrate that the site of reduced activation was distant from the site of structural damage and suggest a functional disintegration between the anterior and posterior temporal cortices. If this is the case, we might expect the posterior temporal region to perform normally in other tasks that do not require input from the anterior temporal region. This has not yet been investigated with the semantic dementia patients. However, an example of how an underresponsive region can respond normally in one task but abnormally in another is given below in the context of patients with damage to Broca's area.

Broca's aphasia was first described at the end of the 19th century (Broca, 1861) in the context of a patient who had impaired speech production but relatively intact speech comprehension following damage to the posterior inferior frontal cortex in the left hemisphere (see above). By scanning such patients during language tasks they are able to perform, the effect of damage to Broca's area on other undamaged cortical regions can be assessed. For this purpose, we (Price, Warburton, et al., 1999) assessed regional activation when four patients with lesions to Broca's area performed a simple visual feature detection task on words, relative to the same task on consonant letter strings. Like the normal controls, all four patients activated a region of the left middle temporal lobe associated with semantic processing (Vandenberghe et al., 1996) but failed to activate Broca's area or a region in the left posterior inferior temporal cortex that is activated when subjects name visual or tactile stimuli (Buechel et al., 1998; Price, 1998).

The lack of activation in Broca's area confirmed that damage to this region had rendered it dysfunctional. More interesting were the abnormal responses in the left posterior inferior temporal cortex. This region is seldom damaged by stroke because it is supplied by the posterior and middle cerebral arteries. Therefore its function has not, until recently, been associated with naming using the lesion deficit model (Raymer et al., 1997; Foundas et al., 1998). Certainly, the effect of damage to Broca's area on the left posterior inferior temporal cortex could not have been inferred without functional neuroimaging. The question that remains concerns whether damage to Broca's area renders the left posterior inferior temporal cortex permanently inactive or whether dysfunctionality depends on the involvement of Broca's area. This was evaluated in two ways. First, we note that it was not simply the case that the left posterior inferior temporal cortex failed to activate; the abnormal responses were characterized by a deactivation. In other words, the responses were determined by the task with decreased activation when interaction with Broca's area was required. The second approach was to scan one of the patients again, using the semantic similarity paradigm described for the patients with semantic dementia (see above). In this paradigm, which emphasizes temporoparietal interactions, the region that showed underactivity during the implicit reading paradigm activated normally (and the interaction between paradigm and pathology was significant). The inference from both accounts is that responses in the left posterior inferior temporal cortex were context dependent, with abnormality expressed only when input from Broca's area was required. In summary, functional neuroimaging can be used to assess the effect of brain damage on brain activity at, and distant from, the site of damage. The context-sensitive abnormalities detected in the left posterior inferior temporal cortex speak to the integrative nature of neuronal architectures.

We turn now to studies of schizophrenia where functional deficits have not been attributed to obvious anatomical damage. Schizophrenia is a psychiatric condition in which patients suffer from the intermittent recurrence of one or more of at least three symptom types: psychomotor poverty (a lack of volition, e.g., to initiate motor movements or speech); reality disorder (hallucinations and delusions) in the context of normal cognition; and disorganized and incoherent speech and thought. Studies that have attempted to correlate the syndrome, or particular symptoms of the syndrome, with changes in cortical responsiveness (see above) have revealed inconsistent results. For instance, some studies have shown reduced responses in the frontal lobes (Weinberger et al., 1988; Berman et al., 1988, 1995), whereas others have shown normal prefrontal responses (Frith et al., 1995; Fletcher et al., 1996).

The inconsistency has been related in part to the finding that hypofrontality correlates only with the expression of psychomotor poverty (Liddle et al., 1992) and in part to the fact that the performance of patients is not always matched with that of normals (Frith et al., 1995). An alternative explanation is that some of the symptoms of schizophrenia do not necessarily reflect a regionally specific pathology; rather, there is abnormal integration between different regions that may function normally when they are not required to interact. This would account for why, in schizophrenia, a region such as the frontal lobe might show normal activity in some contexts and abnormal activity in others: the responsiveness of the frontal region depends on the neuronal architecture and implicitly on the cognitive architecture engendered by the task.

Studies of abnormal functional integration can be assessed by measuring changes in the functional connectivity between regions. Essentially these measurements are based on temporal correlations between activity in distant cortical regions. In electrophysiological studies, which record spike trains of neural activity, the temporal scale is on the order of milliseconds. In functional neuroimaging, which measures hemodynamic changes, the temporal scale is on the order of seconds and a significant correlation simply implies that activity (pooled over the time scale) goes up and down together in distant regions. Such temporal correlations imply functional connectivity that could be of two critically different types. One type results from direct connections between the correlated regions (i.e., activity changes in one region cause activity changes in another region). The second type does not imply direct connections between correlated regions, but different regions may share connections from a region that is the source of correlated activity. The important point of this distinction is that functional connectivity does not necessarily imply direct connections between correlated regions.

Studies of functional connectivity in schizophrenia have shown that there are abnormal correlations between activity in the prefrontal and temporal regions during word generation tasks. More specifically, in normal subjects, activity in bilateral superior temporal cortices during word generation (relative to word repetition) is negatively correlated with activity in the prefrontal cortex, but in three groups of patients with schizophrenia, activity in the left superior temporal cortex was positively correlated with prefrontal activity (see Friston & Frith, 1995). These results, illustrating a complete reversal of the large-scale prefronto-temporal interactions in the schizophrenics, indicate consistent abnormalities in regionally specific functional connectivity. The reversed correlations can be regarded as a failure of prefrontal cortex to suppress activity in the temporal lobes (or vice versa). One behavioral interpretation that has been offered by Friston and Frith (1995) is that the prefrontal regions are necessary for intrinsically generated behavior and the bilateral temporal lobes are sensory perception regions that register the consequences of behavior (Frith et al., 1991). A failure to integrate these two regions may impair (1) intrinsically generated action, as in psychomotor poverty, and (2) perception, as in hallucinations and delusions, when self-induced sensory changes are attributed to an external cause. In other words, coherent interactions between prefrontal cortices and cortices devoted to perceptual representations may be crucial for the integration of intrinsically generated behavior and perception.

Further studies are being conducted to explore the prefronto-temporal disintegration in schizophrenia. As noted above, correlated activity could result from direct causal connections between the frontal and temporal regions or from shared influences from a third region. One hypothesis (Dolan et al., 1995) is that normal frontotemporal integration during the word generation paradigm is modulated by activity in the anterior cingulate (i.e., the anterior cingulate governs the negative correlations between frontal and temporal regions). This hypothesis could be tested with studies of effective connectivity (see Friston et al., 1997) and structural equation modeling. (See chapter 3 in this volume for further details on this sort of network analysis.)

Finally, we consider mechanisms of functional recovery. How patients might recover a lost function is one of the most crucial questions that needs to be addressed by imaging studies of brain-damaged patients. Structural indices of lesions (from conventional use of CT and MRI scanners) do not necessarily imply a complete loss of function, and it is sometimes surprising when a patient with a large lesion makes an unexpectedly good recovery. Functional neuroimaging, by contrast, can detect areas where a degree of functional responsiveness has been maintained even in areas that appear damaged in structural images. Typically these areas are around the region of insult (e.g., peri-infarct tissue) and sometimes within the lesion. Recovery of a lost function results either from the reactivation of tissue that was initially incapacitated (e.g., due to a reduction in edema) or from increases in the capacity of viable tissue until it can support a function that was originally executed by lost cells.

Functional imaging has an important role to play in evaluating the contribution of these mechanisms. However, to date it has probably been grossly underestimated. This is because functional imaging studies have usually been able to make inferences only by pooling data from different patients into one group and then comparing the patient group to a group of normal subjects (e.g., Weiller et al., 1995). Since peri-infarct activity inevitably varies from patient to patient, depending on the size and location of the lesion, it will not be detected in group-to-group comparisons. The demonstration of peri-infarct activity therefore relies on studies where each subject is analyzed individually.

In a study by Warburton et al. (1999), six patients with large left temporoparietal lesions who had lost, and then recovered, the ability to generate words were scanned six times during a word generation task and six times during rest. Data from each patient were analyzed independently and compared to a group of nine control subjects. In normal subjects, the word generation task (relative to rest) consistently activates a widely distributed system of language regions in the left hemisphere (in particular the left prefrontal and posterior temporal cortices). By analyzing data from each subject individually it was possible to ascertain that half the normal subjects also activate the same set of regions in the right hemisphere. All six recovered aphasics also evidenced activation in the left prefrontal regions, all but one activated the damaged left temporal lobe, and half activated the right prefrontal and temporal cortices. The consistent activation in the damaged left temporal lobe in all but one patient demonstrated varying degrees of peri-infarct activity. This left temporal activity was not detected when the patients were pooled together for a group analysis. The conclusions of this study were that activations associated with cued word retrieval in the recovered aphasics were indistinguishable from those of the normal controls, except that in the presence of a lesion the activations were perilesional. Similar results have been obtained in a single case study of a patient who had recovered from auditory agnosia (Engelein et al., 1995). Furthermore, Heiss et al. (1997) have demonstrated, in a longitudinal study, that the recovery from aphasia is related to the reactivation of left hemispheric speech areas surrounding the area of infarction.

In contrast, other studies have suggested that recovery occurs following a laterality shift, with homologous regions in the contralateral cortex assuming the functions of the damaged region (e.g., Weiller et al., 1995; Buckner et al., 1996). Such a mechanism, when a different neuronal architecture sustains the same cognitive architecture, indicates that there may be a duplicated language system in the right hemisphere which can be bought into action, perhaps by disinhibition, following damage to the left hemisphere language system (see "Introduction"). However, there are a number of methodological issues that need to be resolved before such conclusions can be resolved, in particular, whether the patients (1) performed the task using the same cognitive architecture as normal subjects and (2) activated outside the normal range of controls. For example, the Warburton et al. study (1999) illustrated that almost half the normal subjects respond to language tasks by activating the right hemisphere. If these are the subjects who are most likely to recover following damage to the left hemisphere system, then patients who have recovered language abilities should ideally be contrasted to normals who also activate in the right hemisphere. Only when the patients (1) perform like normals and (2) activate more than normals with bilateral language function can inferences regarding disinhibition of a right hemisphere language system be made. To our knowledge, these criteria have not yet been met.

Informing Models of Normal Functional Anatomy

In the "Introduction," we discussed how the lesion deficit model (with neuropsychological patients) is limited because although it is able to identify regions that are necessary to perform a task, it does not establish the premorbid sufficiency of the damaged regions. For instance, a cognitive function can be impaired if the connections between two vital cortical areas are damaged (the connections are necessary for performance but they are not sufficient). In contrast, functional neuroimaging in normal subjects reveals distributed brain systems that can be considered sufficient to perform a task, but it does not distinguish the relative contributions of the subcomponents involved. Some activated regions may be superfluous to the task requirements (Price et al., 1996).

The joint and complementary use of neuroimaging and neuropsychology offers a fundamental advantage over either technique in isolation. Neuroimaging in normal subjects defines the sufficient set of regions (the neural architecture) for performing one task relative to another. Neuropsychology establishes the necessity of component brain areas in one of three ways. The first, most conventional, approach has been described above and involves identifying the lesion site associated with a functional deficit. By implication, this region was necessary for the specified function. The second approach looks at the effect of a lesion on a region identified in a neuroimaging paradigm. For example, a behavioral study of a patient with a right cerebellar infarct (Fiez et al., 1992) was motivated by the observation that functional imaging studies show activity in the right cerebellum during verbal fluency (Petersen et al., 1988). On nonmotor tasks, the patient showed deficits in completing and learning a word generation task but had normal or above normal behavior when performing standardized language tasks. In this instance, a neuroimaging study motivated a neuropsychological study and the neuropsychological study allowed inferences to be made regarding a subcomponent of the language system. The third approach involves inferences from patients who are not functionally impaired on a specified task but nevertheless have damage to parts of the system defined by neuroimaging. Here the damaged regions can be construed as not necessary. By designating each region in the sufficient system as necessary or not necessary, the critical system can be identified. However, the caveat is that some patients may be able to perform a task by activating peri-infarct tissue that appears to be damaged in routine structural imaging (see above). Another possibility is that functionality is preserved due to neuronal reorganization (e.g., involving the homologue region in the contralateral hemisphere; Weiller et al., 1995; Buckner et al., 1996) or cognitive reorganization. To discount these possibilities, functional imaging of the patient is a prerequisite.

Two attempts have been made to harness neuroimaging and neuropsychology in order to investigate the role of the prefrontal cortex in linguistic processing. Neuroimaging studies of patients with frontal lobe lesions are able to determine whether (1) patients retain the ability to perform some linguistic tasks without the left prefrontal cortex; (2) there is peri-infarct activation in the left prefrontal cortex; or (3) there is compensatory activity in the right prefrontal cortex. In one study, Buckner et al. (1996) used functional neuroimaging and a stem completion task (generate words from word stems such as "TRO") to demonstrate that a patient with left frontal lobe damage retained the ability to perform the task by activating the right inferior frontal cortex. In the other study Price, Mummery, et al. (1999) used semantic similarity judgments and found that a patient with a large frontoparietal lesion can perform the task accurately by activating temporoparietal regions in the absence of either left or right frontal activity. By discounting peri-infarct activity in the left frontal cortex and cognitive or neuronal reorganization in the right frontal cortex, this result indicates that the left prefrontal activity, consistently seen in normals, is not necessary to perform the semantic similarity judgment task.

If the left prefrontal activation is not necessary for semantic similarity judgments, why is it activated normally? One possibility is that it relates to implicit memory processes, but to confirm this we would need to show that the patient was less able to remember the stimuli at a later date. Another question that is raised relates to whether other regions of the semantic system are not necessary for task performance. An indication that the left posterior inferior temporal cortex is not required comes from the observation (reported above) that the patients with semantic dementia failed to activate this area during the same task. Is it possible, then, that there is no critical semantic area but, rather, that other components of the system are able to compensate if one area is malfunctioning? This hypothesis needs to be tested explicitly, but it appears that some of the left extrasylvian temporal regions are critical, because damage to the ventral anterior temporal cortex results in semantic deficits (Hodges et al., 1992), and damage to the posterior inferior parietal cortex can result in speech comprehension deficits (Alexander et al., 1989). The set of regions where normals activate, and damage results in an inability to perform semantic tasks, are those which will constitute the necessary and sufficient neural system. Ideally, in order to delineate the complete necessary and sufficient brain system involved in semantic similarity judgments (or any other task), we need to image patients with lesions to each component of the system identified in normal subjects. In this way, functional imaging and neuropsychology can be combined to make inferences about functional anatomy that could not be done with either alone. Figure 11.1 illustrates the inferences that can be drawn from neuropsychology, neuroimaging on normal subjects, and neuroimaging on patients.

The other important ways that functional imaging studies of patients can inform models of normal functional anatomy have been summarized in table 11.2. One relates to the effect that regionally specific brain damage has on the responses in

Lesion associated with speech production deficit

**Neuropsychology /
Lesion deficit model**

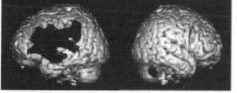

The normal distributed semantic system

**Neuroimaging:
normal subjects**

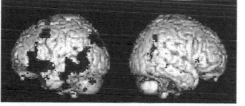

The system sufficient for patient to perform task

**Neuroimaging:
patient**

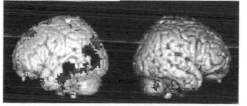

Areas not necessary for performance

**Neuroimaging :
normals - patient**

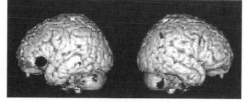

Figure 11.1
Examples of inferences that can be drawn from neuropsychology and the lesion deficit model, neuroimaging studies on normal subjects, and neuroimaging studies on patients. In the top row, the extent of the lesion is illustrated in black on models of the left and right hemispheres. In the second and third rows, respectively, the areas activated when normal subjects and the patient perform semantic similarity judgments relative to perceptual tasks are indicated in black. In the bottom row, the areas that are activated by each normal control but not by the patient are shown in black. Since the patient could perform the task within normal limits, we conclude that the left inferior frontal cortex is not necessary for semantic similarity judgments (see Price, Mummery, et al., 1999).

undamaged areas of the brain. For instance, the finding that the left posterior inferior temporal lobe failed to activate during semantic similarity judgments in the context of anterior temporal damage (Mummery et al., 1999), but not in the context of left frontoparietal damage (Price, Mummery, et al., 1999), indicates that during semantic judgments, inputs to the posterior temporal region come from the anterior temporal region. Similarly, the finding that in the context of left frontoparietal damage the left posterior inferior temporal cortex activated normally during semantic similarity judgments, but not during reading (Price, Warburton, et al., 1999), indicates that this region relies on inputs from the damaged frontal region during reading but not during semantic similarity judgments.

ISSUES

In this section, we address the issues encountered when designing and interpreting experiments that measure the brain function of patients with neuropsychological impairment. The key to interpreting neuroimaging results lies in experimental design and task analysis that allow one to disambiguate between a cognitive change, a neuronal change, or both.

The first consideration in designing experiments to study a brain-damaged patient is how the results are going to inform our understanding of the neuronal and cognitive architectures pertinent to that patient or the normal population. The critical observation in neuropsychological imaging is a differential pattern of activation in the patient relative to a normal group (a subject group-by-task interaction). As described above, this can be attributed to either neuronal or cognitive reorganization.

Distinguishing between Neuronal and Cognitive Reorganization

Neuronal reorganization (or plasticity) refers to the changes in a task-specific neuronal architecture that take place during learning or relearning in the normal or damaged brain. A key distinction can be made between plasticity that is "enduring" (the time course varies from hours to years) and plasticity that is "dynamic" (the time course ranges from several milliseconds to minutes). In the postdevelopmental period both are mediated by changes in the strength of preexisting connections (the efficacy of existing synapses is altered). Dynamic changes in connection strengths can be mediated by factors that are intrinsic or extrinsic to the neuronal processes themselves, such as the recent history of neuronal firing (e.g., facilitation, adaptation, and potentiation) or inputs from other neuronal populations that modulate connection strengths either by postsynaptic mechanisms or, more directly, by release of modulatory neurotransmitters such as noradrenaline. Enduring plastic changes consolidate the dynamic changes into permanent changes. During development, new extrinsic connections (axons that traverse the white matter from area to area) can be formed through axonal sprouting and synaptic remodeling. However, in the mature brain, the gross schema of extrinsic connectivity is thought to be fairly fixed.

The point that neuronal reorganization results from changes in a preexisting system is an important factor for interpreting changes in neuronal activity following brain damage. Another important point is that dynamic plasticity can be expressed in many natural and experimental contexts, ranging from changes that underlie attentional modulation to profound changes in the organization of somatosensory fields shortly after deafferentation. For example, rapid neuronal reorganization can occur when a system is disinhibited following deafferentation of the inhibiting inputs (Buonomano & Merzenich, 1998). It follows that it would be incorrect to ascribe changes in attentional set or disinhibition to substantial remodeling of the anatomical connections. In summary, to demonstrate that neuronal reorganization of a dynamic or enduring nature has occurred, it is necessary to show that the cognitive architecture (including the attentional set and performance level) is the same in both patients and normal subjects. This may not be possible, particularly because the cognitive architecture is likely to change as the neuronal implementation changes. Similarly, if the cognitive architecture changes, the underlying neuronal architecture is likely to change.

Cognitive reorganization takes place when a patient uses a different set of cognitive processes to implement the same task, for instance, when a patient learns a particular strategy to recover the ability to perform a lost function. A more specific example is when dyslexic patients adopt a serial letter-by-letter reading strategy to compensate for a deficit in parallel letter processing. In this case cognitive, but not neuronal, reorganization has taken place. In order to demonstrate, with functional imaging, that patients are using a different cognitive architecture to perform the same task, reorganization at a neuronal level needs to be discounted. This would involve demonstrating that an equivalent activation pattern is elicited in normals when they are forced to use the same cognitive strategy as the patients. To our knowledge this experimental technique has not been explored, and it is likely to be extremely hard to implicate. We are therefore left with a dilemma. In order to demonstrate that differential activations reflect cognitive reorganization, it is necessary to show that there has been no change in the neuronal architecture, and in order to infer neuronal reorganization, it is necessary to exclude a change in the cognitive architecture. The distinction rests on the task analysis. However, a task analysis is seldom sufficiently detailed to ensure a constant cognitive architecture and thereby to demonstrate plasticity. Nevertheless, there is a continuum of task analysis depth—the more detailed the task analysis, the more valid the inferences about changes in neural implementation.

Task Analysis

There are several levels of task specification. At one extreme, there must be a one-to-one mapping between the cognitive architecture and its implementation; at this level, a change in neuronal dynamics implies a respective change in the functional correlates. At progressively coarser levels of analysis, where the elemental operations are less specified, many different functional operations could be employed to achieve the same task performance; a complicated relationship between the cognitive architecture and its neuronal implementation ensues. This may be seen as a one-to-many mapping (the same cognitive process can be implemented by different neuronal systems, e.g., in the right and left hemispheres) or a many-to-one mapping (different cognitive process are implemented by the same neuronal system). The point being made here is that although any task analysis may be valid at its own level of specification, it is useful in discriminating between cognitive and neuronal reorganization only if it is as detailed as possible. If the task analysis is very unspecified in terms of the elemental operations, then implied differences in neuronal implementation (plasticity) between the normals and the patient become specious. We mean this in the sense that although differential activations may emulate a plastic reorganization of the neuronal implementation, this may simply reflect the fact that different subprocesses are being called upon at a cognitive level which have not been addressed in the task analysis.

Unfortunately, in practice, a task analysis will never be as refined or as comprehensive as one would like because certain attributes of cognitive processing are not amenable to measurement. For example, subtle changes in attentional or cognitive set may bring about plastic changes in the neuronal architecture through neuromodulatory mechanisms. One of the more important factors of this sort is time, because performing a given task continuously means that the temporal context is changing, and this may evoke time-dependent plasticity in the neuronal implementation. Another example is incidental and implicit processing that may not be required for a task (see Price et al., 1996). A complete task analysis therefore should include not only the processing components but also all the contextual factors that may influence them.

To summarize, in order to make sense of neuropsychological studies with imaging, one has to have a sufficiently comprehensive task analysis to enable one to say that the cognitive architecture elicited by task performance in the patient and the control group are identical. Only when this is the case does a significant interaction imply that plastic changes in neuronal implementation have occurred. If the cognitive architectures are not demonstrably equivalent, then cognitive reorganization may be an explanation. The nature of this reorganization and the underlying neuronal architecture can be defined when normal subjects are coerced into adopting cognitive strategies that emulate those used by the patient (rendering the cognitive architectures the same). Clearly, demonstrating interactions when the cognitive architectures are not identical is still useful in highlighting candidate brain regions. However, it is logically impossible to ascribe these interactions to plasticity or to change in cognitive strategy unless the constraints described above are applied.

Finally, the interpretation of abnormal activations shown by a particular type of patient will be informative only when the normal functional anatomy of the cognitive task, and all the compensatory measures that might be used to perform it, are understood. The usefulness of patient studies can therefore grow only in relation to our understanding of normal functional anatomy, which in turn depends on neuroimaging studies of normal subjects.

REFERENCES

Alexander, M. P., Hiltbrunner, B., & Fischer, R. S. (1989). Distributed anatomy of transcortical sensory aphasia. *Archives of Neurology* 46, 885–892.

Berman, K. F., Gold, J. M., Noga, J. T., Abi-Dargham, A., Van Horn, J. D., & Weinberger, D. R. (1995). A PET study of working memory in schizophrenia: Effects of performance level. *Society for Neuroscience Abstracts* 21, 260.

Berman, K. F., Illowsky, B. P., & Weinberger, D. R. (1988). Physiological dysfunction of dorsolateral prefrontal cortex in schizophrenia. IV. Further evidence for regional and behavioral specificity. *Archives of General Psychiatry* 45, 616–622.

Broca, P. (1861). Remarques sur le siège de la faculté du langage articulé; suivies d'une observation d'aphémie (perte de la parole). *Bulletin de la Société Anatornigue de Paris* 6, 330–357, 398–407. Translated in R. Herrnstein & E. G. Boring. (1965). *A Source Book in the History of Psychology.* Cambridge, MA: Harvard University Press.

Brunswick, N., McCrory, E., Price, C. J., Frith, C. D., & Frith, U. (1999). Explicit and implicit processing of words and pseudowords by adult developmental dyslexics: A search for Wernicke's Wortschatz. *Brain* 122, 1901–1917.

Buckner, R. L., Corbetta, M., Schatz, J., Raichle, M. E., & Petersen, S. E. (1996). Preserved speech abilities and compensation following prefrontal damage. *Proceedings of the National Academy of Sciences USA* 93, 1249–1253.

Büchel, C., Price, C. J., & Friston, K. J. (1998). A multimodal language area in the ventral visual pathway. *Nature* 394, 274–277.

Buonomano, D. V., & Merzenich, M. M. (1998). Cortical plasticity: From synapses to maps. *Annual Review of Neuroscience* 2, 149–186.

Coltheart, M. (1981). Disorders of reading and their implications for models of normal reading. *Visible Language* 15, 245–286.

Dolan, R. J., Fletcher, P., Frith, C. D., Friston, K. J., Frackowiak, R. S. J., & Grasby, P. J. (1995). Dopaminergic modulation of an impaired cognitive activation in the anterior cingulate cortex in schizophrenia. *Nature* 378, 180–182.

Engelein, A., Silbersweig, D., Stern, E., Huber, W., Doring, W., Frith, C. D., & Frackowiak, R. S. J. (1995). The functional anatomy of recovery from auditory agnosia. *Brain* 118, 1395–1409.

Fiez, J. A., Petersen, S. E., Cheney, M. K., & Raichle, M. E. (1992). Impaired nonmotor learning and error detection associated with cerebellar damage. *Brain* 115, 155–178.

Fletcher, P. C., Frith, C. D., Grasby, P. M., Friston, K. J., & Dolan, R. J. (1996). Local and distributed effects of apomorphine on fronto-temporal function in acute unmedicated schizophrenia. *Journal of Neuroscience* 16, 7055–7062.

Foundas, A. L., Daniels, S. K., & Vasterling, J. J. (1998). Anomia: Case studies with lesion localisation. *Neurocase* 4, 35–43.

Friston, K. J. (1995). Functional and effective connectivity in neuroimaging, A synthesis. *Human Brain Mapping* 2, 56–78.

Friston, K. J., Büchel, C., Fink, G. R., Morris, J., Rolls, E., & Dolan, R. J. (1997). Psychophysiological and modulatory interactions in neuroimaging. *Neuroimage* 6, 218–229.

Friston, K. J., & Frith, C. D. (1995). Schizophrenia, A disconnection syndrome? Clinical Neuroscience 3, 89–97.

Friston, K. J., Frith, C. D., & Frackowiak, R. S. J. (1993). Time-dependent changes in effective connectivity measured with PET. *Human Brain Mapping* 1, 69–79.

Frith, C. D. (1992). *The Cognitive Neuropsychology of Schizophrenia*. Hove, UK: Lawrence Erlbaum.

Frith, C. D., Friston, K. J., Herold, S., et al. (1995). Regional brain activity in chronic schizophrenic patients during the performance of a verbal fluency task. *British Journal of Psychiatry* 167, 343–349.

Frith, C. D., Friston, K. J., Liddle, P. F., Frackowiak, R. S. J. (1991). Willed action and the prefrontal cortex in man: A study with PET. *Proceedings of the Royal Society of London* B244, 241–246.

Goltz, F. (1881). In *Transactions of the 7th International Medical Congress*, W. MacCormac, ed., vol. 1, 218–228. London: Kolkmann.

Heiss, W. D., Karber, H., Weber-Luxenburger, G., Herholz, K., Kessler, J., Pietrzyk, U., & Pawlik, G. (1997). Speech-induced cerebral metabolic activation reflects recovery from aphasia. *Journal of the Neurological Sciences* 145(2), 213–217.

Hodges, J. R., Patterson, K., Oxbury, S., & Funnell, E. (1992). Semantic dementia: Progressive fluent aphasia with temporal lobe atrophy. *Brain* 115, 1783–1806.

Lichtheim, L. (1885). On aphasia. *Brain* 7, 433–484.

Liddle, P. F., Friston, K. J., Frith, C. D., Jones, T., Hirsch, S. R., & Frackowiak, R. S. J. (1992). Patterns of cerebral blood flow in schizophrenia. *British Journal of Psychiatry* 160, 179–186.

Liddle, P. F., & Morris, D. L. (1991). Schizophrenic syndromes and frontal lobe performance. *British Journal of Psychology* 158, 340–345.

Mummery, C. J., Patterson, K., Wise, R. J. S., Vandenberghe, R., Price, C. J., & Hodges, J. R. (1999). Disrupted temporal lobe connections in semantic dementia. *Brain* 122, 61–73.

Petersen, S. E., Fox, P. T., Posner, M. I., Mintun, M., & Raichle, M. E. (1988). Positron emission tomographic studies of the cortical anatomy of single-word processing. *Nature* 331, 585–589.

Price, C. J. (1998). The functional anatomy of word comprehension and production. *Trends in Cognitive Sciences* 2, 281–288.

Price, C. J., Mummery, C. J., Moore, C. J., Frackowiak, R. S. J., & Friston, K. J. (1999). Delineating necessary and sufficient neural systems with functional imaging studies of neuropsychological patients. *Journal of Cognitive Neuroscience* 11, 371–382.

Price, C. J., Warburton, E. A., Moore, C. J., Frackowiak, R. S. J., & Friston, K. J. (1999). Dynamic diaschisis: Anatomically remote and context specific human brain lesions. Under review.

Price, C. J., Wise, R. J. S., & Frackowiak, R. S. J. (1996). Demonstrating the implicit processing of visually presented words and psudowords. *Cerebral Cortex* 6, 62–70.

Raymer, A. M., Foundas, A. L., Maher, L. M., et al. (1997). Cognitive neuropsychological analysis and neuroanatomic correlates in a case of acute anomia. *Brain and Language* 58, 137–156.

Sasanuma, S., & Monoi, H. (1975). The syndrome of gogi (word-meaning) aphasia: Selective impairment of kanji processing. *Neurology* 25, 627–632.

Vandenberghe, R., Price, C. J., Wise, R., Josephs, O., & Frackowiak, R. S. J. (1996). Functional anatomy of a common semantic system for words and pictures [see comments]. *Nature* 383, 254–256.

Warburton, E. A., Price, C. J., Swinburn, K., & Wise, R. J. S. (1999). Mechanisms of recovery from aphasia: Evidence from positron emission tomography studies. *Journal of Neurology, Neurosurgery and Psychiatry* 66, 155–161.

Warrington, E. K. (1975). Selective impairment of semantic memory. *Quarterly Journal of Experimental Psychology* 27, 635–657.

Weiller, C., Insensee, C., Rijntjes, M., Huber, W., Muller, S., Bier, D., et al. (1995). Recovery from Wernicke's aphasia: A positron emission tomography study. *Annals of Neurology* 37, 723–732.

Weinberger, D. R., Berman, K. F., & Illowsky, B. P. (1988). Physiological dysfunction of dorsolateral prefrontal cortex in schizophrenia. III. A new cohort and evidence for monoaminergic mechanism. *Archives of General Psychiatry* 45, 609–615.

Wernicke, C. (1874). *Der aphasiche Symptomenkomplex*. Breslau: Poland: Cohn and Weigert.

Contributors

Jeffrey Binder
Department of Neurology and Cellular
Biology, Neurobiology, and Anatomy
Medical College of Wisconsin
Milwaukee, Wisconsin

Randy L. Buckner
Department of Psychology
Washington University
St. Louis, Missouri

Roberto Cabeza
Center for Cognitive Neuroscience
Duke University
Durham, North Carolina

Mark D'Esposito
Neuroscience Institute and
Department of Psychology
University of California, Berkeley
Berkeley, California

Paul Downing
Department of Brain and Cognitive
Sciences
Massachusetts Institute of Technology
Cambridge, Massachusetts

Russell Epstein
Department of Brain and Cognitive
Sciences
Massachusetts Institute of Technology
Cambridge, Massachusetts

Karl J. Friston
Wellcome Department of Cognitive
Neurology
Institute of Neurology
Queen Square, London, UK

John D. E. Gabrieli
Department of Psychology
Stanford University
Stanford, California

Todd C. Handy
Center for Cognitive Neuroscience
Dartmouth College
Hanover, New Hampshire

Joseph B. Hopfinger
Department of Psychology and Center
for Neuroscience
University of California at Davis
Davis, California

Nancy G. Kanwisher
Department of Brain and Cognitive
Sciences
Massachusetts Institute of Technology
Cambridge, Massachusetts

Alan F. Kingstone
Department of Psychology
University of British Columbia
Vancouver, British Columbia, Canada

Zoe Kourtzi
Department of Brain and Cognitive
Sciences
Massachusetts Institute of Technology
Cambridge, Massachusetts

Jessica M. Logan
Department of Psychology
Washington University
St. Louis, Missouri

George R. Mangun
Center for Cognitive Neuroscience
Duke University
Durham, North Carolina

Alex Martin
Laboratory of Brain and Cognition
National Institute of Mental Health
Bethesda, Maryland

A. R. McIntosh
Department of Psychology
University of Toronto
Toronto, Ontario, Canada

L. Nyberg
Department of Psychology
Umeå University
Umeå, Sweden

Cathy J. Price
Wellcome Department of Cognitive
Neurology
Institute of Neurology
Queen Square, London, UK

Marcus E. Raichle
School of Medicine
Washington University
St. Louis, Missouri

Index

Note: Figures are indicated by an italic *f* after the page number, tables by an italic *t*.

Achromatopsia and semantic memory, 163
Aging
  and attention, 336–337, 338
  and brain activation patterns, 367–369
  and brain atrophy, 333–334
  and central executive control, 338, 351–355, 352*t*
  and cerebral blood flow, 343–346, 345*f*, 358*f*
  and cognitive dysfunction, 63–67, 331–333, 332*f*, 361–364
  cognitive psychology of, 336–338
  and episodic memory, 337–338, 346–351, 355–356, 369–370, 370*f*
  and functional changes of the brain, 334–336
  and hemispheric asymmetry, 358–361
  and inhibitory activity, 339, 355*f*, 356–357
  and Moscovitch's memory model, 341–342
  neurogenic effects of, 332
  and neuroimaging issues, 361–371
  neuroscience of, 340–343, 355–361
  and perception, 344*t*
  and performance measures, 365–366, 366*f*
  and positron emission tomography (PET), 343–346
  and prefrontal cortex, 344–355, 355*f*, 369*f*
  and priming, 337, 346–351, 347*t*, 349*f*
  and processing speed, 338–339
  psychogenic effects of, 332
  and structural changes of the brain, 333–334
  and task design, 363–364
  and visual recognition, 344–346
  and visual tasks, 336–337
  and white matter hyperintensities, 333–334
  and working memory, 338, 351–355, 352*t*, 356, 370
Agnosia, 113–114
Akinetopsia, 163
Alexia, 114
Alzheimer's dementia (AD), 65–66, 66*f*, 333
  and hemispheric asymmetry, 359
Amnesia, global, 255–256
Aphasia, 160–161
Apperceptive agnosia, 110–111, 111*f*
Attention, selective. *See also* Attention, spatial; Attention, visual
  and aging, 336–337, 338, 344*t*
  and frontal cortex, 85–88
  and network analyses, 56–58
  and parietal lobule, 85–88
  processes, functional neuroimaging of, 75–76
  quantitative properties of, 98–99
  and reaction times (RT), 76–77
  and stimulus-unrelated language processing, 191
  and visual input, 75–76

Attention, spatial, 56–58, 57*f*, 60*f*. *See also* Attention, selective; Attention, visual
  activation patterns in, 87–88
  and aging, 336–337, 338, 344*t*
  and Alzheimer's dementia (AD), 66*f*
  cognitive model of, 77
  and event-related potentials (ERPs), 78–82, 79*f*, 91–98
  and functional magnetic resonance imaging (fMRI), 82–84, 88–89
  and fusiform face area (FFA), 90
  limitations in studies of, 90–91
  neural correlates of, 77–82
  and perceptual load, 78–80, 79*f*, 98–103, 102*f*
  and perceptual salience of stimuli, 89–90
  and positron emission tomography (PET), 82–83, 85–88
  and reaction times (RT), 76–77
  and reflexive movements, 85–86, 87
  and retinotopic mapping, 84–85
  and sensory gain, 88–89
  and thalamus, 80–81
  and voluntary movements, 85–86
Attention, visual, 139–140, 141. *See also* Attention, selective; Attention, spatial

Baseline state. *See* Control state
Bilingualism and language processing, 234–235
Biological motion and visual recognition, 133
Blocked task designs, 32–33. *See also* Control state; Task state
  and episodic memory encoding, 36–38
  and functional neuroimaging, 37
Blood flow, cerebral
  and aging, 335, 343–346, 345*f*, 358*f*
  and anesthesia, 20
  and blood oxygen level dependent (BOLD) signal, 11–13
  and event-related potentials (ERPs), 92
  and excitatory activity, 12
  and functional magnetic resonance imaging (fMRI), 11–12
  and glycolysis, 11–12, 14–20
  and inhibitory activity, 12
  and oxygen consumption, 11–12, 14–20, 16*f*
  and perception, attention and language, 56–58
  and positron emission tomography (PET), 8*f*
Blood oxygen level dependent (BOLD) signal, 11, 28–29
  and event-related functional magnetic resonance imaging (fMRI), 33–42
  and functional magnetic resonance imaging (fMRI), 11–12, 15*f*, 34–35

Blood oxygen level dependent (BOLD) signal
  (cont.)
  and language processing, 191–192, 195–198
  and positron emission tomography (PET), 15*f*
Brain
  anatomy changes due to aging, 334–336
  atrophy due to aging, 333–334
  blood flow, 4–20, 8*f*
  and cognitive dysfunction due to aging, 340–343
  damaged patients, 379–397
  functional changes due to aging, 334–336
  hemispheric asymmetry, 358–361, 360*f*
  left hemisphere of, 160–162
  lesion-deficit research, 188, 254, 304, 306,
    379–381, 392, 393*f*
  mapping of neuronal activity, 7–11
  and Moscovitch's memory model, 341–342
  motion during PET and fMRI imaging, 30–31
  and neuropsychology, 379–380
  regions associated with category-related activa-
    tions, 173–176, 176*f*
  regions associated with episodic memory,
    255–259
  regions associated with language processing,
    188–214, 237–238
  regions associated with phonological processing,
    210
  regions associated with semantic memory,
    156–179
  regions associated with spatial attention, 77–82
  regions associated with speech perception,
    198–199
  regions associated with visual recognition, 56–58,
    117–136
  regions associated with working memory,
    296–309
  serotonin in, 334–335
  structural changes due to aging, 333–334
  volume, 333
  and white matter hyperintensities, 333–334
Brain activity
  and blood oxygen level dependent (BOLD)
    signal, 11–12, 28–29, 33–42, 191–198
  in brain-damaged patients, 381–385, 384*t*
  and cognitive subtraction, 298–299, 301
  and control state, 7–8
  and effective connectivity, 50, 50*t*
  and episodic memory encoding, 36–42
  and functional connectivity, 50, 50*t*
  and functional magnetic resonance imaging
    (fMRI), 28–31
  and glycolysis, 14–20
  and hemispheric asymmetry, 358–361, 360*f*
  and hemodynamic changes, 29–30

  and interactions among brain regions, 50–56
  and network analyses, 49–68
  and oxygen consumption, 14–20
  and partial least squares (PLS) analysis, 51–56,
    52*f*
  patterns in aging subjects, 367–369
  and performance measures, 365–366, 366*f*
  and positron emission tomography (PET), 28–
    31
  and schizophrenia, 387–389
  and semantic dementia, 385–387
  and structural equation modeling, 54–62, 55*f*
  and task state, 7–8, 10*f*
Brain regions
  selection of, for partial least squares (PLS) analy-
    sis, 53–54
  and task partial least squares (PLS) analysis,
    51–53, 52*f*
Broca's area. *See also* Cortex, frontal; Gyrus,
  inferior frontal (IFG)
  and neuropsychologically impaired patients,
    386–387
Brodmann cytoarchitectural areas (BA)
  and episodic memory, 260
  and working memory, 297*f*, 302, 303*f*

Central executive system and working memory,
  293–296, 304–306
  and aging, 338, 351–355, 352*t*
Cerebellar diaschisis, 14–15
Cingulate, anterior, 58
Cingulate, posterior, 160
Cognition
  in brain-damaged patients, 382–385, 384*t*
  dysfunction and aging subjects, 63–67, 336–343,
    361–364
  dysfunction and Alzheimer's dementia (AD), 65,
    66*f*, 333
  dysfunction and schizophrenia, 63
  impaired patients and neuropsychology, 379–
    380
  and Moscovitch's memory model, 341–342
  neuroscience of, 340–343
  operations and task design, 31–33
  and priming, 337
  and processing speed, 338–339
  psychology of aging, 336–338
  reorganization, 394–395
  and visual recognition, 138–143
  and working memory, 293–296
Cognitive subtraction, 298–299, 301
Color recognition, 162–167, 163*f*
Computed tomography (CT), 7
Connectivity, effective and functional, 50, 50*t*

Control state, 7–8, 14. *See also* Blocked task
  designs; Task state
  and functional magnetic resonance imaging
    (fMRI), 13*f*
  and phonological tasks, 215–218
  and positron emission tomography (PET), 13*f*
  and semantic memory, 55*f*
Cortex, auditory
  activation patterns in, 203*f*
  and nonword speech sounds, 203
Cortex, cerebral, 12
  and cerebellar diaschisis, 14–15
  and loose task comparisons, 38–39
Cortex, frontal. *See also* Broca's area
  and episodic memory, 257–259
  lateral, and word generation, 230–231
  and selective attention, 85–88
  and semantic memory, 156–162, 157*f*
  and word recognition, 164
Cortex, lateral and inferior occipital (LO),
  116–117
Cortex, medial posterior parietal, 156–162
Cortex, occipital
  and aging, 344–346
  category-related activations of, 170–171, 172*f*
  medial, and letter strings, 206–207
  and semantic memory, 171–174, 172*f*
  and visual character perception, 205
Cortex, posterior parietal, 318–320
Cortex, posterior temporoparietal, 156–162
Cortex, posterior ventral temporal
  and color word generation, 165–166
  and semantic memory, 171–174
Cortex, prefrontal (PFC)
  and aging, 333–334, 334*f*, 344–355, 369*f*
  and central executive control, 304–306, 351–355
  correlations with retrieval performance, 276–277
  dorsolateral, 58
  and encoding of episodic memories, 270–274
  and encoding of episodic memory, 317–318
  and episodic memory, 257–259, 281–283
  functional subdivisions of, 309–310, 309*f*
  and inhibitory activity, 355*f*
  and maintenance tasks, 314–318, 316*f*
  and manipulation tasks, 314–318, 316*f*
  organization by content, 310–314
  organization by process, 314–318
  and retrieval manipulations, 277–278
  and retrieval of episodic memories, 274–279
  and semantic memory, 156–167
  and spatial versus nonspatial working memory,
    310–314, 311*f*, 313*f*
  specificity of, for working memory, 307–309
  and stimulus comparisons, 275–276

and task difficulty, 306–307
  and working memory, 293–304, 297*f*
Cortex, premotor
  and object identification, 176–178
  and working memory, 320–321
Cortex, visual, 61–62. *See also* Visual recognition;
  Visual tasks
  and occipitoparietal activations, 115–116
  and retinotopic mapping, 84–85
  and spatial attention, 82–84
Cortical specialization, 136–143

Dementia, semantic, 160–162, 385–387
Dyslexia, developmental, 67

Echoplanar imaging (EPI), 36–42, 195–196, 196*f*
Encoding of episodic memory
  and aging, 348–351
  experimental comparisons of, 260–262
  and functional magnetic resonance imaging
    (fMRI), 260–263
Event-related functional magnetic resonance imaging (fMRI), 33–42
  and blood oxygen level dependent (BOLD) signal
    hemodynamic response, 34–35
  and presentation rates, 34–36
  and spatial versus nonspatial working memory,
    314
  and working memory, 299–302, 300*f*, 301*f*
Event-related potentials (ERPs)
  and cerebral blood flow, 92
  and electrophysiology, 92–95
  experimental design for, 91–92
  and positron emission tomography (PET), 92–95,
    94*f*
  and spatial attention, 78–82, 79*f*
  and steady-state visual evoked potentials, 95–96
  and striate modulation, 96–97
  and systematic covariation, 97–98, 98*f*
Excitatory activity, 12
  and functional magnetic resonance imaging
    (fMRI), 29
  and positron emission tomography (PET), 29

Face recognition. *See* Fusiform face area (FFA);
  Visual recognition
Frontal lobes, 188–214
Functional neuroimaging. *See also* Magnetic resonance imaging, functional; Positron emission
  tomography (PET)
  and aging subjects, 41–43, 342–346, 361–371
  and brain blood flow, 8*f*, 9*f*
  of brain-damaged patients, 379–397
  and control state, 7–8

Functional neuroimaging (cont.)
  future of, 20–21
  and hemispheric asymmetry, 358–361
  history of, 3–11
  of language processes, 188–191
  limitations of, 42–43
  and network analyses, 49–68
  of neuropsychologically impaired patients,
    385–397
  and neuropsychology, 385–394, 393f
  paradigms, 39–41
  and partial least squares (PLS) analysis, 51–56,
    52f
  and positron emission tomography (PET), 13f
  and semantic memory, 153–179
  and task state, 7–8, 10f
Fusiform face area (FFA), 90, 117–120, 118f, 119f,
    122f. See also Visual recognition; Visual tasks
  and emotional expression, 123
  and face recognition, 123–128
  and face selectivity, 120–123
  and prosopagnosia, 128
  and visual expertise, 125–128

Gender and language processing, 235–237, 237f
Genetics and language processing, 233–237
Glycolysis and brain blood flow, 11–12, 14–20, 16f
Gyrus, angular
  and Alzheimer's dementia (AD), 65–66
  and developmental dyslexia, 67
  and semantic memory, 227–228, 228f
Gyrus, fusiform
  and category-related activations, 173–174, 173f
  and color word generation, 165
  and semantic memory, 156–162, 157f
Gyrus, inferior frontal (IFG). See also Broca's
    area
  and perceptual tasks, 220–221
  and phonological tasks, 211–212
  and semantic memory, 226–227
Gyrus, inferior temporal (ITG)
  and semantic memory, 156–162, 222–225
Gyrus, middle temporal (MTG)
  and nonword speech sounds, 202–204
  and semantic memory, 222–225
  and speech perception, 199
Gyrus, superior temporal (STG)
  and language processing, 193–194, 194f
  and nonword speech sounds, 202–204
  and semantic memory, 225
  and speech perception, 198–199, 200
Gyrus, supramarginal, 212–214

Habituation to stimuli, 18, 20
Hemispheric asymmetry, 358–361, 360f

Hemodynamic changes and brain activity, 29–30
  and blood oxygen level dependent (BOLD)
    signal, 34–35
  neuroimaging of, 75–103
Hippocampus, 256–257
  and aging, 333–334, 334f, 348
  and episodic memory, 59–60

Inhibitory activity, 12
  and aging, 339, 355f, 356–357
  and functional magnetic resonance imaging
    (fMRI), 29
  and positron emission tomography (PET), 29

Lactate and neuronal activity, 17
Language processing, 65–67. See also Word
    retrieval
  and bilingualism, 234–235
  and blood oxygen level dependent (BOLD)
    signal, 195–198
  brain regions associated with, 188–214, 237–238
  components of, 187–188
  cortical regions associated with, 134–136
  and developmental dyslexia, 67
  and echoplanar imaging (EPI), 195–196, 196f
  functional imaging of, 188–191
  and functional magnetic resonance imaging
    (fMRI), 191–198, 193f
  gender and, 235–237, 237f
  genetic and developmental influences on, 233–237
  and inferior frontal gyrus (IFG), 226–227
  and inferior temporal gyrus (ITG), 222–225
  and lesion-deficit research, 188
  and letters, 205
  and linguistic subsystems, 187, 188–189
  and middle temporal gyrus (MTG), 199, 222–225
  and neuropsychology, 391–392
  and nonlinguistic tasks, 218–220
  and nonword speech sounds, 202–204
  and orthographic stimuli, 206–209, 207f
  and phonological tasks, 209–214
  and positron emission tomography (PET), 191–
    194, 193f
  and preattentive processing, 189–190, 190f
  and pronounceable versus unpronounceable
    letter strings, 206–208
  and semantic memory, 214–229, 219f
  and speech sounds versus nonspeech sounds,
    199–202
  and speech sound versus nonspeech sounds, 201f
  and spoken speech perception, 198–204
  stimulus-unrelated, 190–191
  and Stroop effect, 189
  and superior temporal gyrus (STG), 198–199
  and superior temporal sulcus (STS), 200–202

and visual character perception, 204–209
and word generation, 189–190, 190*f*, 229–233, 232*f*
Lesion-deficit research, 188, 379–381
  and episodic memory, 254
  limitations of, 380–381
  and neuropsychology, 392, 393*f*
  and working memory, 304, 306
Letters
  pronounceable versus unpronounceable strings of, 206–208
  visual recognition of, 205
Lexical regions, 208–209
  and language processing, 187
  and semantic memory, 221–223
Linguistic subsystems, 187, 188–189
Loose task designs, 37–39

Magnetic resonance imaging (MRI), functional. *See also* Functional neuroimaging
  and aging, 353
  and blocked designs, 32–33, 37
  and blood oxygen level dependent (BOLD) signal, 11–12, 15*f*
  of brain-damaged patients, 383
  and brain motion, 30–31
  and category-related activations, 174–175
  and cognitive subtraction, 298–299
  and control state, 13*f*
  development of, 3–4, 10–11
  and encoding of episodic memories, 260–263
  and episodic memory, 259–260, 279–281
  event-related (ER), 33–43
  and excitatory activity, 29
  and fusiform face area (FFA), 124–125
  and inhibitory activity, 29
  and language processing, 191–198, 193*f*
  limitations of, 28–31, 28*f*
  and network analyses, 50
  physiological basis of, 28–31
  and prefrontal cortex, 309–314, 313*f*
  and presentation rates, 34–36
  and retrieval of episodic memories, 263–264
  and semantic memory, 159
  and semantic processing, 216–217*f*
  and spatial attention, 82–84, 88–91
  and striate modulation, 96–97
  and task design, 31–33
  and task state, 13*f*
  and visual recognition, 138–143
  and visual tasks, 57–58
Memory, episodic
  and aging, 337–338, 341, 346–351, 347*t*, 355–356, 370*f*
  brain regions associated with, 255–259

definition of, 253–255
  encoding, 36–42, 260–263
  and frontal cortex, 257–259
  and functional magnetic resonance imaging (fMRI), 259–260, 279–281
  and global amnesias, 255–256
  and hippocampus, 59–60
  and medial temporal lobes (MTL), 59–61, 255–257, 266–270, 279–281
  and positron emission tomography (PET), 259–260
  and priming, 337, 346–351, 347*t*, 349*f*
  and retrieval, 263–266
  versus semantic memory, 153–154
  and thinking, 227–229
Memory, long-term, 58–62
  and aging, 358–359
  and visual tasks, 61–62
Memory, nondeclarative, 59
Memory, semantic, 153–179
  and angular gyrus, 227–228, 228*f*
  and aphasia, 160–162
  and association tasks, 159–162
  brain regions associated with, 218–220
  and category-related activations, 171–179
  and color recognition, 162–167
  control tasks using word or picture stimuli, 220–221
  decisions and language processing, 210–214
  definition of, 153–156
  and difficulties in object naming, 156–158
  and difficulties in word reading, 156–158
  dysfunction, 155–156
  versus episodic memory, 153–154
  and frontal cortex, 156–162, 157*f*
  and functional magnetic resonance imaging (fMRI), 159, 216–217*f*
  and fusiform gyrus, 156–162, 157*f*
  and inferior temporal gyrus (ITG), 222–225
  and language processing, 214–229
  and middle temporal gyrus (MTG), 222–225
  neuroanatomy of, 162–167
  and nonlinguistic tasks, 218–220
  and nonsemantic tasks, 227–229, 228*f*, 229*f*
  and object category-specific disorders, 167–170
  and object identification, 56–58, 57*f*, 60*f*
  and occipital cortex, 171–174, 172*f*
  and perceptual tasks, 220–221
  and phonological tasks, 221–223
  and positron emission tomography (PET), 216–217*f*
  processes, 214–229, 216–217*f*, 219*f*
  and semantic association tasks, 159–162
  and semantic decision, 159–162
  and semantic dementia, 160–162, 385–387

Memory, semantic (cont.)
  and semantic fluency, 158–159
  and spatial location, 56–58, 57*f*, 60*f*
  and temporal lobes, 156–162, 157*f*
  and thinking, 227–229
  and visual tasks, 160–162
  and word generation, 229–233, 232*f*
Memory, working, 58–62
  and active maintenance process, 296–304
  and aging, 338, 351–355, 352*t*, 356
  and Brodmann's area, 297*f*, 302, 303*f*
  central executive system and, 293–296, 304–306
  and cognitive subtraction, 298–299, 301
  definition of, 293–296
  and dual-task performance, 304–307
  and event-related functional magnetic resonance
    imaging (fMRI), 299–302, 300*f*, 301*f*, 314
  functional imaging of, 296–309
  functional subdivisions of prefrontal cortex
    (PFC) for, 309–310, 309*f*
  and inhibitory activity, 339
  and maintenance tasks, 314–318, 316*f*
  and manipulation tasks, 314–318, 316*f*
  and positron emission tomography (PET), 302
  and posterior parietal cortex, 318–320
  and prefrontal cortex organization by process,
    314–318
  and prefrontal cortex (PFC), 293–321
  and premotor areas, 320–321
  and processing speed, 338–339
  representational, 195
  role of non-prefrontal cortex regions in, 318–321
  spatial versus nonspatial, 310–314, 311*f*, 313*f*
  specificity of prefrontal cortex (PFC) for,
    307–309
  and structural equation modeling, 59–60
  and task difficulty, 306–307
Mental imagery, 141–142
Moscovitch's memory model, 341–342

Network analyses
  and aging subjects, 63–67
  and Alzheimer's dementia (AD), 65, 66*f*
  and effective connectivity, 50
  and functional connectivity, 50
  introduction to, 49–56
  and long-term memory, 58–62
  and object identification, 56–58, 57*f*
  and partial least squares (PLS) analysis, 50*t*,
    51–56, 52*f*
  and perception, attention and language, 56–58
  and schizophrenia, 63
  and sensory-sensory associative learning, 61–62,
    62*f*

  and spatial location, 56–58, 57*f*
  and structural equation modeling, 50*t*, 54–62, 55*f*
  techniques for, 50–56, 50*t*
  theoretical basis for, 49
  and working memory, 58–62
Neurocognitive aging. *See* Aging
Neuronal activity
  and functional magnetic resonance imaging
    (fMRI), 28–31
  and glycolysis, 16–20
  and positron emission tomography (PET), 28–31
  reorganization, 394–395
Neuropsychology
  definition of, 379–380
  and functional neuroimaging, 385–394, 393*f*
  and functional neuroimaging of impaired
    patients, 385–397
  and informing abnormal models of functional
    anatomy, 385–390
  and informing normal models of functional
    anatomy, 390–394
  and lesion-deficit research, 379–381, 392, 393*f*
Nonlinguistic stimuli, 218–220

Object identification, 56–58, 57*f*, 60*f*
  and Alzheimer's dementia (AD), 66*f*
  versus face recognition, 128–132
  and semantic memory, 167–170
  and visual recognition, 109–113
Occipital lobes and color recognition, 162–167,
  163*f*
Occipitoparietal activations, 115–116
Optic aphasia, 112
Orthographic stimuli, 187
  frontal lobe activation by, 208–209
  and nonorthographic stimuli, 206–209, 207*f*
Oxygen consumption and brain blood flow, 11–12,
  14–20
  and cerebellar diaschisis, 14–15

Palsy, supranuclear, 80
Parahippocampal place area (PPA), 130*f*
  and episodic memory, 256–257
  and face recognition, 128–132
Parietal lobule, 85–88
Parkinson disease (PD), 341
Partial least squares (PLS), 50*t*, 51–56, 52*f*
Perception
  and aging, 336–337, 344*t*
  attention and language, 56–58
  and inferior frontal gyrus (IFG), 220–221
  and perceptual load, 98–103, 102*f*
  quantitative properties of, 98–99
  and salience of stimuli, 89–90

Phonetics, 187
Phonology, 187
 and aging, 338
 brain regions associated with, 211–212
 and inferior frontal gyrus (IFG), 211–212
 and language processing, 209–211
 and semantic memory, 221–223
 and short-term memory, 213–214
 and supramarginal gyrus, 212–214
Place recognition, 131–132
Positron emission tomography (PET). *See also*
    Functional neuroimaging
 and aging, 343–346
 and blood oxygen level dependent (BOLD)
    signal, 15*f*
 and brain blood flow, 8*f*
 of brain-damaged patients, 383
 and central executive control, 304–306
 and control state, 13*f*
 development of, 3–4, 7
 and episodic memory, 259–260
 and episodic memory encoding, 37
 and event-related potentials (ERPs), 92–95, 94*f*
 and excitatory activity, 29
 and hemodynamic changes, 29–30
 and inhibitory activity, 29
 and language processing, 191–194, 193*f*
 limitations of, 28–31, 28*f*
 and loose task comparisons, 37–39
 and network analyses, 50, 67–68
 physiological basis of, 28–31
 and posterior parietal cortex, 318–320
 and semantic processing, 216–217*f*
 and spatial attention, 82–83, 85–88, 90–91
 and task design, 31–33
 and task state, 13*f*
 and working memory, 302
Priming, 337, 346–351, 347*t*, 349*f*
Prosopagnosia, 113–115
 and fusiform face area (FFA), 128
Pyruvate and neuronal activity, 17

Reaction times (RT), 76–77
Reading. *See* Language processing; Word retrieval
Retinotopic mapping, 84–85
Retrieval of episodic memories
 experimental comparisons of, 265–266
 and functional magnetic resonance imaging
    (fMRI), 263–264

Schizophrenia, 63, 387–389
Semantics, 187
Sensory-sensory associative learning, 61–62, 62*f*
Shape analysis, 116–117

Speech perception, 195
 brain regions associated with, 198–199
 and nonspeech sounds, 199–202, 201*f*
 and nonword speech sounds, 202–204
 and Wernicke's area, 198
Striate modulation and event-related potentials
    (ERPs), 96–97
Stroke, 14–15
Stroop effect, 189
Structural equation modeling, 50*t*, 54–62, 55*f*
 and aging subjects, 63–67
 and developmental dyslexia, 67
 and network analyses, 67–68
 and sensory-sensory associative learning, 61–62,
    62*f*
 and working memory, 59–60
Sulcus, intraparietal, 86–87
Sulcus, superior temporal (STS)
 and biological motion stimuli, 133
 and letters, 206–208
 and nonword speech sounds, 202–204
 and object-related visual motion, 173–174
 and speech perception, 200–202
Syntax, 187
Systematic covariation and event-related
    potentials (ERPs), 97–98, 98*f*

Task state, 7–8, 9*f*, 10*f. See also* Blocked task
    designs; Control state; Visual tasks
 and aging subjects, 363–364
 and blocked designs, 32–33, 37
 and functional magnetic resonance imaging
    (fMRI), 13*f*, 31–33
 and loose task comparisons, 37–39
 and neuropsychologically impaired patients,
    396–397
 and partial least squares (PLS) analysis, 51–56,
    52*f*
 and positron emission tomography (PET), 13*f*,
    31–33
 and semantic processing, 55*f*, 214–229
 and sequential performance of two tasks, 304–306
 and structural equation modeling, 54–62, 55*f*
 and task design, 31–33
 and word retrieval, 162–167
 and working memory, 306–307
Temporal lobes
 and aging, 357–358
 and category-related activations, 173*f*
 and category-specific disorders, 170–171
 and color recognition, 164
 and language processing, 224–225
 posterior ventral, and word generation, 232
 and semantic memory, 156–162, 157*f*

Temporal lobes, medial (MTL)
  and encoding of episodic memories, 266–269
  and episodic memory, 59–61, 255–256
  and retrieval of episodic memories, 269–270
  and semantic memory, 156–162
  structure of, 256–257
Thalamus, 80–81
Transcranial magnetic stimulation (TMS), 67–68

Visual evoked potentials, steady-state (SSVEP),
    95–96
Visual recognition. *See also* Cortex, visual;
    Fusiform face area (FFA); Visual tasks
  and aging, 344–346
  and agnosia, 113–114
  and alexia, 114
  and apperceptive agnosia, 110–111, 111*f*
  of biological motion stimuli, 133
  category-specific mechanisms for, 113–115
  cognitive theory of, 109–110
  cortical regions associated with, 134–136, 136*f*
  and cortical specialization, 136–143
  dissociable stages in, 110–113, 111*f*
  and face selectivity, 120–125
  and functional magnetic resonance imaging
    (fMRI), 138–143
  and fusiform face area (FFA), 117–128, 118*f*,
    119*f*, 122*f*
  and language processing, 134–136, 204–209
  of letters, 205
  of living versus nonliving things, 114–115,
    132–133
  and mental imagery, 141–142
  neuroimaging of, 115–116
  versus object identification, 128–132
  and occipitoparietal activations, 115–116
  and parahippocampal place area (PPA), 128–132,
    130*f*
  and place recognition, 131–132
  and prosopagnosia, 113–115
  and semantic memory, 112–113
  and shape analysis, 111, 111*f*, 116–117
Visual tasks. *See also* Cortex, visual; Fusiform face
    area (FFA); Visual recognition
  and aging, 336–337
  and functional magnetic resonance imaging
    (fMRI), 57–58
  and long-term memory, 61–62
  and reflexive movements, 85–86
  and selective attention, 57–58, 75–76
  and semantic memory, 160–162
  and sensory-sensory associative learning, 61–62,
    62*f*
  and spatial attention, 76–82

and structural equation modeling, 56–58
and voluntary movements, 85–86

Wernicke's area
  of brain-damaged patients, 381–382
  and speech perception, 198
Word retrieval. *See also* Language processing
  cortical regions associated with, 134–136
  in language processing, 189–190
  and semantic memory, 162–167, 229–233, 232*f*